MW00677724

James H. Taylor
P. O. Box 141, Hwy. 172
Hubert, N.C. 28539

NANCY L. CAROLINE, M.D.

Visiting Professor of Critical Care Medicine,
University of Pittsburgh School of Medicine, Pittsburgh

AMBULANCE CALLS

REVIEW PROBLEMS FOR THE PARAMEDIC

Third Edition

LITTLE, BROWN AND COMPANY, BOSTON/TORONTO/LONDON

Grateful acknowledgment to David Ladd, Paul Ahearn, John Bilotas, Pete Brown, Carlos Grau, and George Murphy of the City of Boston EMS service for their help in preparing the cover.

Library of Congress Catalog Card No. 91-61049

ISBN 0-316-12889-9

Printed in the United States of America

MV-NY

TO THE AUTHOR OF THE AUTHOR: ZELDA CAROLINE, WHO HAS ALWAYS MANAGED THE EMERGENCIES AND NONEMERGENCIES OF THE LIVES AROUND HER WITH SINGULAR WISDOM AND COMPASSION

CONTENTS

PREFACE

This is a book of adventures. Clinical adventures. For nowhere in medicine is the element of adventure and challenge so powerful as in the sphere of prehospital emergency care. The doctor, nurse, or paramedic who ventures out into the field to render initial treatment at the scene of emergencies has to like surprises, for one never knows what the next call will bring. Until the moment of arrival at the scene, one cannot be certain whether the door will open upon a lonely old woman with a mild respiratory infection or a middle-aged man dead on the floor.

This kind of work requires a special sort of temperament. Hours may pass without a call, and then, right at the end of the shift, there are three cardiac arrests in a row, followed by an emergency childbirth and a child who got his finger stuck in a bubble gum machine. One must be able to switch gears rapidly; to confront the bizarre and the routine in quick succession; to run like mad up five flights of stairs for a resuscitation and to sit and talk for half an hour with a depressed, suicidal patient; to perform effectively under the most difficult conditions possible; to improvise, to learn, to laugh, to care.

Thus it demands a lot, this maverick branch of medicine. But it gives a lot too. In no other branch of medicine can one gain so much insight into the patient as a unique individual. Here one encounters the patient on *his* turf, among his family, friends, or business associates, and one sees him in a way that is not possible in the hospital setting, where patients are stripped of the surroundings that form part of their individual identities. Furthermore, in no other branch of medicine can one's timely arrival on the scene make such a crucial difference. The mobile intensive care unit patrols the perimeter between life and death, and there is no feeling quite like that which an ambulance team experiences after saving a human life in the field.

It takes a great deal of study to become a paramedic. But you can't learn it all in the classroom. Until you are actually out there, trying to deliver a baby in section 11 of the football stadium or do a resuscitation at the community bingo game, you haven't passed the course. For the real education of a paramedic takes place on the streets. No textbook can substitute for that experience, and no textbook should try to do so.

The present text attempts to review the basic principles of emergency care in the field and to convey a bit of the mood and pace of that branch of medicine. In the first section, we go back quickly over some fundamentals: terminology, physiology, fluids and electrolytes, pharmacology, and the like—just to touch base with the theoretic core of emergency medical care. And then we head out for the streets and take the calls as they come, each with its own unique challenges and dilemmas. In this third edition, the reader will also find extensive, up-to-date references to guide the inquisitive to further reading on any given subject. For those who wish to reminisce after completing the ambulance calls herein, a general index is included at the end of the book. An instructors' index is also provided, keyed to the segments of the National Training Course for Emergency Medical Technician–Paramedic, so that this book can be used in conjunction with paramedic training courses.

The cases presented in this book are fictitious, yet they are faithful to reality. Get any group of paramedics together and you will hear tales much stranger and more wondrous than those presented here. They are adventure stories, all of them, and adventures of the highest order—in the service of human life.

N. L. C.

ACKNOWLEDGMENTS

Emergency medicine covers a lot of territory, and no one—especially the present author—knows it all. Thus I am grateful to Dr. Mordechai Gerstein and to the late Professor Ron Rozin, both of whom took a great deal of time and care to review the original manuscript of this book. I am indebted as well to my former editor, Sarah Boardman, with whom the idea for this book originated. To my brother, Peter Caroline, I owe particular thanks for the very expressive cartoons he drew to illustrate this volume. Finally, I must acknowledge my debt to all the paramedics with whom I have worked over the years and with whom I have shared adventures such as those recounted here.

BASICS

FROM THE FIRST HELLO TO THE LAST GOOD-BYE

You have transported an unconscious patient to the emergency room of the base hospital. The emergency room staff are all preoccupied with the care of a group of patients who were brought in from a highway accident. You and your crew should

a. Transfer the patient onto an empty bed in the emergency room, and get back into service immediately.
b. Transfer the patient onto an empty bed in the emergency room, notify the receptionist about the patient, and then get back into service.
c. Transfer the patient onto an empty bed in the emergency room, and find a bystander from the waiting room to stay with the patient before you go back into service.
d. Leave the patient in the ambulance, and get a cup of coffee until things calm down in the emergency room.
e. Remain with the patient in the emergency room until there is a physician or nurse free to receive your report and take over responsibility for the patient's care.

A1 The correct answer is **e**: You should remain with the patient until there can be an orderly transfer of responsibility to qualified medical personnel in the emergency room.

Once a medical professional has assumed responsibility for the care of a patient, he may not terminate his care of the patient (assuming the patient continues to require care) until he has formally transferred his responsibility to another qualified individual. Failure to do so can be regarded as "abandonment," a very serious charge in a court of law.

Our patient clearly had a need of continuing care; he was unconscious and thus unable to care for himself or to call attention to his own distress. And in a busy emergency room where the staff is preoccupied with a multicasualty road accident, such a patient can easily die unnoticed if simply transferred to a cart and left off in a corner (answer a). Notifying the receptionist about the patient (answer b) is not sufficient; the receptionist is not medically qualified to take over the patient's care, nor is a bystander from the waiting room (answer c). Leaving the patient unattended in the ambulance while you relax in the hospital cafeteria (answer d) is clearly just as negligent as leaving him unattended in the emergency room, if not more so.

In summary, whenever you take responsibility for a patient—which is essentially every time you respond to a call—you must remain with that patient at all times until you have formally transferred him to the care of another medical professional and have fully informed that medical professional of all pertinent details regarding the patient's findings and management.

FURTHER READING

Ansell DA, Schiff RL. Patient dumping: Status, implications and policy recommendations. *JAMA* 257:1500, 1987.
Caroline NL. *Emergency Care in the Streets* (4th ed.). Boston: Little, Brown, 1991, Ch. 3.
Chayet NL. *Legal Implications of Emergency Care.* New York: Appleton-Century-Crofts, 1969.
Curran WJ. Economic and legal considerations in emergency care. *N Engl J Med.* 312:374, 1985.
Frew SA. *Street Law: Rights and Responsibilities of the EMT.* Reston, Va.: Reston Publishing, 1983.
George J. *Law and Emergency Care.* St. Louis: Mosby, 1980.
Goldberg RJ et al. A review of prehospital care litigation in a large metropolitan EMS system. *Ann Emerg Med* 19:557, 1990.
Goldstein AS. *EMS and the Law.* Bowie, Md: Brady, 1983.
Henry GL. Legal Rounds. Problem: What constitutes negligence? *Emerg Med* 17(13):67, 1985.
Henry GL. Legal Rounds. Problem: Preventing malpractice suits. *Emerg Med* 18(13):53, 1986.
Mosher CB. The EMT and the law. *Emerg Med Serv* 6(5):44, 1977.
Shanaberger CJ. Protect yourself: Avoiding the claim of abandonment. *JEMS* 15(1):143, 1990.

Medical information should always be communicated to the physician in the same order, regardless of the order in which the information was obtained. Arrange the following categories of information in the correct order for transmission to the physician:

a. Patient's vital signs
b. Patient's chief complaint
c. Patient's state of consciousness and degree of distress
d. Pertinent physical findings, in head-to-toe order
e. History of the present illness
f. Patient's medications, allergies, and significant past illnesses

1. _____
2. _____
3. _____
4. _____
5. _____
6. _____

Communicating medical information in the proper sequence is as important as making sure the information is accurate and complete, for medical professionals are accustomed to hearing data presented in a specific order; when the order is altered, some of the data may not be well heard because the doctor is expecting to hear something else.

The traditional format for presentation of medical information is as follows:

1. __b__ Patient's chief complaint (a brief statement, usually in the patient's own words, of what is bothering him)
2. __e__ History of the present illness (an amplification of the chief complaint)
3. __f__ Patient's medications, allergies, and significant past illnesses
4. __c__ Patient's state of consciousness and degree of distress
5. __a__ Patient's vital signs
6. __d__ Pertinent physical findings, in head-to-toe order

FURTHER READING

Boyd DR. Record keeping. *EMT J* 1(1):54, 1977.
Caroline NL. *Emergency Care in the Streets* (4th ed.). Boston: Little, Brown, 1991, Ch. 13.
Caroline NL. *Emergency Medical Treatment: A Text for EMT-As and EMT-Intermediates* (3rd ed.). Boston: Little, Brown, 1991, Ch. 12.

A, YOU'RE ADORABLE; B, YOU'RE SO BEAUTIFUL; C, ...

List the following steps in evaluating and managing an unconscious patient in the correct sequence:

a. Cover any open wounds.
b. Determine if the patient has a pulse.
c. Transport to the hospital.
d. Determine if the patient is breathing.
e. Splint any fractures.
f. Open the patient's airway.
g. If there is no pulse, start cardiac compressions.
h. If the patient isn't breathing, start artificial ventilation.
i. Arrest hemorrhage.

1. _____
2. _____
3. _____
4. _____
5. _____
6. _____
7. _____
8. _____
9. _____

A3   By the time a paramedic gets to be a paramedic, he should be able to recite the ABCs of emergency care in his sleep:

A is for AIRWAY
B is for BREATHING
C is for CIRCULATION (i.e., presence or absence of pulse; presence or absence of profuse bleeding)

The management of EVERY unconscious patient ALWAYS proceeds in that order: ABC. Once those factors are adequately controlled, we determine whether a load-and-go situation exists. If so, transport is begun. If not, we turn our attention to lesser wounds, and then to fractures. When the patient has been stabilized as best as possible, transport to the hospital is undertaken.

1. __f__ Open the patient's AIRWAY.
2. __d__ Determine if the patient is BREATHING.
3. __h__ If the patient isn't breathing, start artificial ventilation.
4. __b__ Determine if the patient has a pulse (CIRCULATION).
5. __g__ If there is no pulse, start cardiac compressions.
6. __i__ Arrest hemorrhage (CIRCULATION).
7. __a__ Cover any open WOUNDS.
8. __e__ Splint any FRACTURES.
9. __c__ Transport to the hospital.

FURTHER READING

Aprahamian C et al. Traumatic cardiac arrest: Scope of paramedic services. *Ann Emerg Med* 14:583, 1985.
Caroline NL. *Emergency Care in the Streets* (4th ed.). Boston: Little, Brown, 1991, Chs. 6, 20.
Compton J et al. Role of the intensive care ambulance in the transport of accident victims. *Aust NZ J Surg* 53:435, 1983.
Copass MK et al. Prehospital cardiopulmonary resuscitation of the critically injured patient. *Am J Surg* 148:20, 1984.
Gervin AS et al. The importance of prompt transport in salvage of patients with penetrating heart wounds. *J Trauma* 22:443, 1982.
Jacobs LM et al. Prehospital advanced life support: Benefits in trauma. *J Trauma* 24:8, 1984.
Pepe PE, Stewart RD, Copass MK. Prehospital management of trauma: A tale of three cities. *Ann Emerg Med* 15:1484, 1986.
Pilcher DB, Gettinger CE, Goss JR. Too much or too little: Assessment at the scene of the injury. *EMT J* 1(2):28, 1977.
Potter D et al. A controlled trial of prehospital advanced life support in trauma. *Ann Emerg Med* 17:582, 1988.
Reines HD et al. Is advanced life support appropriate for victims of motor vehicle accidents? The South Carolina highway trauma project. *J Trauma* 28:563, 1988.
Smith JP et al. Prehospital stabilization of critically injured patients: A failed concept. *J Trauma* 25:65, 1985.
Trunkey DD. Is ALS necessary for pre-hospital trauma care? *J Trauma* 24:86, 1984.

EVERY TIME I TRIED TO TELL YOU, THE WORDS JUST CAME OUT WRONG . . .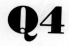

Match the following medical terms with the phrase that best fits each:

a. Dyspnea
b. Arthritis
c. Hemiplegia
d. Hyperglycemia
e. Hematoma

f. Bradycardia
g. Pneumonectomy
h. Anuria
i. Myalgia
j. Neuropathy

1. _____ Absence of urine flow
2. _____ High blood sugar level
3. _____ Paralysis on one side of the body
4. _____ Slow heart rate (below 60/min)
5. _____ Difficulty breathing
6. _____ Collection of blood beneath the skin
7. _____ Inflammation of the joints
8. _____ Disease affecting nerves
9. _____ Surgical removal of a lung
10. _____ Pain in muscles

A4

Much of medical terminology is constructed from Latin or Greek prefixes and suffixes, and familiarity with these prefix and suffix roots enables one to figure out the meaning of the majority of medical terms. In our exercise, we have used the following roots:

a-	absence of
arthro-	joint
brady-	slow
cardio-	heart
dys-	disordered, painful, difficult
glyco-	sugar
hema- or hemato-	blood
hemi-	half
hyper-	above, excess
myo-	muscle
neuro-	nerve
pneumo-	lung
-algia	pain
-ectomy	surgical removal
-emia	pertaining to the blood
-itis	inflammation
-oma	tumor, swelling
-pathy	disease
-plegia	paralysis
-pnea	breathing
-uria	urine

Putting these together, we have our answers:

1. __h__ Absence of urine flow (an- + -uria)
2. __d__ High blood sugar (hyper- + glyco- + -emia)
3. __c__ Paralysis on one side of the body (hemi- + -plegia)
4. __f__ Slow heart rate (brady- + -cardia)
5. __a__ Difficulty breathing (dys- + -pnea)
6. __e__ Collection of blood beneath the skin (hemato- + -oma)
7. __b__ Inflammation of the joints (arthro- + -itis)
8. __j__ Disease affecting nerves (neuro- + -pathy)
9. __g__ Surgical removal of a lung (pneumo- + -ectomy)
10. __i__ Pain in the muscles (myo- + -algia)

FURTHER READING

Caroline NL. *Emergency Care in the Streets* (4th ed.). Boston: Little, Brown, 1991, Ch. 5.
Caroline NL. *Emergency Medical Treatment: A Text for EMT-As and EMT-Intermediates* (3rd ed.). Boston: Little, Brown, 1991, Ch. 3.
Frenay AC. *Understanding Medical Terminology* (6th ed.). St. Louis: Catholic Health Association, 1977.
Prendergast A. *Medical Terminology: A Text/Workbook* (2nd ed.). Reading, MA: Addison-Wesley, 1983.
Smith GL, Davis PE. *Medical Terminology: A Programmed Text* (4th ed.). New York: Wiley, 1981.

Identify the following according to whether each is a

a. Symptom
b. Sign

1. _____ Chest pain
2. _____ Rapid pulse
3. _____ Pale, clammy skin
4. _____ Nausea
5. _____ Dizziness
6. _____ Tachypnea
7. _____ Ecchymoses
8. _____ Headache

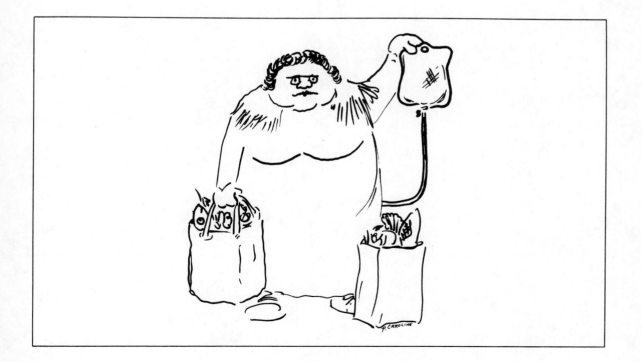

A5 Recall that a SYMPTOM (a) is some bodily discomfort that the patient *feels* and that is reported in the history of the present illness. A SIGN (b) is a physical abnormality that you *observe* and that forms part of the physical examination. One can learn all of the patient's symptoms without ever seeing him, simply by talking with him over the telephone. His signs, on the other hand, can all be determined even if he is entirely uncommunicative.

1. __a__ Chest pain
2. __b__ Rapid pulse
3. __b__ Pale, clammy skin
4. __a__ Nausea
5. __a__ Dizziness
6. __b__ Tachypnea
7. __b__ Ecchymoses
8. __a__ Headache

FURTHER READING

Caroline NL. *Emergency Care in the Streets* (4th ed.). Boston: Little, Brown, 1991, Ch. 11.
Caroline NL. *Emergency Medical Treatment: A Text for EMT-As and EMT-Intermediates* (3rd ed.). Boston: Little, Brown, 1991, Ch. 12.

1. Distention of the external jugular veins in a patient sitting at a 45-degree angle is suggestive of

   a. Right heart failure
   b. Hypovolemia
   c. Muscular development of the neck
   d. Left heart failure
   e. Neurogenic shock

2. Drainage of clear fluid or blood from the ear of a patient who has sustained multiple trauma is suggestive of

   a. Ear infection
   b. Orbital fracture
   c. Mandibular fracture
   d. Basilar skull fracture
   e. Usually of no clinical significance

A6

1. The correct answer is **a: right heart failure.**

When the right heart fails, i.e., no longer pumps blood out efficiently, blood backs up behind the right heart, into the systemic circuit; thus the systemic veins, of which the external jugular is the most easily visible, become engorged and distended.

By contrast, when the left heart fails (answer d), blood backs up into the pulmonary circuit, and serum extravasates into the lungs, producing the clinical sign of rales.

In hypovolemia (answer b) or neurogenic shock (answer e), there is no distention of neck veins; to the contrary—as anyone who has ever tried to start an IV on a hypovolemic patient can testify—the veins of such a patient are quite dramatically collapsed.

Muscular development of the neck (answer c) does not produce either distention or collapse of neck veins.

2. The correct answer is **d: basilar skull fracture.**

In a patient with head injury, clear fluid draining from the ear must be presumed to be cerebrospinal fluid (CSF) from a basilar skull fracture until proved otherwise. Blood draining from the ear is also highly suggestive of basilar skull fracture. The ear should be covered *lightly* with a sterile dressing, but no attempt should be made to dam up the flow of fluid.

An ear infection (answer a), when associated with drainage, usually involves pus rather than clear fluid. Orbital fractures (answer b) are characterized by ecchymoses around the eyes and sometimes drainage of clear fluid (CSF) from the *nose* if the cribiform plate of the skull has been fractured as well. Mandibular fracture (answer d) presents as instability and deformity of the lower jaw.

The drainage of fluid from an ear, bloody or otherwise, should *always* be considered clinically significant (answer e), and you should call the attention of emergency room personnel to this finding when you make your report on the patient.

FURTHER READING
Caroline NL. *Emergency Care in the Streets* (4th ed.). Boston: Little, Brown, 1991, Ch. 12.
Caroline NL. *Emergency Medical Treatment: A Text for EMT-As and EMT-Intermediates* (3rd ed.). Boston: Little, Brown, 1991, Ch. 11.

Match the following terms with the phrase that best describes each:

a. Stridor
b. Rales
c. Rhonchi
d. Wheezes
e. Snoring

1. _____ Rattling noises, often caused by partial obstruction of the upper airways by mucus.
2. _____ Gurgling noise produced by partial *upper* airway obstruction.
3. _____ Harsh, high-pitched sound heard on inhalation, characteristic of tight *upper* airway obstruction, as in laryngeal edema.
4. _____ Whistling sound heard diffusely in asthma and some cases of pulmonary edema, caused by narrowing of the smaller airways.
5. _____ Fine, moist sounds, sometimes crackling or bubbling in quality, associated with fluid in the smaller airways.

A7 It has often been observed that the most important part of the stethoscope is the part that fits between the two earpieces. There is little point in auscultating a patient's chest if the examiner cannot identify the sounds he hears and describe those sounds in a manner understandable to another medical professional. Sick lungs manifest all sorts of squeaks and gurgles, but most of the abnormal respiratory sounds can be adequately described with the terminology listed in the question.

1. ___c___ Rattling noises, often caused by partial obstruction of the upper airways by mucus (= **rhonchi**).

2. ___e___ Gurgling noise produced by partial *upper* airway obstruction (= **snoring**).

The secret of eliminating snoring is simply to tilt the snorer's head back (or, in extreme cases, perform a triple airway maneuver: backward tilt of the head, forward displacement of the mandible while opening the mouth with your thumbs)—a simple technique that could save many a marriage.

3. ___a___ Harsh, high-pitched sound heard on inhalation, characteristic of tight *upper* airway obstruction, as in laryngeal edema (= **stridor**).

Stridor is one of the most alarming of abnormal respiratory sounds, often audible from another room without a stethoscope. It is heard in croup, a respiratory infection in children, and may bear a striking resemblance to the barking of a very small but determined dog.

4. ___d___ Whistling sound heard diffusely in asthma and some cases of pulmonary edema, caused by narrowing of the smaller airways (= **wheezes**).

Wheezing occurs whenever there is bronchospasm for any reason. It may occur in persons with normal lungs after inhalation of smoke or toxic fumes. Wheezing localized to one area of the chest usually suggests that there is a foreign body obstructing the airway in that region.

5. ___b___ Fine, moist sounds, sometimes crackling or bubbling in quality, associated with fluid in the smaller airways (= **rales**).

Rales are often described as "fine" or "coarse," depending upon their character. They are heard in pulmonary edema and usually become evident initially at the bases of the lungs; thus it is important always to listen over all lung fields when auscultating the chest.

FURTHER READING
Caroline NL. *Emergency Care in the Streets* (4th ed.). Boston: Little, Brown, 1991, Chs. 12, 22.
Caroline NL. *Emergency Medical Treatment: A Text for EMT-As and EMT-Intermediates* (3rd ed.). Boston: Little, Brown, 1991, Ch. 11.

Match the following conditions with the physical findings most characteristic of each:

a. Moderate asthmatic attack
b. Pulmonary edema
c. Tension pneumothorax on the right
d. Hemothorax on the right

1. _____ Breath sounds poorly heard on the right; right chest hyperresonant to percussion; left chest normal.
2. _____ Loud, crackling rales heard in both lungs, from the diaphragm about halfway up the chest, and frequently throughout the whole chest.
3. _____ Diffuse wheezing; all lung fields hyperresonant to percussion.
4. _____ Breath sounds poorly heard on the right; right chest dull to percussion; left chest normal or with slightly diminished breath sounds.

A8

1. __c__ Breath sounds poorly heard on the right; right chest hyperresonant to percussion; left chest normal or with slightly diminished breath sounds.

TENSION PNEUMOTHORAX ON THE RIGHT. Because the right lung is collapsed, no air is moving through it, so the only breath sounds audible over the right chest are those being transmitted from the left side. Hyperresonance is present because there is air, rather than lung tissue, beneath the chest wall. Breath sounds on the left side may be slightly diminished because of a mediastinal shift to the left with consequent compression of left lung tissue.

2. __b__ Loud, crackling rales heard in both lungs, from the diaphragm about halfway up the chest, and frequently throughout the whole chest.

PULMONARY EDEMA. The rales are indicative of fluid in the alveoli and smaller airways.

3. __a__ Diffuse wheezing; all lung fields hyperresonant to percussion.

MODERATE ASTHMATIC ATTACK. While wheezing may be heard in congestive heart failure (pulmonary edema), hyperresonance is not. In asthma, hyperresonance of the chest occurs because of progressive air-trapping in the lungs, which have relatively less difficulty inhaling than exhaling. Thus, during each breath, slightly less air is exhaled than was inhaled, and the result is progressive accumulation of air within the lungs.

4. __d__ Breath sounds poorly heard on the right; right chest dull to percussion; left chest normal.

HEMOTHORAX ON THE RIGHT. Breath sounds are poorly heard because there is an insulating layer of blood between the chest wall and the lungs. Dullness to percussion occurs for the same reason.

FURTHER READING

Caroline NL. *Emergency Care in the Streets* (4th ed.). Boston: Little, Brown, 1991, Chs. 17, 22.
Caroline NL. *Emergency Medical Treatment: A Text for EMT-As and EMT-Intermediates* (3rd ed.). Boston: Little, Brown, 1991, Chs. 15 and 19.

Label the following statements from a patient's history according to whether they are part of the

a. Chief complaint
b. History of the present illness
c. Past medical history
d. Physical examination
e. Treatment

1. _____ The patient was pale, diaphoretic, and in considerable distress.
2. _____ Oxygen was given at 6 liters per minute by nasal cannula.
3. _____ He had been hospitalized 10 years ago for ulcer disease.
4. _____ The patient is a 45-year-old man who called for an ambulance because of severe pain in his chest.
5. _____ He is allergic to penicillin.
6. _____ Pulse was 110 and weak, blood pressure was 100/60, and respirations were 20 and labored.
7. _____ The pain was squeezing in nature, radiating into the left arm, and had been present for 1 hour.
8. _____ There was no jugular venous distention, lungs were clear, and there was no pedal edema.
9. _____ He denied shortness of breath.
10. _____ He is not known to have cardiac disease.

Now retell the story in the correct order!

A9 The CHIEF COMPLAINT is the reason that the patient sought medical help. It is usually stated in a word or short phrase, such as "headache," or "fell down."

The HISTORY OF THE PRESENT ILLNESS is an elaboration of the chief complaint. If the chief complaint is pain, what kind of pain? How long has it been present? Does it relate to some known, ongoing disease process (e.g., chest pain in a patient with long-standing heart disease)? Has the patient taken anything for his symptoms? Etc.

The PAST MEDICAL HISTORY reviews other problems (unrelated to the chief complaint) that the patient has suffered. In addition, information about the patient's allergies, usual medications, and previous surgery is generally reported as part of the past medical history, unless those allergies, medications, or previous operations are relevant to the present illness. For example, in a patient whose chief complaint is "abdominal pain," the fact that he had ulcers in the past and currently takes antacids would be included in the history of the present illness, since that information is relevant to his present complaint, but the fact that he is allergic to penicillin or takes Dilantin for seizures would be part of the past medical history.

The PHYSICAL EXAMINATION includes all information obtained from direct *observation* of the patient, irrespective of what he says. Did he appear in distress? restless? pale? What were the vital signs? What did you hear upon auscultating the lungs?

The TREATMENT includes anything you did for the patient. Did you put him in a sitting position? Did you administer oxygen? Did you start an IV?

Thus, the answers:

1. __d__ The patient was pale, diaphoretic, and in considerable distress.
2. __e__ Oxygen was given at 6 liters per minute by nasal cannula.
3. __c__ He had been hospitalized 10 years ago for ulcer disease.
4. __a__ The patient is a 45-year-old man who called for an ambulance because of *severe pain in his chest.*
5. __c__ He is allergic to penicillin.
6. __d__ Pulse was 110 and weak, blood pressure was 100/60, and respirations were 20 and labored.
7. __b__ The pain was squeezing in nature, radiating down the left arm, and had been present for 1 hour.
8. __d__ There was no jugular venous distention, lungs were clear, and there was no pedal edema. (Note the "pertinent negatives.")
9. __b__ He denied shortness of breath. (Again, a "pertinent negative.")
10. __b__ He is not known to have cardiac disease. (Another "pertinent negative.")

THE STORY
The patient is a 45-year-old man who called for an ambulance because of severe pain in his chest. The pain was squeezing in nature, radiating into the left arm, and had been present for 1 hour. He denied shortness of breath. He is not known to have cardiac disease. He had been hospitalized 10 years ago for ulcer disease. He is allergic to penicillin. (On physical examination) the patient was pale, diaphoretic, and in considerable distress. Pulse was 110 and weak, blood pressure was 100/60, and respirations were 20 and labored. There was no jugular venous distention, lungs were clear, and there was no pedal edema. Oxygen was given at 6 liters per minute by nasal cannula.

Question: What do you think is wrong with this patient? What other problems might be causing the same symptoms?

FURTHER READING
Caroline NL. *Emergency Care in the Streets* (4th ed.). Boston: Little, Brown, 1991, Ch. 13.
Caroline NL. *Emergency Medical Treatment: A Text for EMT-As and EMT-Intermediates* (3rd ed.). Boston: Little, Brown, 1991, Ch. 12.

Which of the following statements relating to osmosis is NOT true?

a. If seawater is aspirated into the lungs, fluid from the blood vessels will tend to move into the lungs because the seawater is hypertonic with respect to plasma.
b. Ringer's solution is nearly isotonic with plasma.
c. Water tends to move from a solution of higher solute concentration to a solution of lower solute concentration.
d. Fresh water aspirated into the lungs will rapidly be absorbed into the bloodstream, since fresh water is hypotonic with respect to plasma.
e. A hypertonic solution is one having a higher solute concentration than that inside the cells.

A10

Answer **c** is NOT true. If two solutions of different concentrations are separated by a semipermeable membrane (such as a cell wall), water will always move in a direction that will tend to equalize the concentration of solution on both sides of the membrane, i.e., *from* a solution of lower solute concentration (making that solution more concentrated as water leaves) *to* a solution of higher solute concentration (making that solution less concentrated as water enters). The movement of water will continue until the solutions on both sides of the membrane are at the same solute concentration.

Answer **a** is true. Seawater has a higher solute concentration than plasma (i.e., it is *hypertonic* with respect to plasma). Thus seawater in the lungs will tend to "draw" water from the less concentrated fluid (plasma) in the surrounding blood vessels. Conversely, as stated in answer d, fresh water has a solute concentration lower than that in the plasma (i.e., it is *hypotonic* with respect to plasma); thus fresh water aspirated into the lungs will quickly move across blood vessel walls into the plasma, and the lungs will remain "dry," at least temporarily.

Answer **b** is true. Ringer's solution is designed to mimic extracellular fluid in order that infusion of Ringer's solution will not cause large fluid shifts either into or out of cells. The same is true of normal saline solution.

Answer **e** is a correct definition of a hypertonic solution, i.e., a solution having a higher solute concentration than that inside body cells. Recall that a solution having a *lower* solute concentration than that inside body cells (e.g., ½ normal saline) is called *hypotonic,* while one having a solute concentration equivalent to that inside body cells (e.g., normal saline or Ringer's solution) is called *isotonic.*

FURTHER READING

Caroline NL. *Emergency Care in the Streets* (4th ed.). Boston: Little, Brown, 1991, Ch. 9.
Lindeman RD, Papper S. Therapy of fluid and electrolyte disorders. *Ann Int Med* 82:64, 1975.
Travenol Laboratories. *The Fundamentals of Body Water and Electrolytes.* Deerfield, IL: Travenol, 1973.
Weldy NJ. *Body Fluids and Electrolytes.* St. Louis: Mosby, 1982.

Match the following terms with the situation each best describes:

a. Respiratory acidosis
b. Metabolic acidosis
c. Respiratory alkalosis
d. Metabolic alkalosis

1. _____ A diabetic patient with an excess of organic acids in his blood.
2. _____ A patient with ulcer disease who has been taking large quantities of baking soda to relieve his pain.
3. _____ A nervous young man who is hyperventilating and complaining of tingling sensations in his hands and feet and cramping pains in his chest.
4. _____ An unconscious patient who is breathing shallowly 3 times per minute.

A11 Recall the meanings of the words associated with disturbances in acid-base balance. A *respiratory acidosis* is a condition in which the body fluids become acidotic because of a failure in the respiratory system—specifically, a failure to blow off sufficient quantities of carbon dioxide. A *metabolic acidosis* is a condition in which the body fluids become acidotic because of an increased load of organic acids in the body, either because the body is producing more organic acids than normal (as in diabetes or shock) or because the long-term mechanisms of getting rid of these acids, through the kidneys, have broken down (as in renal failure). A *respiratory alkalosis* refers to the situation in which the pH of body fluids rises because carbon dioxide is being blown off by the lungs in excessive quantities, and the level of carbonic acid in the body consequently falls below normal. A *metabolic alkalosis* occurs when there is an increased load of base (or alkali) in the body, such as when one inadvertently gives too much bicarbonate during a resuscitation attempt.

Now, let us look at our cases:

1. __**b**__ A diabetic patient with an excess of organic acids in his blood.

This is, by definition, a METABOLIC ACIDOSIS, for there is an excess of acid in the body fluids (hence acidosis), and the source of this acid is the body's own overproduction (i.e., a metabolic source).

2. __**d**__ A patient with ulcer disease who has been taking large quantities of baking soda to relieve his pain.

Baking soda is sodium bicarbonate, and like the patient in cardiac arrest who receives too much bicarbonate, the patient who ingests too much antacid is likely to raise his body fluid pH and develop a METABOLIC ALKALOSIS.

3. __**c**__ A nervous young man who is hyperventilating and complaining of tingling sensations in his hands and feet and cramping pains in his chest.

Primary hyperventilation, i.e., hyperventilation that is *not* a compensatory response to metabolic acidosis, is a classic cause of RESPIRATORY ALKALOSIS. As the patient hyperventilates, he blows off carbon dioxide, and his blood levels of carbon dioxide (and thus carbonic acid) fall, leading to alkalosis. Since the cause of this case is respiratory, it is a respiratory alkalosis.

4. __**a**__ An unconscious patient who is breathing shallowly 3 times per minute.

Any patient hypoventilating to this degree will not be able to blow off the carbon dioxide produced by the body's metabolism; hence, carbon dioxide will accumulate, levels of carbonic acid in the blood will rise, and the patient will become acidotic. Since the source of this acidosis is a defect in the respiratory system (failure to breathe sufficiently deeply and rapidly), it is termed a RESPIRATORY ACIDOSIS.

FURTHER READING
Abbot Laboratories. *Acid-base balance* (pamphlet). North Chicago: Abbot, 1974.
Caroline NL. *Emergency Care in the Streets* (4th ed.). Boston: Little, Brown, 1991, Ch. 9.
Flomenbaum N. Acid-base disturbances. *Emerg Med* 16(3):59, 1984.
Hazard PB et al. Calculation of sodium bicarbonate requirement in metabolic acidosis. *Am J Med Sci* 283:18, 1982.
Hazard PB, Griffin JP. Sodium bicarbonate in the management of systemic acidosis. *South Med J* 73:1339, 1980.
Kassirer JP. Serious acid-base disorders. *N Engl J Med* 291:773, 1974.
Miller WC. The ABCs of blood gases. *Emerg Med* 16(3):37, 1984.
Stein JM. Interpreting arterial blood gases. *Emerg Med* 18(1):61, 1986.

Which of the following statements about shock is NOT true?

a. One of the earliest signs of shock is a falling blood pressure.
b. The adequacy of perfusion to vital organs may be roughly gauged in the field by the patient's state of consciousness.
c. Urinary output falls when the kidneys are not adequately perfused with blood.
d. Restlessness, diaphoresis, and confusion may be early warning signs of shock.
e. Shock may develop as a consequence of widespread burns because of large fluid losses across damaged skin.

A12 Answer **a** is NOT true. Falling blood pressure is a very LATE sign of shock, for the blood pressure does not begin to fall significantly until all of the body's compensatory mechanisms have been overwhelmed. The *earliest* signs of shock are often nonspecific, such as restlessness, diaphoresis, and confusion (answer d); by the time the patient becomes hypotensive, it may be too late to save him.

Shock is defined as a state of inadequate perfusion of vital tissues, and perhaps the most vital of these tissues are those in the brain, the heart, and the kidneys. The adequacy of perfusion of the brain can be gauged by a patient's state of consciousness (answer b), while kidney perfusion can be monitored by measuring a patient's urine output (answer c); inadequate perfusion of the coronary arteries may produce chest pain or cardiac dysrhythmias.

Any condition that results in a profound loss of fluids can lead to shock. Thus, in a patient with widespread burns, shock may rapidly develop because of massive fluid losses across the damaged skin (answer e), for burned skin is no longer able to function effectively as a barrier against fluid loss from the body.

FURTHER READING

Adams SL et al. Absence of a tachycardic response to intraperitoneal hemorrhage. *J Emerg Med* 4:383, 1986.
Barber JM. EMT checkpoint: Early detection of hypovolemic states. *EMT J* (2(2):72, 1978.
Caroline NL. *Emergency Care in the Streets* (4th ed.). Boston: Little, Brown, 1991, Ch. 9.
Caroline NL. *Emergency Medical Treatment: A Text for EMT-As and EMT-Intermediates* (3rd ed.). Boston: Little, Brown, 1991, Chs. 8, 9.
Garvin JM. Keeping shock simple. *Emerg Med Serv* 9(5):49, 1980.
Geelhoed GW. Shock and its management. *Emerg Med Serv* 5(6):42, 1976.
Wilson RF. Science and shock: A clinical perspective. *Ann Emerg Med* 14:714, 1985.

Label the following statements about military antishock trousers (MAST) according to whether each is true or false:

a. The MAST is useful in the treatment of patients with pulmonary edema.

TRUE   FALSE

b. The MAST should not be used in patients with suspected pelvic fractures.

TRUE   FALSE

c. The MAST should not be deflated before adequate volume replacement has been achieved.

TRUE   FALSE

d. The MAST must be removed before x-rays can be taken.

TRUE   FALSE

e. In deflating the MAST, the leg sections should be deflated before the abdominal section.

TRUE   FALSE

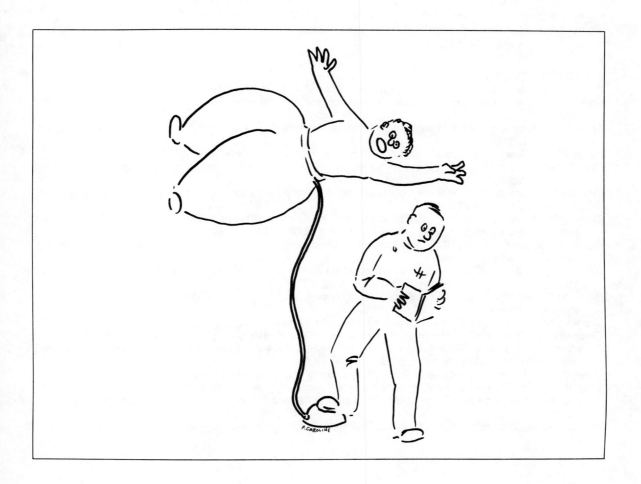

A13

a. The MAST is useful in the treatment of patients with pulmonary edema.

FALSE! The MAST is *contraindicated* in patients with pulmonary edema. Such patients already have a circulatory overload, and they certainly do NOT need another 2 to 4 units of blood pumped into their central circulation. Indeed, the measures we take to treat pulmonary edema are intended to accomplish precisely the opposite of what the MAST accomplishes. We sit the patient up, with legs dangling, so that blood will pool in the legs. And sometimes we even remove a unit of blood (phlebotomy) in order to decrease the circulating blood volume further.

b. The MAST should not be used in patients with suspected pelvic fractures.

FALSE! Pelvic fracture is the most definitive indication for the use of the MAST because the MAST provides an excellent splint to stabilize the pelvis and promotes hemostasis by pressure on the pelvic area.

c. The MAST should not be deflated before adequate volume replacement has been achieved.

TRUE! Even after fluid replacement, the MAST should be deflated slowly and cautiously, segment by segment, with careful monitoring of the pulse and blood pressure at each stage. The moment the pulse begins to rise or the blood pressure begins to fall, fluids must be infused rapidly and, if necessary, the MAST reinflated.

d. The MAST must be removed before x-rays can be taken.

FALSE! The MAST garment is transparent to x-rays and may be left in place while x-rays are being taken. Many patients in unstable shock will have to remain in the MAST until they reach the operating room.

e. In deflating the MAST, the leg sections should be deflated before the abdominal section.

FALSE! If the leg sections are deflated first, the abdominal section remains as a tourniquet, preventing blood from returning to the legs. The abdominal section is always deflated first. If vital signs remain stable, one of the leg sections is then slowly deflated. Then, after careful monitoring over several minutes to make certain the blood pressure is not falling, the second leg section may be deflated.

FURTHER READING

Abraham E et al. Effect of pneumatic trousers on pulmonary function. *Crit Care Med* 10:754, 1982.

Abraham E et al. Cardiorespiratory effects of pneumatic trousers in critically ill patients. *Arch Surg* 119:912, 1984.

Aprahamian C et al. Effect of circumferential pneumatic compression devices on digital flow. *Ann Emerg Med* 13:1092, 1984.

Bartlett L. An overview of military antishock trousers. *Emerg Med Serv* 14(6):23, 1985.

Bass RR et al. Thigh compartment syndrome without lower extremity trauma following application of pneumatic antishock trousers. *Ann Emerg Med* 12:382, 1983.

Bickell WH et al. Effect of antishock trousers on the trauma score: A prospective analysis in the urban setting. *Ann Emerg Med* 14:218, 1985.

Bickell WH et al. Randomized trial of pneumatic antishock garments in the prehospital management of penetrating abdominal injuries. *Ann Emerg Med* 16:653, 1987.

Bircher N, Safar P, Stewart RD. A comparison of standard, MAST-augmented, and open chest CPR in dogs. *Crit Care Med* 8:147, 1980.

Bivens HG et al. Blood volume displacement with inflation of antishock trousers. *Ann Emerg Med* 11:409, 1982.

Brotman S, Browder B, Cox E. MAS trousers improperly applied causing a compartment syndrome in lower extremity trauma. *J Trauma* 22:598, 1982.

Caroline NL. *Emergency Care in the Streets* (4th ed.). Boston: Little, Brown, 1991, Ch. 9.

Chipman CD. The MAST controversy. *Emerg Med* 15(3):206, 1983.

Christiansen KS. Pneumatic antishock garments (PASG): Do they precipitate lower-extremity compartment syndromes? *J Trauma* 26:1102, 1986.

Civetta JM et al. Prehospital use of the military antishock trouser (MAST). *JACEP* 5:581, 1976.

Cogbill TH et al. Pulmonary function after military antishock trouser inflation. *Surg Forum* 32:302, 1981.

Crile, GW. *Hemorrhage and Transfusion: An Experimental and Clinical Research*. New York: Appleton, 1909, p. 139.

Flint, LM et al. Definite control of bleeding from severe pelvic fracture. *Ann Surg* 189:709, 1979.

Gaffney FA et al. Hemodynamic effects of medical antishock trousers (MAST garment). *J Trauma* 21:931, 1981.

Goldsmith SR. Comparative hemodynamic effects of antishock suit and volume expansion in normal human beings. *Ann Emerg Med* 12:348, 1983.

Gustafson RA et al. The use of the MAST suit in ruptured abdominal aortic aneurysms. *Am Surg* 49:454, 1983.

Hanke BK et al. Antishock trousers: A comparison of inflation techniques and inflation pressures. *Ann Emerg Med* 14:636, 1985.

Hauswalk M, Greene ER. Aortic blood flow during sequential MAST inflation. *Ann Emerg Med* 15:1297, 1986.

Lee HR et al. MAST augmentation of external cardiac compression: Role of changing intrapleural pressure. *Ann Emerg Med* 10:560, 1981.

Lee HR et al. Venous return in hemorrhagic shock after application of military anti-shock trousers. *Am J Emerg Med* 1:7, 1983.

Lilja GP, Long RS, Ruiz E. Augmentation of systolic blood pressure during external cardiac compression by the use of the MAST suit. *Ann Emerg Med* 10:182, 1981.

Lilja GP et al. MAST usage in cardiopulmonary resuscitation. *Ann Emerg Med* 13:833, 1984.

Lloyd S. MAST and IV infusion: Do they help in prehospital trauma management? *Ann Emerg Med* 16:565, 1987.

Ludewig RM, Wangensteen SL. Effect of external counterpressure on venous bleeding. *Surgery* 65:515, 1969.

Mahoney BD, Mirick MJ. Efficacy of pneumatic trousers in refractory prehospital cardiopulmonary arrest. *Ann Emerg Med* 12:8, 1983.

Mannering D et al. Application of the medical anti-shock trouser (MAST) increases cardiac output and tissue perfusion in simulated mild hypovolaemia. *Intensive Care Med* 12:143, 1986.

Mattox KL. Prospective randomized evaluation of antishock MAST in post-traumatic hypotension. *J Trauma* 26:779, 1986.

Mattox KL et al. Prospective MAST study in 911 patients. *J Trauma* 29:1104, 1989.

McBride G. One caution in pneumatic anti-shock garment use. *JAMA* 247:112, 1982.

McCabe JB, Seidel DR, Jagger JA. Antishock trouser inflation and pulmonary vital capacity. *Ann Emerg Med* 12:290, 1983.

McSwain NE. Pneumatic anti-shock garment: State of the art 1988. *Ann Emerg Med* 17:506, 1988.

McSwain NE. Pneumatic anti-shock garment: Does it work? *Prehosp Disaster Med* 4(1):42, 1989.

McSwain NE. PASG—holding on for dear life. *Emergency* 22(8):39, 1990.

Oertel T, Loehr M. Bee-sting anaphylaxis: The use of medical antishock trousers. *Ann Emerg Med* 13:459, 1984.

Pepe PE, Bass RR, Mattox KL. Clinical trials of the pneumatic antishock garment in the urban prehospital setting. *Ann Emerg Med* 15:1407, 1986.

Polando G et al. PASG use in pelvic fracture immobilization. *JEMS* 15(3):48, 1990.

Pricolo VE et al. Trendelenburg versus PASG application: Hemodynamic response in man. *J Trauma* 26:718, 1986.

Ransom KJ, McSwain NE. Physiologic changes of antishock trousers in relationship to external pressure. *Surg Gynecol Obstet* 158:488, 1984.

Rockwell DD et al. An improved design of the pneumatic counter-pressure trousers. *Am J Surg* 143:377, 1982.

Sanders AB, Meislin HW. Alterations in MAST suit pressure with changes in ambient temperature. *J Emerg Med* 1:37, 1983.

Sanders AB, Meislin HW. Effect of altitude change on MAST suit pressure. *Ann Emerg Med* 12:140, 1983.

Savino JA et al. Overinflation of pneumatic antishock garments in the elderly. *Am J Surg* 155:572, 1988.

Wangensteen SL et al. The effect of external counterpressure on arterial bleeding. *Surgery* 64:922, 1968.

Wayne MA, MacDonald SC. Clinical evaluation of the antishock trouser: Prospective study of low-pressure inflation. *Ann Emerg Med* 12:285, 1983.

Wayne MA, MacDonald SC. Clinical evaluation of the antishock trouser: Retrospective analysis of five years of experience. *Ann Emerg Med* 12:342, 1983.

Williams TM, Knopp R, Ellyson JH. Compartment syndrome after antishock trouser use without lower extremity trauma. *J Trauma* 22:595, 1982.

Which of the following statements about a person with type O blood is NOT true?

a. He may donate blood to a person with type AB blood.
b. He may receive blood from a person with type O blood.
c. He may donate blood to a person with type B blood.
d. He may receive blood from a person with type AB blood.
e. He may donate blood to a person with type A blood.

A14

Answer **d** is NOT true.

Recall that the individual with type O blood has red blood cells that do not carry either A antigens or B antigens. Thus he is considered a "universal donor," for his red blood cells will not be agglutinated by the serum containing antibodies to A (i.e., the serum of a type B recipient), by serum containing antibodies to B (i.e., the serum of a type A recipient), or by serum containing both anti-A and anti-B antibodies (a type O recipient). The individual with type AB blood, on the other hand, is called the "universal recipient," for this individual has neither anti-A nor anti-B antibodies in his serum and can thus receive blood from any donor.

Answers a, c, and e are all true: The person with type O blood can *donate* blood to an AB, A, or B recipient. Answer b is also true, for in principle one can always receive blood from someone of the same blood type. However, the person with O blood may NOT receive blood from a person with type AB blood (answer d), because the red cells from a type AB donor carry both A antigens and B antigens, and the type O recipient has antibodies to *both* those antigens in his own serum. If he were to receive a transfusion of AB blood, the antibodies in his serum would cause the red blood cells being infused to agglutinate, and a transfusion reaction would ensue.

These concepts are summarized in Tables 1 and 2.

Table 1. ABO System of Blood Typing

Blood Type	Antigen Present on RBC	Antibody Present in Serum
A	A	Anti-B
B	B	Anti-A
AB	A & B	None
O	None	Anti-A & anti-B

Table 2. Compatibility Among ABO Blood Groups

Cells of donor	Reaction with Serum of Recipient			
	O	A	B	AB
O	−	−	−	−
A	+	−	+	−
B	+	+	−	−
AB	+	+	+	−

+ indicates agglutination; − indicates nonagglutination.

FURTHER READING

Berkman SA. The spectrum of transfusion reactions. *Hospital Practice* 19(6):205, 1984.
Brzica SM. Trouble with transfusions. *Emerg Med* 15(20):115, 1983.
Collins ML, Kafer ER. Using blood components: I. *Emerg Med* 17(11):131, 1985.
Gervin AS et al. Resuscitation of trauma patients with type-specific uncrossmatched blood. *J Trauma* 24:327, 1984.
Iserson KV. Whole blood in trauma resuscitations. *Am J Emerg Med* 3:358, 1985.
Kafer ER, Collins ML. Using blood components: II. *Emerg Med* 17(14):46, 1985.

BREATHING HIS LAST

You are caring for a patient with status epilepticus, and you administer 10 mg of diazepam (Valium) IV in an attempt to terminate his seizures. Approximately 5 minutes later, the patient's respiratory rate falls to 4 per minute. After several minutes in this condition, the patient would probably develop

a. Metabolic acidosis
b. Metabolic alkalosis
c. Respiratory acidosis
d. Respiratory alkalosis

The immediate treatment for this problem is

a. Administration of 50 ml of sodium bicarbonate IV.
b. Administration of oxygen by nasal cannula.
c. Administration of epinephrine, 0.5 ml of a 1:1,000 solution SQ.
d. Assisted ventilation with a bag-valve-mask or demand valve.
e. There is no need for treatment.

A15 A patient whose respiratory rate falls to 4 per minute will soon develop **RESPIRATORY ACIDOSIS** (answer c). Why? Recall the reasons why we breathe. First of all, we breathe in order to obtain oxygen from the outside world. But equally important, we also breathe in order to excrete the carbon dioxide (CO_2) that our bodies are continuously producing in the normal processes of metabolism. Thus if our respirations become depressed or stop altogether, our excretion of CO_2 cannot keep up with the body's production, and CO_2 begins to accumulate, leading to acidosis. It is a *respiratory* acidosis because the defect leading to this condition is in the respiratory system.

If a patient isn't breathing sufficiently to keep his arterial CO_2 levels in the normal range, how do we manage him? We have to try to help him breathe, i.e., answer **d (assisted ventilation with a bag-valve-mask or demand valve).** Sodium bicarbonate (answer a) won't help, for his problem is not an excess of organic acids that need to be neutralized; indeed, the CO_2 that dissociates from sodium bicarbonate will only worsen the situation, by adding to the CO_2 overload. Oxygen is always a nice idea (answer b), but blowing O_2 over the face of a patient who is scarcely breathing won't raise his arterial O_2 level very much, and it won't do anything at all to lower his arterial CO_2 concentration. In order to excrete CO_2, one must have a good respiratory rate and a good tidal volume (the product of which equals the minute volume). Administration of epinephrine (answer c), a drug that stimulates the heart and promotes bronchodilation, is uncalled for here; this patient's problem is not bronchospasm—as far as we know, his bronchi are wide open. His problem is respiratory depression secondary to a drug.

Answer e is completely incorrect: Without assisted ventilation, this patient will die from respiratory acidosis and hypoxemia. You got him into this mess; you gave him the Valium that caused his respiratory depression. So now it's your job to sit there squeezing the bag and breathing for him until he recovers sufficiently to breathe adequately on his own. (P.S. Don't overdo it just because you're feeling guilty. Hyperventilation, with the lowering of the arterial PCO_2 below normal levels, can lower the seizure threshold as well, and this patient has already had more than enough seizures for one afternoon. So just ventilate him at a normal respiratory rate, about 12 to 15 times per minute.)

FURTHER READING

Abbot Laboratories. *Acid-base balance* (pamphlet). North Chicago: Abbot, 1974.
Caroline NL. *Emergency Care in the Streets* (4th ed.). Boston: Little, Brown, 1991, Chs. 8, 22.
Flomenbaum N. Acid-base disturbances. *Emerg Med* 16(3):59, 1984.
Hazard PB et al. Calculation of sodium bicarbonate requirement in metabolic acidosis. *Am J Med Sci* 283:18, 1982.
Hazard PB, Griffin JP. Sodium bicarbonate in the management of systemic acidosis. *South Med J* 73:1339, 1980.
Kassirer JP. Serious acid-base disorders. *N Engl J Med* 291:773, 1974.
Miller WC. The ABCs of blood gases. *Emerg Med* 16(3):37, 1984.
Stein JM. Interpreting arterial blood gases. *Emerg Med* 18(1):61, 1986.

Match the following intravenous solutions with the situations in which each would be the preferred solution:

a. Normal saline solution
b. 5% dextrose in water (D5W)

1. _____ A patient in congestive heart failure
2. _____ A patient who has been vomiting for 36 hours
3. _____ A patient with severe injury to the abdomen, rapid pulse, and pale, clammy skin
4. _____ A patient with edema who needs a "keep-open" line
5. _____ A patient with extensive burns
6. _____ A patient who collapsed because of the heat and is found with cool, clammy skin and a rapid, thready pulse
7. _____ A patient with chest pain and frequent PVCs

A16

Recall that glucose crosses cell membranes much more rapidly than does sodium; thus a solution of glucose and water will equilibrate between the vascular space and the rest of the extracellular fluid much more rapidly than will a solution of normal saline. For that reason, salt-containing solutions like normal saline or Ringer's solution are preferred when one wishes to expand the intravascular volume, as in cases of dehydration or shock; glucose solutions without salt are preferred in instances where one wishes to avoid a large fluid load, i.e., for keep-open lines.

1. __b__ A patient in congestive heart failure

   This patient certainly does NOT need a fluid load; he already has an excess of fluid on board. What he does need is an IV lifeline, through which medications can be injected, and, as noted above, D5W is preferred for keep-open lines.

2. __a__ A patient who has been vomiting for 36 hours

   It's a good bet that this patient is severely dehydrated and does need volume, so normal saline solution is the ticket.

3. __a__ A patient with severe injury to the abdomen, rapid pulse, and pale, clammy skin

   This is a patient in hemorrhagic shock; he needs volume.

4. __b__ A patient with edema who needs a "keep-open" line

5. __a__ A patient with extensive burns

   Remember, patients with extensive burns may lose massive amounts of fluid across the damaged skin and are very liable to go into shock. Burned patients therefore also need volume.

6. __a__ A patient who collapsed because of the heat and is found with cool, clammy skin and a rapid, thready pulse

   Heat exhaustion is caused by the loss of salt and water, so salt and water is what you have to replace.

7. __b__ A patient with chest pain and frequent PVCs

   The patient with possible acute myocardial infarction needs an IV line chiefly as a route for medications. Unless he is in shock, large volumes of fluid should be avoided (and even in cardiogenic shock, fluids should be given judiciously), for he may be in borderline congestive heart failure. Use D5W at a keep-open rate.

FURTHER READING

Aeder MI et al. Technical limitations in the rapid infusion of intravenous fluids. *Ann Emerg Med* 14:307, 1985.

Bickell WH, Shaftan GW, Mattox K. Intravenous fluid administration and uncontrolled hemorrhage (editorial). *J Trauma* 29:409, 1989.

Chudnofsky CR et al. Intravenous fluid therapy in the prehospital management of hemorrhagic shock: Improved outcome with hypertonic saline/6% dextran 70 in a swine model. *Am J Emerg Med* 7:357, 1989.

Cone JB et al. Beneficial effects of a hypertonic solution for resuscitation in the presence of acute hemorrhage. *Am J Surg* 154:585, 1987.

Cross JS et al. Hypertonic saline attenuates the hormonal response to injury. *Ann Surg* 209:684, 1989.

Data JL, Nies AS. Dextran 40. *Ann Intern Med* 81:500, 1974.

Dula DJ et al. Rapid flow rates for the resuscitation of hypovolemic shock. *Ann Emerg Med* 14:303, 1985.

Greenfield RH, Bessen HA, Henneman PL. Effect of crystalloid infusion on hematocrit and intravascular volume in healthy, nonbleeding subjects. *Ann Emerg Med* 18:51, 1989.

Maningas PA et al. Hypertonic sodium chloride solutions for the prehospital management of traumatic hemorrhagic shock: A possible improvement in the standard of care? *Ann Emerg Med* 15:1411, 1986.

Mazzoni MC et al. The efficacy of iso- and hyperosmotic fluids as volume expanders in fixed-volume and uncontrolled hemorrhage. *Ann Emerg Med* 19:350, 1990.

Moss GS et al. Colloid or crystalloid in the resuscitation of hemorrhagic shock: A controlled clinical trial. *Surgery* 89:434, 1981.

Peters RM et al. Comparison of isotonic and hypertonic fluids in resuscitation from hypovolemic shock. *Surg Gynecol Obstet* 163:219, 1986.

Shoemaker WC. Comparison of emergency resuscitation with colloids and crystalloids. *Disaster Med* 1:10, 1983.

Shoemaker WC et al. Fluid therapy in emergency resuscitation: Clinical evaluation of colloid and crystalloid regimens. *Crit Care Med* 9:367, 1981.

Traverso LW et al. Fluid resuscitation after an otherwise fatal hemorrhage: I. Crystalloid solutions. *J Trauma* 26:168, 1986.

Traverso LW et al. Fluid resuscitation after an otherwise fatal hemorrhage: II. Colloid solutions. *J Trauma* 26:176, 1986.

Weil MH, Rackow EC. A guide to volume repletion. *Emerg Med* 16(8):101, 1984.

Indicate which of the following statements about administration of drugs are true and which are false:

a. The most rapidly effective route of administration of a medication is the intravenous route.

TRUE   FALSE

b. Patients in shock should receive medications through the intramuscular route.

TRUE   FALSE

c. Medications administered orally are absorbed more rapidly than when administered subcutaneously.

TRUE   FALSE

d. Epinephrine, atropine, and lidocaine are the only resuscitation drugs that may be given through an endotracheal tube.

TRUE   FALSE

e. Intracardiac injections may cause laceration of a coronary artery.

TRUE   FALSE

A17

a. The most rapidly effective route of administration of a medication is the intravenous route.

   TRUE. The intravenous route is the most effective and reliable route for administration of medications, for the medication is delivered directly to the bloodstream, whence it is carried swiftly to its various target organs. Medications administered by any other route must first be absorbed into the bloodstream, imposing variable and sometimes unpredictable delays.

b. Patients in shock should receive medications through the intramuscular route.

   FALSE! Shock is characterized by poor perfusion of peripheral tissues, including muscles. And a medication injected into a poorly perfused muscle will be absorbed into the bloodstream in an erratic and unpredictable fashion. Large amounts of the medication may remain in the muscle, only to be released suddenly into the circulation hours later, when perfusion improves. As a general rule, the intramuscular route is not used in the field because it is so difficult to predict the rate at which the injected drug will be absorbed and hence when the effective dose will actually be delivered to the target organs. For that reason, the intravenous route (where the dose injected = the effective dose delivered) is preferred in the field situation.

c. Medications administered orally are absorbed more rapidly than when administered subcutaneously.

   FALSE! Absorption of medication from the stomach is much slower than from a subcutaneous site, and many factors—such as the nature of the medication itself, food in the stomach, or pain (which slows emptying of the stomach)—may slow this absorption even further. For these reasons, the oral route is not used for administration of drugs in an emergency situation. In shock, *both* the gastrointestinal tract and subcutaneous tissues are very poorly perfused, slowing down absorption from those sites to an even greater extent and thus compromising the effectiveness of drugs administered by those routes.

d. Epinephrine, atropine, and lidocaine are the only resuscitation drugs that may be given through an endotracheal tube.

   TRUE. Epinephrine, atropine, and lidocaine are rapidly absorbed across mucous membranes, such as the membranes lining the bronchi, and thus can be effectively administered through an endotracheal tube in situations where it has not been possible to start an IV line. That is NOT true, however, of other resuscitation drugs, such as verapamil. Remember: Among the drugs used for resuscitation, ONLY EPINEPHRINE, ATROPINE, AND LIDOCAINE MAY BE GIVEN THROUGH AN ENDOTRACHEAL TUBE. (Naloxone and diazepam, which are used in circumstances other than CPR, may also be given via endotracheal tube.)

e. Intracardiac injections may cause laceration of a coronary artery.

   TRUE. There is considerable controversy concerning the use of intracardiac injection during cardiopulmonary resuscitation, and certainly any person using this technique should be aware of its potential hazards, which include (1) laceration of a coronary artery, (2) pneumothorax, and (3) inadvertent injection into cardiac muscle rather than into one of the cardiac chambers, which can cause refractory dysrhythmias. Those who oppose the technique also argue that intracardiac injection requires interruption of external cardiac compressions and artificial ventilation.

FURTHER READING

American Heart Association. Standards and guidelines for cardiopulmonary resuscitation (CPR) and emergency cardiac care (ECC). *JAMA* 255:2905, 1986.

Amey BD et al. Paramedic use of intracardiac medications in prehospital sudden cardiac death. *JACEP* 7:130, 1978.

Boster SR et al. Translaryngeal absorption of lidocaine. *Ann Emerg Med* 11:461, 1982.

Caroline NL. *Emergency Care in the Streets* (4th ed.). Boston: Little, Brown, 1991, Ch. 10.

Chernow B et al. Epinephrine absorption after intratracheal administration. *Anesth Analg* 63:829, 1984.

Davison R et al. Intracardiac injections during cardiopulmonary resuscitation—a low risk procedure. *JAMA* 244:1110, 1980.

Hao-Hui C. Closed-chest intracardiac injection. *Resuscitation* 9:103, 1981.

McDonald JL. Serum lidocaine levels during cardiopulmonary resuscitation after intravenous and endotracheal administration. *Crit Care Med* 13:914, 1985.

Roberts JR et al. Blood levels following intravenous and endotracheal epinephrine administration. *JACEP* 8:53, 1979.

Roberts JR, Greenberg JI, Baskin SI. Endotracheal epinephrine in cardiorespiratory collapse. *JACEP* 8:515, 1979.

Sabin HI et al. Accuracy of intracardiac injections determined by a post-mortem study. *Lancet* 2:1054, 1983.

Ward JT. Endotracheal drug therapy. *Amer J Emerg Med* 1:71, 1983.

You have been instructed by the base station physician to administer a lidocaine infusion at a rate of 2 mg per minute. You have an ampule containing 0.5 gm of lidocaine and a 250-ml bag of D5W. Your microdrip infusion set delivers 60 drops per milliliter.

At what rate, in drops per minute, must you run the infusion in order to deliver 2 mg per minute of lidocaine?

A18

Did you answer **60 drops per minute**? If not, you'd better review the steps in calculating doses:

FIRST, we need to determine the concentration of lidocaine in our solution:

$$\text{CONCENTRATION} = \frac{\text{mg of lidocaine added to the bag}}{\text{ml of solution in the bag}}$$

We have added 0.5 gm of lidocaine (=500 mg) to a bag containing 250 ml of solution. Thus our equation looks like this:

$$\text{CONCENTRATION} = \frac{500 \text{ mg}}{250 \text{ ml}} = 2 \text{ mg/ml}$$

So we know that in every milliliter of solution in the IV bag, there is 2 mg of lidocaine. We have been instructed to administer 2 mg per minute:

$$\text{ml to be administered} = \frac{\text{desired dose}}{\text{concentration on hand}} = \frac{2 \text{ mg/min}}{2 \text{ mg/ml}} = 1 \text{ ml/min}$$

How many drops per minute constitute 1 ml per minute? Our administration set is constructed to deliver 60 drops per milliliter:

$$\begin{aligned} \text{Drops/min} &= \text{drops/ml} \times \text{desired ml/min} \\ &= 60 \text{ drops/ml} \times 1 \text{ ml/min} \\ &= 60 \text{ drops/min} \end{aligned}$$

Got it?

OK, then, let's try another one, just for practice. This time, the physician orders you to administer 1 mg per minute of lidocaine. You have an ampule containing 1 gm of lidocaine and an IV bag containing 250 ml of D5W. Once again, you are using a microdrip infusion set, which delivers 60 drops per milliliter. How many drops should the patient receive in order to receive 1 mg of lidocaine per minute? (The answer is at the bottom of the page.)

FURTHER READING
Caroline NL. *Emergency Care in the Streets* (4th ed.). Boston: Little, Brown, 1991, Ch. 10.

ANSWER: 15 drops per minute

Match the following dosages with the drug to which each applies:

a. 0.01 to 0.02 mg per kilogram IV
b. 0.1 mg per kilogram by slow IV titration
c. 1.0 mg per kilogram IV push
d. 50 ml IV push
e. 5 ml of a 1:10,000 solution IV or by intracardiac injection
f. 1 to 3 mg per minute IV
g. 0.3 to 0.5 ml of a 1:1,000 solution SQ

1. _____ Continuous *infusion* of LIDOCAINE for ventricular dysrhythmias
2. _____ Single dose of ATROPINE for bradycardias
3. _____ Single dose of 50% GLUCOSE for a patient in coma
4. _____ Single dose of EPINEPHRINE for a mild asthmatic attack or a mild anaphylactic reaction
5. _____ Dose of MORPHINE for pulmonary edema
6. _____ Dose of EPINEPHRINE for asystole
7. _____ Minimum single dose of LIDOCAINE for ventricular dysrhythmias

A19

The paramedic should be able to recite in his sleep the correct dosage of every drug he uses in the field because the base station physician—whom you may contact at 3:00 in the morning for instructions—*is* frequently reciting his orders in his sleep, and being human, he can sometimes make a mistake. The paramedic must know enough about the drugs he uses in the field to question an order that seems in any way inappropriate ("Uh, Doctor, are you certain you want me to give 10—I repeat, 10—milligrams of atropine?"). Remember: THE PARAMEDIC IS AS MUCH RESPONSIBLE FOR THE ADMINISTRATION OF A DRUG AND ITS POSSIBLE CONSEQUENCES AS THE PHYSICIAN WHO GIVES THE ORDER. So learn those dosages.

1. __f__ Continuous *infusion* of LICOCAINE for ventricular dysrhythmias

   1 to 3 mg per minute IV. Make sure you use a microdrip infusion set for this and any other titrated, continuous infusions.

2. __a__ Single dose of ATROPINE for bradycardias

   0.01 to 0.02 mg per kilogram IV. That works out to 0.75 to 1.5 mg for the 75-kg man. (In emergency care, however, it is preferable always to give a *minimum* initial dose of 1 mg of atropine to an adult.)

3. __d__ Single dose of 50% GLUCOSE for a patient in coma

   50 ml IV push. Be certain you have a good, freely flowing IV line, for 50% glucose can cause significant local tissue damage if it inadvertently infiltrates.

4. __g__ Single dose of EPINEPHRINE for a mild asthmatic attack or a mild anaphylactic reaction

   0.3 to 0.5 ml of a 1:1,000 solution SQ. Use a 25-gauge needle for subcutaneous injections.

5. __b__ Dose of MORPHINE for pulmonary edema

   0.1 mg per kilogram by slow IV titration. That works out to about 7.5 mg for the 75-kg patient. Administer morphine only a few milligrams at a time, starting with 4 to 5 mg, and monitor the patient carefully for a fall in blood pressure.

6. __e__ Dose of EPINEPHRINE for asystole

   5 ml of a 1:10,000 solution IV or by intracardiac injection. If intracardiac injections are not authorized or attempts to start an IV have been unsuccessful, this dose may be delivered through the endotracheal tube.

7. __c__ Minimum single dose of LIDOCAINE for ventricular dysrhythmias

   1.0 mg per kilogram IV push, which works out to 75 mg for the famous 75-kg man. A loading dose is followed by a lidocaine infusion, so prepare the infusion ahead of time, label the bag, and piggyback the infusion in after you have administered the bolus.

FURTHER READING

American Heart Association. Standards and guidelines for cardiopulmonary resuscitation (CPR) and emergency cardiac care (ECC). *JAMA* 255:2905, 1986.

Caroline NL. *Emergency Care in the Streets* (4th ed.). Boston: Little, Brown, 1991, Drug Handbook.

Remember the autonomic nervous system and its two main subdivisions (the parasympathetic and sympathetic nervous systems)? The heart remembers. The heart gets most of its instructions through the autonomic nervous system, and a considerable number of the drugs used in the field interact with this system.

Indicate whether each of the following conditions or medical interventions would be expected to

a. Increase the heart rate
b. Decrease the heart rate

1. _____ Carotid sinus massage
2. _____ Administration of isoproterenol (Isuprel)
3. _____ Valsalva maneuver
4. _____ Administration of atropine
5. _____ Fright
6. _____ Abrupt rise in blood pressure
7. _____ Administration of propranolol (Inderal)
8. _____ Hemorrhage of 4 units of blood
9. _____ Acute hypoxemia
10. _____ Straining to have a bowel movement

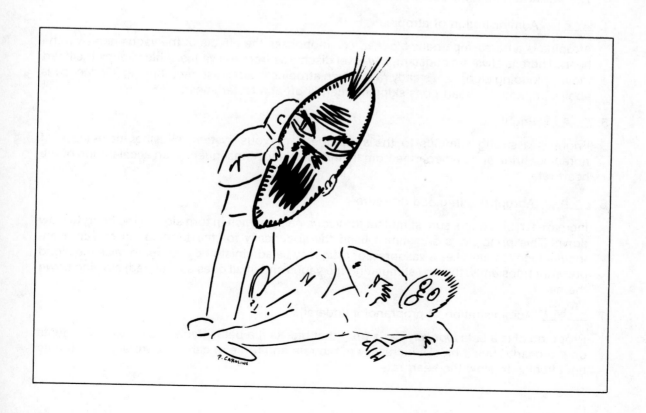

If you're a whiz on the autonomic nervous system, you can skip the next few paragraphs and go on to check your answers. But if you feel a bit shaky on the details, pause here and review a moment.

The autonomic, or involuntary, nervous system is divided into two major subdivisions: the parasympathetic nervous system and the sympathetic nervous system. The parasympathetic system, which is concerned largely with maintaining so-called vegetative functions, sends its signals to the heart through the vagus nerve. When the vagus nerve is stimulated, through whatever means, the heart slows down. Certain drugs, such as atropine, interfere with the action of the parasympathetic nervous system and block its messages from reaching the heart.

The sympathetic nervous system—or "fight-flight system"—prepares the body to respond to stress. It is mediated through chemicals released at nerve endings (norepinephrine) or by the adrenal gland (epinephrine), both of which, through their interaction with beta receptors in the myocardium, stimulate the heart to beat faster and more forcefully. Beta blockers, i.e., drugs that block the beta effects of sympathetic drugs or stimulation, have the opposite effect.

Now, let's look at the factors that (a) increase the heart rate or (b) decrease the heart rate:

1. __b__ Carotid sinus massage

Pressure or massage over the carotid sinus is a potent stimulus to the vagus nerve, i.e., a *parasympathetic* stimulus. The vagus, in turn, increases its output, and the heart receives a very emphatic command to slow down. For that reason, carotid sinus massage is used to terminate certain tachyarrhythmias.

2. __a__ Administration of isoproterenol (Isuprel)

Isoproterenol is a beta *sympathetic* drug. Hence it stimulates the heart to beat more rapidly and more forcefully.

3. __b__ Valsalva maneuver

The Valsalva maneuver is performed by straining to exhale against a closed glottis, and it represents another potent stimulus to the *vagus* nerve. Some patients with recurrent tachycardias of a type known as PAT (paroxysmal atrial tachycardia) will instinctively perform a Valsalva maneuver—by making themselves gag—in an attempt to terminate the dysrhythmia. The Valsalva maneuver acts by the same mechanism as carotid sinus massage.

4. __a__ Administration of atropine

Atropine is a parasympathetic *blocker,* i.e., it opposes the effects of the vagus nerve on the heart. There is always a constant, low-level discharge from the vagus, which keeps the heart mostly plodding along at a steady rate. When atropine is administered, the vagal influence is abolished, and the heart goes skipping merrily off at a faster speed.

5. __a__ Fright

Fright is a strong stimulus to the *sympathetic* nervous system, causing the release of norepinephrine and epinephrine from their depots and, consequently, an acceleration of the heart rate.

6. __b__ Abrupt rise in blood pressure

Increases in blood pressure stimulate the *vagus* nerve, which in turn signals the heart to slow down. This principle is sometimes used therapeutically for the termination of supraventricular tachycardias, i.e., a vasopressor drug may be administered in order to raise the blood pressure transiently, thereby stimulating the vagus and (if all goes as planned) slowing down the heart.

7. __b__ Administration of propranolol (Inderal)

Propranolol is a beta *blocker,* i.e., a drug that blocks the beta effects of *sympathetic* agents on the heart. Thus it blocks increases in the rate and force of cardiac contractions, and its net effect is to slow the heart rate.

8. __a__ Hemorrhage of 4 units of blood

Rapid blood loss provides a stimulus to the *sympathetic* nervous system, which attempts to compensate for the loss both through beta effects (increase in heart rate to increase cardiac output) and alpha effects (vasoconstriction).

9. __a__ Acute hypoxemia

Another stimulus to the *sympathetic* nervous system. When a person is deprived of oxygen, the O_2 levels in his blood rapidly decline, and the tissues begin to feel the effects of O_2 deprivation. They send out a distress signal, which activates the sympathetic nervous system to speed up the heart. After all, if each milliliter of blood is carrying only half the O_2 it should, the heart is going to have to pump out twice as much blood per minute to keep the tissues supplied with O_2 at the normal rate. That is to say, the heart must increase its output to compensate for the relative O_2 desaturation of the blood.

10. __b__ Straining to have a bowel movement

This is simply another Valsalva maneuver. It is important to know about because there are situations in which it is undesirable that a person's heart rate should slow down abruptly, such as in the wake of myocardial infarction. In such circumstances, the heart may respond to a sudden bradycardia by developing PVCs or ventricular tachycardia, and that is something we don't like to see happen. For this reason, it is standard policy on many coronary care units to give patients stool softeners and mild laxatives—in an attempt to prevent cardiac arrests on the commode.

FURTHER READING
Caroline NL. *Emergency Care in the Streets* (4th ed.). Boston: Little, Brown, 1991, Ch. 23.

Your patient is a 55-year-old man who takes propranolol (Inderal) at home for his angina. Which of the following drugs might you expect to be less effective in this patient on account of the propranolol he is taking?

a. Atropine
b. Furosemide (Lasix)
c. Isoproterenol (Isuprel)
d. Phenylephrine (Neo-Synephrine)
e. Sodium bicarbonate

A21 The correct answer is **c: isoproterenol.** If you missed it, let's go over the relevant features of the autonomic nervous system once again, just to be sure we get it straight.

Propranolol is a BETA BLOCKER, i.e., it acts by blocking the effects of beta-stimulating drugs on beta receptors. As you recall, drugs that affect the *sympathetic* nervous system can be classified as alpha drugs and beta drugs. ALPHA DRUGS (such as phenylephrine and norepinephrine) interact with alpha receptors in the blood vessels to produce vasoconstriction. BETA DRUGS (such as isoproterenol and epinephrine) act on beta receptors in the heart to increase the rate and force of cardiac contractions, they act on beta receptors in the arteries to produce vasodilation, and they act on beta receptors in the lungs to produce bronchodilation. When a beta *blocking* drug, such as propranolol, is administered, it occupies the beta receptors and prevents beta-stimulating drugs from doing their work.

Of the list of drugs presented, only isoproterenol (answer c) is a beta-stimulating drug, and therefore only isoproterenol would be blocked by propranolol. Atropine (answer a) is a blocking drug that acts (remember?) on the *parasympathetic* nervous system; specifically, it counteracts the effects of vagal stimulation. Furosemide (answer b) is of a different class of drugs altogether: It is a diuretic, which acts on the kidneys to promote excretion of urine. Phenylephrine (answer d) *is* a sympathetic agent, but it is an *alpha* agent, and therefore its effects will not be disturbed by a drug that blocks only beta receptors. Finally, sodium bicarbonate (answer e) is a buffer, which acts to minimize changes in the pH of a solution, and its actions are not affected by sympathomimetic drugs (i.e., drugs that act on the sympathetic nervous system).

FURTHER READING
Caroline NL. *Emergency Care in the Streets* (4th ed.). Boston: Little, Brown, 1991, Ch. 23.
Morrelli HF. Propranolol. *Ann Intern Med* 78:913, 1973.
Shand DG. Propranolol. *N Engl J Med* 293:280, 1975.
Zharadwajak, Promisloff R. Clinical pharmacology of propranolol. *Drug Ther Bull* 3:22, 1977.

The following are among the drugs commonly stocked on mobile intensive care ambulances, and the paramedic must be thoroughly familiar with the indications for each. Match the drugs in the list below with the condition for which each is most appropriately administered.

a. Epinephrine 1:1,000, 0.4 ml SQ
b. Lidocaine, 100 mg slowly IV followed by 2 mg per minute IV infusion
c. Atropine, 1.0 to 1.5 mg IV push
d. Morphine, 5 to 10 mg by slow IV titration
e. Sodium bicarbonate, 50 ml IV

1. _____ A 40-year-old man with chest pain and multifocal PVCs.
2. _____ A 60-year-old man in severe left heart failure, coughing up foamy sputum.
3. _____ A 58-year-old man found in the street in cardiac arrest; bystanders state that he collapsed 4 minutes earlier. Cardiopulmonary resuscitation has been initiated, an IV line has been inserted, and CPR has been ongoing for 25 minutes.
4. _____ A 24-year-old man with a moderately severe asthmatic attack.
5. _____ A 40-year-old man with severe chest pain and sinus bradycardia at a rate of 32 per minute.

Which of the above patients should receive oxygen?

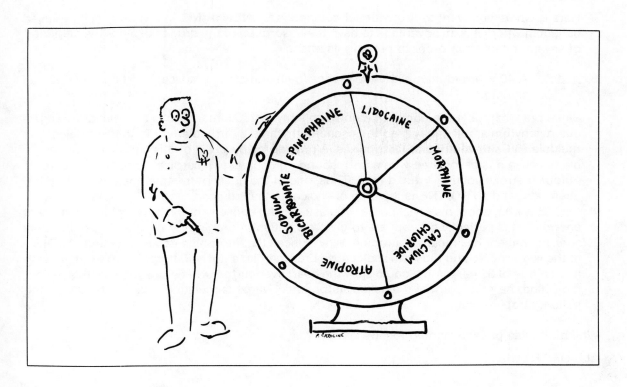

A22

1. __b__ A 40-year-old man with chest pain and multifocal PVCs.

LIDOCAINE is the drug of choice for PVCs, and this patient's PVCs are particularly worrisome—first, because they are occurring in the context of a probable myocardial infarction, and second, because they are multifocal, indicating widespread ventricular irritability. When lidocaine is administered, it should always be given *first* by bolus (75–100 mg slowly IV), followed up by a constant infusion (1–4 mg/min); the bolus provides an immediate therapeutic blood level, which is then sustained by the infusion. If the bolus were not given, it would take hours to reach a therapeutic blood level with an infusion alone; conversely, if the bolus is not followed up with an infusion, the effects of the bolus will wear off after several minutes, and repeated boluses will be required.

2. __d__ A 60-year-old man in severe left heart failure, coughing up foamy sputum.

From the list provided, **MORPHINE** is the drug of choice for the treatment of left heart failure with pulmonary edema. Morphine acts both to decrease venous return to the heart and to allay anxiety. It must be given in carefully titrated doses, starting with 4 to 5 mg and then a few milligrams at a time, until the desired therapeutic effect is achieved or the blood pressure begins to fall toward hypotensive levels.

3. __f__ A 58-year-old man found in the street in cardiac arrest; bystanders state he collapsed 4 minutes earlier. Cardiopulmonary resuscitation has been initiated, an IV line has been inserted, and CPR has been ongoing for 25 minutes.

A patient who has been in cardiac arrest for 25 minutes will almost certainly be at least moderately acidotic. One begins dealing with the acidosis by initiating artificial ventilation. The acidosis may also require **SODIUM BICARBONATE,** which should be administered only on a doctor's order.

Perhaps you answered "a" to this question: You wanted to give epinephrine. While it is true that epinephrine will usually be required in the resuscitation of an unwitnessed cardiac arrest, the dosage and route of administration of epinephrine listed in answer a—0.4 ml of a 1:1,000 solution SQ—are entirely inappropriate for cardiac arrest, for which IV administration of a 1:10,000 solution is required. PAY ATTENTION TO DOSAGE! The wrong dosage of the right drug can be just as lethal as using the wrong drug.

4. __a__ A 24-year-old man with a moderately severe asthmatic attack.

Here is where you want to use your subcutaneous **EPINEPHRINE,** in a young, well-perfused patient in whom it is an advantage to have the absorption of the drug take place over a period of several minutes, in order to prolong its effect.

5. __c__ A 40-year-old man with severe chest pain and sinus bradycardia at a rate of 32 per minute.

Sinus bradycardia in the context of a probable myocardial infarction is a potentially dangerous dysrhythmia, for it may lead to "escape" rhythms by irritable foci in the ventricles, i.e., multiple PVCs or ventricular tachycardia. A marked bradycardia of this sort is also undesirable because it is associated with a corresponding decrease in cardiac output (since cardiac output = stroke volume × heart rate). Thus, one of the goals of treatment is to speed up the heart rate, and **ATROPINE** is the drug of choice for that purpose.

"But what about his chest pain?" you ask, having chosen answer d, morphine, instead of answer c. It is perfectly appropriate to give this patient morphine for his chest pain, but only *after* the patient has received atropine. Why? Recall that morphine can be a potent stimulant to the vagus nerve and thus can itself cause bradycardia; a dose of morphine to a patient with a heart rate of 32 per minute could slow the heart even further. So before you give this patient morphine, be sure you have blocked its potential vagal stimulating effects—by giving the patient atropine first.

Which of these patients should receive oxygen?

ALL OF THEM!

FURTHER READING

American Heart Association. Standards and guidelines for cardiopulmonary resuscitation (CPR) and emergency cardiac care (ECC). *JAMA* 255:2905, 1986.

Appel D et al. Comparative effect of epinephrine and aminophylline in the treatment of asthma. *Lung* 159:243, 1981.

Baron DW et al. Protective effect of lidocaine during regional myocardial ischemia. *Mayo Clin Proc* 57:442, 1982.

Ben-Zvi Z et al. An evaluation of repeated injections of epinephrine for the initial treatment of acute asthma. *Am Rev Resp Dis* 127:101, 1983.

Bishop RL, Weisfeldt ML. Sodium bicarbonate administration during cardiac arrest. *JAMA* 235:506, 1976.

Dauchot P, Gravenstein JS. Bradycardia after myocardial ischemia and its treatment with atropine. *Anesthesiology* 44:501, 1976.

Elenbaas RM et al. Subcutaneous epinephrine vs. nebulized metaproterenol in acute asthma. *Drug Intell Clin Pharm* 19:567, 1985.

Gotz VP et al. Bronchodilatory effect of subcutaneous epinephrine in acute asthma. *Ann Emerg Med* 10:518, 1981.

Granstetter RD et al. Optimal dosing of epinephrine in acute asthma. *Am J Hosp Pharm* 37:1326, 1980.

Karetzy MS. Acute asthma: The use of subcutaneous epinephrine in therapy. *Ann Allergy* 44:12, 1980.

Koster RW, Dunning AJ. Intramuscular lidocaine for prevention of lethal arrhythmias in the prehospitalization phase of acute myocardial infarction. *N Engl J Med* 313:1105, 1985.

Mattar JA et al. Cardiac arrest in the critically ill: II. Hyperosmolal status following cardiac arrest. *Am J Med* 56:162, 1974.

Pliss LB et al. Aerosol vs. injected epinephrine in acute asthma. *Ann Emerg Med* 10:353, 1981.

Robin ED, Cross CE, Zelis R. Pulmonary edema. *NEMJ* 288:239, 1973.

Valentine PA et al. Lidocaine in the prevention of sudden death in the prehospital phase of acute infarction. *N Engl J Med* 291:1327, 1974.

Waller ES. Appropriate lidocaine doses: Science added to the art. *Tex Med* 77:55, 1981.

Wennerblom B et al. Antiarrhythmic efficacy and side-effects of lidocaine given in the prehospital phase of acute myocardial infarction. *Eur Heart J* 3:516, 1982.

Weil MH et al. Sodium bicarbonate during CPR: Does it help or hinder? *Chest* 88:487, 1985.

White BC, Tintinalli JE. Effects of sodium bicarbonate administration during cardiopulmonary resuscitation. *JACEP* 6:187, 1977.

White RD. Lidocaine. *EMT J* 4(3):64, 1980.

Wilson RF. Sodium bicarbonate administration during cardiopulmonary resuscitation (editorial). *JACEP* 6:331, 1977.

Which of the following statements about epinephrine is NOT true?

a. Epinephrine is *primarily* an alpha drug.
b. The initial therapeutic dose of epinephrine in cardiac arrest is 5 ml of a 1:10,000 solution by intracardiac injection or IV.
c. Epinephrine must be used with great caution in patients with known angina pectoris or hypertension.
d. Epinephrine is the primary drug in the treatment of anaphylaxis.
e. Epinephrine is used in asthma for its bronchodilating effects.

A23

Answer **a** is NOT true. While it is the case that epinephrine has some alpha properties, which become evident at high doses, epinephrine is *primarily* a beta drug and is used because of its beta effects, i.e., to increase the rate and force of cardiac contractions and to bring about bronchodilation (note answers d and e).

In cardiac arrest, one uses epinephrine to stimulate the cardiac muscle, and one usually begins with a dose of 5 ml of a 1 : 10,000 solution (answer b). In asthma, one is interested chiefly in the bronchodilating effects of the drug (answer e), while in anaphylaxis both the cardiotonic and bronchodilating effects of epinephrine are important (answer d).

Epinephrine must be used with great caution in patients with known angina pectoris or hypertension (answer c). Because it increases the rate and force of cardiac contractions, epinephrine also increases cardiac work, and this may precipitate an angina attack in patients suffering from ischemic heart disease. The alpha effects of epinephrine can lead to vasoconstriction with resultant elevations in blood pressure, which can be dangerous in a patient whose blood pressure is already at high levels, e.g., a patient with chronic hypertension.

FURTHER READING

American Heart Association. Standards and guidelines for cardiopulmonary resuscitation (CPR) and emergency cardiac care (ECC). *JAMA* 255:2905, 1986.

Appel D et al. Comparative effect of epinephrine and aminophylline in the treatment of asthma. *Lung* 159:243, 1981.

Barach EM et al. Epinephrine for the treatment of anaphylactic shock. *JAMA* 251:218, 1984.

Ben-Zvi Z et al. An evaluation of repeated injections of epinephrine for the initial treatment of acute asthma. *Am Rev Resp Dis* 127:101, 1983.

Chernow B et al. Epinephrine absorption after intratracheal administration. *Anesth Analg* 63:829, 1984.

Davison R et al. Intracardiac injections during cardiopulmonary resuscitation—a low risk procedure. *JAMA* 244:1110, 1980.

Elenbaas RM et al. Subcutaneous epinephrine vs. nebulized metaproterenol in acute asthma. *Drug Intell Clin Pharm* 19:567, 1985.

Gonzales ER et al. Dose-dependent vasopressor response to epinephrine during CPR in human beings. *Ann Emerg Med* 19:322, 1990.

Gotz VP et al. Bronchodilatory effect of subcutaneous epinephrine in acute asthma. *Ann Emerg Med* 10:518, 1981.

Granstetter RD et al. Optimal dosing of epinephrine in acute asthma. *Am J Hosp Pharm* 37:1326, 1980.

Hao-Hui C. Closed-chest intracardiac injection. *Resuscitation* 9:103, 1981.

Karetzy MS. Acute asthma: The use of subcutaneous epinephrine in therapy. *Ann Allergy* 44:12, 1980.

Michael JR et al. Mechanisms by which epinephrine augments cerebral and myocardial perfusion during cardiopulmonary resuscitation in dogs. *Circulation* 69:822, 1984.

Otto CW, Yakaitis RW, Blitt CD. Mechanism of action of epinephrine in resuscitation from asphyxial arrest. *Crit Care Med* 9:321, 1981.

Pearson JW, Redding JS. Epinephrine in cardiac arrest. *Am Heart J* 66:210, 1963.

Peppers MP. Updating epinephrine. *Emergency* 22(3):18, 1990.

Pliss LB et al. Aerosol vs. injected epinephrine in acute asthma. *Ann Emerg Med* 10:353, 1981.

Roberts JR et al. Blood levels following intravenous and endotracheal epinephrine administration. *JACEP* 8:53, 1979.

Roberts JR, Greenberg JI, Baskin SI. Endotracheal epinephrine in cardiorespiratory collapse. *JACEP* 8:515, 1979.

Rothenberg MA. Reviewing high-dose epinephrine. *JEMS* 15(4):43, 1990.

Sabin HI et al. Accuracy of intracardiac injections determined by a post-mortem study. *Lancet* 2:1054, 1983.

Ward JT. Endotracheal drug therapy. *Am J Emerg Med* 1:71, 1983.

Yakaitis RW, Otto CW, Blitt CD. Relative importance of alpha and beta adrenergic receptors during resuscitation. *Crit Care Med* 7:293, 1979.

Which of the following statements about atropine is NOT true?

a. Administration of atropine to a conscious patient may cause blurring of vision, dryness of the mouth, flushing of the skin, and urinary retention.

b. Atropine blocks the action of the vagus nerve.

c. In severe sinus bradycardia with signs of poor peripheral perfusion, one should give 0.01 to 0.02 mg per kilogram of atropine IV.

d. Atropine should not be given to a patient who develops severe bradycardia as a result of the administration of morphine.

e. Atropine should not be given to a patient who has atrial fibrillation with a rapid pulse.

A24

Answer **d** is NOT true. It is not uncommon for patients to develop bradycardia following administration of morphine, because of morphine's stimulating effect on the vagus nerve; atropine is the drug of choice to counteract this effect because atropine works by blocking the action of the vagus nerve (answer b). The therapeutic dose of atropine is 0.01 to 0.02 mg per kilogram, with a miniumum dose of 1.0 mg rapidly IV for the average adult male (answer c). Be sure to give atropine rapidly and in a sufficient dose, for slow administration or the administration of an inadequate dose may have a paradoxical effect (i.e., it may *slow* the heart rate rather than speed it up), and ventricular escape rhythms may result.

Common side effects of atropine administration include blurring of vision, dryness of the mouth, flushing of the skin, urinary retention (especially in older, male patients), headache, and pupillary dilatation (answer a). The patient should be informed that he may experience some of these side effects and that they are part of the usual, expected reaction to the drug.

Atropine should not be given to patients who have atrial fibrillation with a rapid ventricular response (answer e). By blocking the action of the vagus nerve on the atrioventricular node, atropine may permit more atrial impulses to pass from the atria to the ventricles and thereby cause the ventricular rate to increase even further, which is not desirable in a patient who already has a tachycardia.

FURTHER READING

American Heart Association. Standards and guidelines for cardiopulmonary resuscitation (CPR) and emergency cardiac care (ECC). *JAMA* 255:2905, 1986.

Averill JH, Lamb LE. Less commonly recognized actions of atropine on cardiac rhythm. *Am J Med Sci* 237:304, 1959.

Bray BM et al. Tracheal vs. intravenous atropine: A comparison of the effects on heart rate. *Anaesthesia* 42:1188, 1987.

Brown DC, Lewis AJ, Criley JM. Asystole and its treatment: The possible role of the parasympathetic nervous system in cardiac arrest. *JACEP* 8:448, 1979.

Coon GA et al. Use of atropine for brady-asystolic prehospital cardiac arrest. *Ann Emerg Med* 10:462, 1981.

Cooper MJ, Abinader EG. Atropine-induced ventricular fibrillation: Case report and review of the literature. *Am Heart J* 97:255, 1979.

Dauchot P, Gravenstein JS. Bradycardia after myocardial ischemia and its treatment with atropine. *Anesthesiology* 44:501, 1976.

Greenberg MI et al. Endotracheal administration of atropine sulfate. *Ann Emerg Med* 11:546, 1982.

Howard RF et al. Endotracheal compared with intravenous administration of atropine. *Arch Dis Child* 64:449, 1990.

Kottmeier CA, Gravenstein JS. The parasympathomimetic action of atropine and atropine methylbromide. *Anesthesiology* 29:1125, 1968.

Massumi RA et al. Ventricular fibrillation and tachycardia after intravenous atropine for treatment of bradycardias. *N Engl J Med* 287:336, 1972.

Myerburg RJ et al. Outcome of resuscitation from bradyarrhythmic or asystolic prehospital cardiac arrest. *J Am Coll Cardiol* 4:1118, 1984.

Steuven HA et al. Atropine in asystole: Human studies. *Ann Emerg Med* 13:815, 1984.

Which of the following statements about lidocaine is NOT true?

a. Lidocaine should be given immediately to any patient with multifocal PVCs.
b. High doses of lidocaine may cause seizures.
c. Lidocaine is given after successful defibrillation to prevent a recurrence of ventricular fibrillation.
d. Lidocaine can decrease the force of cardiac contractions, leading to a decrease in cardiac output and blood pressure.
e. Lidocaine is given for third-degree heart block in order to stabilize the ventricles.

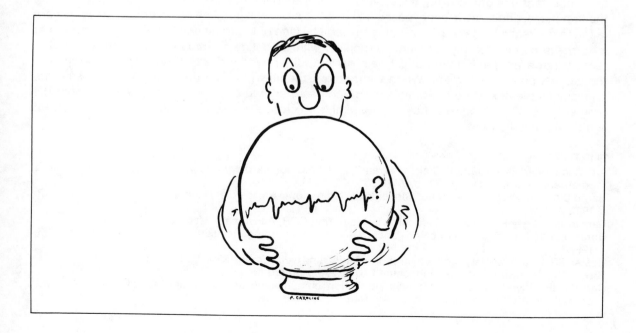

A25

Answer **e** is NOT true. Emphatically not true.

In third-degree heart block, there is complete dissociation between the atria and the ventricles, and thus, in a manner of speaking, *every* ventricular beat is an ectopic beat. Now suppose you administered a bolus of lidocaine to suppress these "ectopic" beats; there is every possibility you might succeed, and the ventricles would stop contracting altogether. Those "ectopic" beats in complete heart block are the only source of cardiac output. So don't reach for the lidocaine every time you see widened or bizarre QRS complexes; check first to make sure you're not dealing with complete heart block. LIDOCAINE IS CONTRAINDICATED IN THIRD-DEGREE HEART BLOCK.

Answer a is true. Some authorities have favored giving lidocaine to any patient with chest pain, as a prophylactic measure against the development of PVCs, although there is no convincing evidence that doing so improves the ultimate outcome of the patient. But nearly all cardiologists would agree that there are certain categories of PVCs that are intrinsically dangerous and should be treated whether or not they occur in the context of acute myocardial infarction. Those PVCs include (1) multifocal PVCs (which can be recognized because they have different sizes and shapes); (2) PVCs that fall on top of the T wave (R–on–T phenomenon), when the ventricle is most vulnerable to fibrillation; and (3) PVCs occurring in salvos (two or more in succession). All of those situations bespeak extreme irritability of the ventricles and identify a patient in considerable danger of developing ventricular tachycardia or ventricular fibrillation. Such a patient warrants immediate treatment with lidocaine to suppress the PVCs *before* they progress to life-threatening dysrhythmias.

Answers b and d refer to two of the potential untoward side effects of lidocaine, namely seizures and hypotension. Seizures are a relatively rare side effect of lidocaine therapy and tend to occur only with excessively rapid administration, very high doses, or high cumulative doses. The latter situation may develop unnoticed in a patient with chronic right heart failure, for in such patients the liver—being chronically congested with blood—may not function with full efficiency to metabolize injected drugs. Thus blood levels of lidocaine gradually build up, and even a therapeutic dose (such as 4 mg/min) can, over a period of hours, lead to the accumulation of toxic levels of the drug in the bloodstream. A grand mal seizure may be the first indication that this has occurred, but usually the seizure is preceded by other symptoms, such as numbness, drowsiness, and confusion, and frequently twitching of the skeletal muscles. Lidocaine may also cause hypotension because it decreases the force of ventricular contraction and sometimes decreases peripheral resistance as well. The lesson in all this is: KNOW THE PROPERTIES OF THE DRUGS WITH WHICH YOU WORK. WHEN YOU ADMINISTER ANY DRUG, BE ALERT FOR ITS POTENTIAL SIDE EFFECTS.

Because it stabilizes the ventricles, lidocaine is frequently given after successful defibrillation to prevent a recurrence of ventricular fibrillation (answer d). That is an entirely appropriate and important use of the drug. It was ventricular irritability that sent the heart into fibrillation in the first place, and there is every possibility that the heart will fibrillate again unless measures are taken to decrease the level of ventricular irritability. One of the most important of such measures is to make certain the myocardium is supplied with an optimum amount of oxygen; that is the reason that every patient with chest pain or ventricular dysrhythmias should receive oxygen at the earliest possible moment. When ventricular irritability persists after oxygen administration, lidocaine is the next drug to administer. Blood gases should be checked at the earliest possible moment after the patient reaches the hospital, for acidosis is also a frequent cause of recurrent ventricular dysrhythmias.

FURTHER READING

American Heart Association. Standards and guidelines for cardiopulmonary resuscitation (CPR) and emergency cardiac care (ECC). *JAMA* 255:2905, 1986.

Baron DW et al. Protective effect of lidocaine during regional myocardial ischemia. *Mayo Clin Proc* 57:442, 1982.

Barsan WG, Levy RC, Weir H. Lidocaine levels during CPR. *Ann Emerg Med* 10:73, 1981.

Borak J et al. Prophylactic lidocaine: Uncertain benefits in emergency settings. *Ann Emerg Med* 11:493, 1982.

Boster SR et al. Translaryngeal absorption of lidocaine. *Ann Emerg Med* 11:461, 1982.

Brown DL, Skiendzielewski JJ. Lidocaine toxicity. *Ann Emerg Med* 9:627, 1980.

Carruth JE, Silverman ME. Ventricular fibrillation complicating acute myocardial infarction: Reasons against the routine use of lidocaine. *Am Heart J* 104:545, 1982.

Chow MSS et al. Antifibrillatory effects of lidocaine and bretylium immediately postcardiopulmonary resuscitation. *Am Heart J* 110:938, 1985.

Dunn HM et al. Prophylactic lidocaine in the early phase of suspected myocardial infarction. *Am Heart J* 110:353, 1985.

Harrison DC et al. Should prophylactic antiarrhythmic drug therapy be used in acute myocardial infarction? *JAMA* 247:2019, 1982.

Harrison EE. Lidocaine in prehospital countershock refractory ventricular fibrillation. *Ann Emerg Med* 10:420, 1981.

Koster RW, Dunning AJ. Intramuscular lidocaine for prevention of lethal arrhythmias in the prehospitalization phase of acute myocardial infarction. *N Engl J Med* 313:1105, 1985.

Levy DB. Update on lidocaine. *Emergency* 20(9):15, 1988.

Lie KI. Pre- and in-hospital antiarrhythmic prevention of ventricular fibrillation complicating acute myocardial infarction. *Eur Heart J* 5(Suppl B):95, 1984.

Lie KI et al. Lidocaine in the prevention of primary ventricular fibrillation. *N Engl J Med* 291:1324, 1974.

Lopez LM et al. Optimal lidocaine dosing in patients with myocardial infarction. *Ther Drug Monit* 4:271, 1982.

MacMahon S et al. Effects of prophylactic lidocaine in acute myocardial infarction: An overview of results from the randomized, controlled trials. *JAMA* 260:1910, 1988.

McDonald JL. Serum lidocaine levels during cardiopulmonary resuscitation after intravenous and endotracheal administration. *Crit Care Med* 13:914, 1985.

Valentine PA et al. Lidocaine in the prevention of sudden death in the prehospital phase of acute infarction. *N Engl J Med* 291:1327, 1974.

Waller ES. Appropriate lidocaine doses: Science added to the art. *Tex Med* 77:55, 1981.

Wennerblom B et al. Antiarrhythmic efficacy and side-effects of lidocaine given in the prehospital phase of acute myocardial infarction. *Eur Heart J* 3:516, 1982.

White RD. Lidocaine. *EMT J* 4(3):64, 1980.

Wyse DG, Kellen J, Rademaker AW. Prophylactic vs. selective lidocaine for early ventricular arrhythmias of myocardial infarction. *J Am Coll Cardiol* 12:507, 1988.

Which of the following statements about administration of sodium bicarbonate is NOT true?

a. Sodium bicarbonate is a buffer used to treat metabolic acidosis.
b. Sodium bicarbonate is used in the treatment of hypokalemia to raise the level of potassium in the blood.
c. Sodium bicarbonate can worsen the condition of a patient in congestive heart failure because it provides salt to a patient who is already overloaded with salt and water.
d. It is no longer recommended to give sodium bicarbonate at the outset of CPR.
e. Effective ventilation must accompany administration of sodium bicarbonate in order to blow off the excess carbon dioxide generated in the blood.

A26 Answer **b** is NOT true. The administration of sodium bicarbonate will LOWER serum potassium levels, and for that reason it is sometimes used in the emergency treatment of *hyper*kalemia. When given to a patient who is already *hypo*kalemic (e.g., a patient on chronic diuretic therapy who has not been taking adequate potassium replacement), sodium bicarbonate may drop the potassium to dangerously low levels, causing ventricular fibrillation and death. For that reason, sodium bicarbonate should be administered with extreme caution to any patient suspected on clinical grounds (e.g., history of diuretic intake) or electrocardiographic grounds (prominent U wave, prolonged P–R interval, S–T depression) of hypokalemia.

The principal use of sodium bicarbonate is as a buffer in the treatment of metabolic acidosis (answer a). In cardiac arrest, it is no longer recommended to give sodium bicarbonate at all at the outset of CPR (answer d). Whether to give bicarbonate later in the resuscitation procedure is left to the discretion of the physician, but even then, doses are best titrated according to arterial blood gas measurements, when available, for research has shown that there is a tendency to use too much bicarbonate during resuscitation procedures. If blood gases are not available, as during a long resuscitation in the field, one ampule (50 ml) of sodium bicarbonate administered after 15 minutes of CPR will probably suffice.

The administration of sodium bicarbonate causes a transient increase in the arterial PCO_2 because of the dissociation of sodium bicarbonate as follows:

$$NaHCO_3 \rightarrow H_2O + CO_2$$

Thus good artificial ventilation must accompany administration of sodium bicarbonate in order to blow off the excess carbon dioxide generated by its administration (answer e).

Each ampule of sodium bicarbonate contains approximately 45 mEq of sodium, i.e., the same amount of sodium that is contained in ⅓ liter of (isotonic) normal saline. In other words, the administration of 3 ampules of sodium bicarbonate is equivalent, in terms of the salt load imposed, to the administration of 1 liter of normal saline. That can be very dangerous to patients who have difficulty tolerating salt loads, such as patients in borderline congestive heart failure (answer c).

FURTHER READING

American Heart Association. Standards and guidelines for cardiopulmonary resuscitation (CPR) and emergency cardiac care (ECC). *JAMA* 255:2905, 1986.
Berenyi KJ, Wolk M, Killip T. Cerebrospinal fluid acidosis complicating therapy of experimental cardiopulmonary arrest. *Circulation* 52:319, 1975.
Bersin RM et al. Metabolic and hemodynamic consequences of sodium bicarbonate administration in patients with heart disease. *Am J Med* 87:7, 1989.
Bicarbonate. *Emerg Med* 8(6):226, 1976.
Bishop RL, Weisfeldt ML. Sodium bicarbonate administration during cardiac arrest. *JAMA* 235:506, 1976.
Cooper DJ et al. Bicarbonate does not improve hemodynamics in critically ill patients who have lactic acidosis. *Arch Intern Med* 112:492, 1990.
Graf H et al. The use of sodium bicarbonate in the therapy of organic acidosis. *Intensive Care Med* 12:285, 1986.
Grundler W et al. The paradox of venous acidosis and arterial alkalosis during CPR. *Chest* 86:282, 1984.
Mattar JA et al. Cardiac arrest in the critically ill: II. Hyperosmolal status following cardiac arrest. *Am J Med* 56:162, 1974.
Sanders AB et al. The role of bicarbonate and fluid loading in improving resuscitation from prolonged cardiac arrest with rapid manual chest compression CPR. *Ann Emerg Med* 19:1, 1990.
Weil MH et al. Sodium bicarbonate during CPR: Does it help or hinder? *Chest* 88:487, 1985.
White BC, Tintinalli JE. Effects of sodium bicarbonate administration during cardiopulmonary resuscitation. *JACEP* 6:187, 1977.
Wilson RF. Sodium bicarbonate administration during cardiopulmonary resuscitation (editorial). *JACEP* 6:331, 1977.

Which of the following statements about morphine sulfate is NOT true?

a. Morphine may cause a fall in blood pressure.
b. Morphine is indicated in the treatment of left heart failure with pulmonary edema.
c. The usual dose of morphine is 1 mg per kilogram of body weight.
d. Morphine may depress respirations.
e. Morphine may cause bradycardia due to a stimulating effect on the vagus nerve.

A27 Answer **c** is NOT true. The therapeutic dose of morphine is 0.1 mg per kilogram of body weight; the dose listed in answer c is 10 times too high and would kill the patient! KNOW YOUR DOSAGES: A DECIMAL POINT CAN BE THE DIFFERENCE BETWEEN RESUSCITATION AND MURDER!

The paramedic must also be thoroughly familiar with the potential side effects of any drug he administers. Morphine may cause hypotension (answer a), respiratory depression (answer d), and nausea, vomiting, and bradycardia due to stimulation of the vagus nerve (answer e). The last complication is more likely to occur in the context of an inferior wall myocardial infarction, and for that reason, some physicians prefer to withhold morphine when the ECG shows S–T changes in the inferior leads. When bradycardia does occur after morphine administration, the treatment is atropine, which should always be drawn up and ready for administration whenever morphine is given.

Morphine is an excellent drug for the treatment of pulmonary edema secondary to left heart failure (answer b) because morphine—by the same mechanism through which it causes hypotension—decreases venous return to the heart; blood pools in the periphery due to vasodilatation, and the circulatory overload on the heart is thereby relatively relieved. That effect is sometimes referred to as an "internal phlebotomy" or a "pharmacologic phlebotomy," since it produces the same results as actually withdrawing a unit or two of blood from the patient's circulation. Another drug that can produce an "internal phlebotomy" is nitroglycerin, and for that reason nitroglycerin is also sometimes used in the management of acute pulmonary edema.

FURTHER READING

Alderman EL. Analgesics in the acute phase of myocardial infarction. *JAMA* 229:1646, 1974.

Hoffman JR, Reynolds S. Comparison of nitroglycerin, morphine, and furosemide in treatment of presumed pre-hospital pulmonary edema. *Chest* 92:586, 1987.

Lowenstein EL et al. Cardiovascular response to large doses of intravenous morphine in man. *N Engl J Med* 281:1389, 1969.

Robin ED, Cross CE, Zelis R. Pulmonary edema. *N Engl J Med* 288:239, 1973.

Semenkovich CF, Jaffe AS. Adverse effects due to morphine sulfate. *Am J Med* 79:325, 1985.

Zelis R et al. The cardiovascular effects of morphine. *J Clin Invest* 54:1247, 1974.

Combinations of 50% oxygen and 50% nitrous oxide are coming into increasing use by ambulance teams for the management of pain. Indicate in which of the following situations the use of N_2O/O_2 combinations is CONTRAINDICATED:

a. A 48-year-old victim of an automobile accident suspected of having suffered a pneumothorax; he is conscious and alert.
b. A 52-year-old man with symptoms and signs of acute myocardial infarction.
c. A 62-year-old woman in acute pulmonary edema.
d. An 18-year-old youth who was struck over the head with a chair during an altercation; he is groggy, but responds to verbal stimuli.
e. A 60-year-old woman with a history of 4 hours of severe abdominal pain.

Note: There may be more than one correct answer.

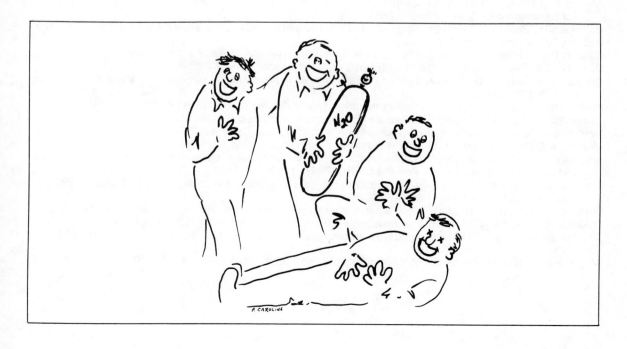

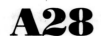

A28 Nitrous oxide/oxygen combinations are contraindicated in patients **a, c, d,** and possibly **e.**

Let's take a look at our patients one by one.

The use of N_2O/O_2 combinations is contraindicated in patient a because he is suspected of having suffered a pneumothorax. Nitrous oxide tends to collect in dead air spaces—such as the space between the visceral and parietal pleura in a patient with a pneumothorax—and for that reason would tend to enlarge a pneumothorax, not a desirable side effect!

Patient b is a very good candidate for N_2O/O_2 therapy, for nitrous oxide has been shown to be effective in providing pain relief in myocardial infarction, and the 50-50 combination with oxygen still enables one to deliver a relatively high oxygen concentration.

Our 62-year-old woman with pulmonary edema (patient c), on the other hand, should not receive the N_2O/O_2 combination. To begin with, she needs an inhaled oxygen concentration much higher than 50%. In the second place, this is one situation where morphine is clearly indicated because of its action in decreasing venous return to the heart. Besides, the patient is not in pain. She simply can't breathe. So there is no reason to give her an analgesic anyway.

The most important sign to monitor in a head-injured patient, such as our young man who had a chair smashed over his skull (patient d), is the state of consciousness. For that reason, nitrous oxide would be contraindicated, since it commonly produces drowsiness and thus might mask the very signs we are trying to monitor.

Our 60-year-old lady with severe abdominal pain (patient e) would seem to be the best candidate of all for nitrous oxide analgesia. On the one hand, the surgeons will be very upset with you if you give her morphine or a similar narcotic, for strong parenteral analgesics may mask the patient's symptoms for hours and thereby make it very difficult for the surgeons in the emergency room to reach a diagnosis. On the other hand, it isn't very pleasant for you to stand there doing nothing while a patient is in terrible pain. To provide relief of suffering is one of the most fundamental missions of any health care professional, and you would like to be able to ease this woman's distress. Nitrous oxide seems like the ideal compromise: It provides rapid and effective relief of pain, but its effects dissipate within minutes of stopping the inhalation. Thus you can keep this woman comfortable throughout transport but still ensure that when the surgeons descend upon her in the emergency room to poke at her belly her clinical signs will not be masked. The problem is that if the woman has an acute abdomen and peristalsis has ceased (so-called ileus), nitrogen will collect in her bowel just as in any other dead air space. So inhaling nitrous oxide for any period of time may lead to potentially dangerous degrees of abdominal distention. For belly pain, therefore, consult medical command before giving N_2O.

FURTHER READING

Amey BD et al. Prehospital administration of nitrous oxide for control of pain. *Ann Emerg Med* 10:279, 1981.

Ancker K et al. Nitrous oxide analgesia during ambulance transportion: Airborne levels of nitrous oxide. *Acta Anaesthesiol Scand* 24:497, 1980.

Ballinger JA. Experience with prehospital administration of nitrous oxide. *Emerg Med Serv* 8(5):14, 1979.

Baskett PJ. Entonox. *Proc R Soc Med* 65:7, 1972.

Baskett PJ, Withnell A. Use of Entonox in the ambulance service. *Br Med J* 2:41, 1970.

Doen N et al. Pre-hospital analgesia with Entonox. *Can Anaesth Soc J* 29:275, 1982.

Gamis AS, Knapp JF, Glenski JA. Nitrous oxide analgesia in a pediatric emergency department. *Ann Emerg Med* 18:177, 1989.

Kunkel DB. Nitrous oxide: Not a laughing matter anymore. *Emerg Med* 21(3):117, 1989.

James MFM et al. Nitrous oxide analgesia and altitude. *Anaesthesia* 37:285, 1982.

McKinnon DDL et al. Nitrous oxide analgesia in emergency care. *Can Fam Physician* 26:83, 1980.

McKinnon DDL. Prehospital analgesia with nitrous oxide/oxygen. *Can Med Assoc J* 125:836, 1981.

Mitchell MM et al. Nitrous oxide does not induce myocardial ischemia in patients with ischemic heart disease and poor ventricular function. *Anesthesiology* 7:526, 1989.

Stewart RD et al. Patient-controlled inhalation analgesia in prehospital care: A study of side effects and feasibility. *Crit Care Med* 11:851, 1983.

Stewart RD. Nitrous oxide sedation/analgesia in emergency medicine. *Ann Emerg Med* 14:139, 1985.

Thal ER et al. Self-administered analgesia with nitrous oxide. *JAMA* 242:2418, 1979.

Thompson PL, Lown B. Nitrous oxide as an analgesic in acute myocardial infarction. *JAMA* 235:924, 1976.

Wright PM Jr. Nitrous oxide: An analgesic for field use. *Emerg Med Serv* 13(3):61, 1984.

Which of the following statements about calcium chloride is NOT true?

a. Calcium chloride is useful in the treatment of digitalis overdose.
b. Calcium chloride increases myocardial contractility.
c. Calcium chloride is used as an antidote to magnesium sulfate.
d. Calcium chloride should not be mixed with sodium bicarbonate in an infusion, since the two will combine to form an insoluble precipitate of calcium carbonate.

A29 Answer **a** is NOT true. Indeed, it couldn't be farther from the truth. CALCIUM CHLORIDE ADMINISTERED TO PATIENTS WHO ARE TAKING DIGITALIS CAN BE LETHAL! Sudden death has been reported after the intravenous injection of calcium even into patients with therapeutic blood levels of digitalis; patients with toxic blood levels of digitalis are at even greater risk. These facts point to yet another aspect of pharmacology with which you must be familiar: For any drug you use in the field, you must be thoroughly familiar with its *potential interactions with other drugs.* The potentially fatal interaction of calcium and digitalis is but one example. Another is the untoward effect of mixing calcium and sodium bicarbonate in the same solution (answer d), which results in the formation of small crystals of calcium carbonate (otherwise known as marble)—something you definitely do not want floating in your IV solution!

Calcium chloride does increase the contractility of a normal heart muscle (answer b), and for that reason it was previously recommended that calcium be given for asystole and electromechanical dissociation. The idea was to try to improve the contractility of a heart in cardiac arrest. Clinical studies, however, failed to show any benefit from using calcium preparations for those conditions—indeed, the effects of calcium on the heart in cardiac arrest often seemed harmful. So calcium chloride has been dropped from the list of first-line resuscitation drugs. It is still useful, however, in opposing the effects of magnesium sulfate (answer c) when that drug has been given in excessive doses.

FURTHER READING
Dembo DH. Calcium in advanced life support. *Crit Care Med* 9:358, 1981.
Harrison EE et al. Use of calcium in electromechanical dissociation. *Ann Emerg Med* 13:844, 1984.
Hughes WG et al. Should calcium be used in cardiac arrest? *Am J Med* 81:285, 1986.
Morris DL et al. Calcium infusion for reversal of adverse effects of intravenous verapamil. *JAMA* 249:3212, 1983.
Redding JS, Haynes RR, Thomas JD. Drug therapy in resuscitation from electromechanical dissociation. *Crit Care Med* 11:681, 1983.
Steuven HS et al. Calcium chloride: Reassessment of use in asystole. *Ann Emerg Med* 13:820, 1984.
Steuven HS et al. The effectiveness of calcium chloride in refractory electromechanical dissociation. *Ann Emerg Med* 14:626, 1985.
Steuven HS et al. Lack of effectiveness of calcium chloride in refractory asystole. *Ann Emerg Med* 14:630, 1985.
Steuven HS et al. Use of calcium in prehospital cardiac arrest. *Ann Emerg Med* 12:136, 1983.
Woie L et al. Successful treatment of suicidal verapamil poisoning with calcium gluconate. *Eur Heart J* 12:239, 1981.

In which of the following situations would it be worthwhile to administer 50% glucose (D50)?

a. Cardiac arrest
b. Coma of undetermined etiology
c. Shock
d. In all of the above situations
e. In none of the above situations

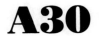 **A30** Answer **b** is correct: D50 is worthwhile in **coma of unknown etiology.**

EVERY patient in coma of unknown etiology should receive D50 (answer b), even if the patient is not known to be a diabetic. Often it is impossible at the scene to obtain enough information to know whether the patient has a diabetic history, and besides, hypoglycemic coma is not limited to diabetics. Alcoholism, the ingestion of certain poisons, and other metabolic disorders all predispose people to hypoglycemia. So when in doubt, administer D50.

"But what if the patient is in *hyper*glycemic coma?" you ask. "He certainly doesn't need any more glucose if his blood sugar is already 800 mg%." That is true, to be sure, but the amount of sugar you will administer in 50 ml of D50 (25 gm, to be exact) is trivial in comparison to the patient's current blood levels and is not likely to do any further harm. On the other hand, withholding glucose from the patient in *hypo*glycemia can lead to irreversible brain damage. So if there is even the slightest doubt as to whether the patient is suffering from hyperglycemia or hypoglycemia, err on the side of caution and GIVE HIM GLUCOSE!

Previous recommendations to administer glucose for cardiac arrest (answer a) and shock (answer c) have not been substantiated by research.

FURTHER READING

Andrade R et al. Hypoglycemic hemiplegic syndrome. *Ann Emerg Med* 13:529, 1984.
Baker FJ et al. Diabetic emergencies: Hypoglycemia and ketoacidosis. *JACEP* 5:119, 1976.
Cox DJ et al. Symptoms and blood glucose levels in diabetics (letter). *JAMA* 253:1558, 1985.
Hypoglycemia: Arrest on suspicion. *Emerg Med* 5(5):226, 1973.
Iscovich AL. Sudden cardiac death due to hypoglycemia. *Amer J Emerg Med* 1:28, 1983.
Kunian L, Wasco J, Hulefeld L. Sweets for the alcoholic. *Emerg Med* 5(a):45, 1973.
Stapczynski JS, Haskell RJ. Duration of hypoglycemia and need for intravenous glucose following intentional overdoses of insulin. *Ann Emerg Med* 13:505, 1984.
Thurston JH. Blood glucose: How reliable an indicator of brain glucose? *Hosp Pract* 11:123, 1976.

How did you do on those questions about calculation of doses? If you still feel a bit shaky with the math, here are a couple of more exercises to work on:

1. The therapeutic dose of atropine is 0.02 mg per kilogram of body weight. If atropine comes in a solution of 1 mg per milliliter, what *volume* of atropine must you administer to a 132-pound woman?
2. You are instructed to start a dopamine infusion at 5 μg/kg/min for a 176-pound man. You add an ampule containing 200 mg of dopamine to an IV bag containing 250 ml of D5W. Assuming you have a microdrip infusion set, which delivers 60 drops per milliliter, at how many drops per minute should you run the infusion to deliver 5 μg/kg/min?

(Hint: Don't forget to convert pounds to kilograms!)

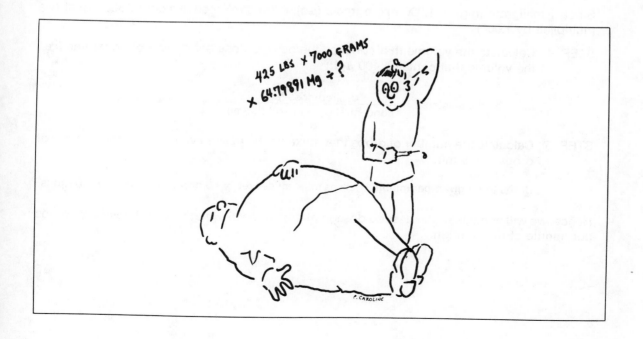

75

A31

1. First, the atropine problem. The correct answer is **0.6 ml.**

   STEP 1: Calculate the woman's weight in kilograms:

   $$\text{Weight in kg} = \frac{\text{weight in lb}}{2.2 \text{ lb/kg}} = \frac{132 \text{ lb}}{2.2 \text{ lb/kg}} = 60 \text{ kg}$$

   STEP 2: Calculate the correct dosage for a 60-kg patient:

   $$\text{Correct dosage} = 0.02 \text{ mg/kg} \times 60 \text{ kg} = 1.2 \text{ mg}$$

   STEP 3: Calculate the volume that contains 1.2 mg:

   $$\text{ml to be administered} = \frac{\text{desired dose (in mg)}}{\text{concentration on hand (in mg/ml)}} = \frac{1.2 \text{ mg}}{1.0 \text{ mg/ml}} = 1.2$$

   (Remember, the *minimum* initial dose of atropine for treating bradycardia in an adult is 1.0 mg IV.)

2. The dopamine question is a bit trickier but basically follows the same steps. The correct answer is **30 drops per minute**. Did you get it right?

   STEP 1: Calculate the man's weight in kilograms:

   $$\text{Weight in kg} = \frac{\text{weight in lb}}{2.2 \text{ lb/kg}} = \frac{176 \text{ lb}}{2.2 \text{ lb/kg}} = 80 \text{ kg}$$

   STEP 2: Calculate the correct dosage for an 80-kg patient:

   $$\text{Correct dosage} = 5 \text{ } \mu g/kg/min = \frac{5 \text{ } \mu g/kg \times 80 \text{ kg}}{min} = 400 \text{ } \mu g/min$$

   STEP 3: Calculate the concentration of dopamine in your infusion:

   $$\text{Concentration of dopamine} = \frac{\text{amount of dopamine added to bag (mg)}}{\text{volume of the bag (ml)}}$$

   $$= \frac{200 \text{ mg}}{250 \text{ ml}} = 0.8 \text{ mg/ml}$$

   Since 1 milligram (mg) = 1,000 micrograms (μg), 0.8 mg/ml is equivalent to 800 μg/ml (we multiplied by 1,000).

   STEP 4: Calculate the volume that contains the desired dose per minute of dopamine (i.e., the volume that contains 400 μg):

   $$\text{ml to be administered} = \frac{\text{desired dose (}\mu g\text{)}}{\text{concentration on hand (}\mu g/ml\text{)}} = \frac{400 \text{ } \mu g}{800 \text{ } \mu g/ml} = 0.5 \text{ ml}$$

   STEP 5: Calculate the number of drops that make up the desired volume (i.e., the number of drops in 0.5 ml):

   $$\text{Drops to be given per minute} = \text{drops/ml} \times \text{ml desired} = 60 \text{ drops/ml} \times 0.5 \text{ ml} = 30 \text{ drops}$$

   Hence, we will administer the desired dosage of dopamine (5 μg/kg/min) by infusing 30 drops per minute of the solution.

RECONNOITERING IN THE MEDICINE CABINET

The following are medications that patients may be taking at home, and knowing what these medications are used for can provide clues to the patient's underlying medical problems. Match the medications in the list below with the condition for which each may be prescribed:

a. Digitalis
b. Nitroglycerin
c. Procainamide (Pronestyl)
d. Phenytoin sodium (Dilantin)
e. Tolbutamide (Orinase)
f. Methyldopa (Aldomet)

1. _____ Angina pectoris
2. _____ Diabetes mellitus
3. _____ Chronic heart failure
4. _____ Hypertension
5. _____ Seizures
6. _____ Chronic PVCs

A32

1. __b__ Angina pectoris

NITROGLYCERIN is taken by many patients to relieve the pain of angina. It is one of the few medications that is usually taken sublingually (under the tongue) rather than swallowed, and its effects are usually felt within 3 to 5 minutes.

2. __e__ Diabetes mellitus

TOLBUTAMIDE (Orinase) is one of several oral hypoglycemic agents that may be prescribed to patients with stable, adult-onset diabetes mellitus. Like insulin, oral hypoglycemic agents may cause dangerous falls in blood sugar.

3. __a__ Chronic heart failure

DIGITALIS is often part of the therapeutic regimen for chronic heart failure because it increases the strength of cardiac contractions and thereby improves cardiac output. Digitalis may also be prescribed for control of rapid atrial dysrhythmias, such as atrial flutter or atrial fibrillation. Thirty to forty percent of patients taking digitalis develop some signs of toxicity from the drug, such as loss of appetite, nausea, abdominal pain, headache, blurred vision, and a variety of cardiac dysrhythmias. Such potential toxic effects of digitalis should be kept in mind when evaluating the symptoms of any patient taking this drug. One should also bear in mind that toxicity from digitalis is *very* frequent when the drug is taken together with quinidine, and this combination should be looked for when evaluating the patient's medications.

4. __f__ Hypertension

METHYLDOPA (Aldomet) is frequently prescribed for control of hypertension. Many patients taking methyldopa will also be taking diuretic medications, and a specific inquiry should be made about other drugs routinely taken. The side effects of methyldopa may include drowsiness, dryness of the mouth, mild gastrointestinal symptoms, and postural hypotension (i.e., a drop in blood pressure upon standing up, often manifested as dizziness upon standing up). The drug may also cause dizziness and temporary loss of consciousness even when the patient is lying down.

5. __d__ Seizures

PHENYTOIN SODIUM (Dilantin) is prescribed to patients with recurrent seizures; it is often prescribed together with phenobarbital and is taken 3 to 4 times a day. Just because you find Dilantin in the patient's medicine cabinet, however, do not take for granted that he uses the medication regularly, especially if his chief complaint is another seizure. One of the most common causes of recurrent seizures is failure to take prescribed antiseizure medications as directed. So whenever your investigations into the medicine cabinet turn up a significant drug, be sure to inquire how regularly it is taken.

6. __c__ Chronic PVCs

PROCAINAMIDE (Pronestyl) is an antiarrhythmic agent very similar to lidocaine in its actions, but it has the advantage, in terms of chronic administration, that it can be taken by mouth. It is most commonly prescribed for treatment of chronic PVCs or recurrent ventricular tachycardia, but it may occasionally be prescribed for control of supraventricular dysrhythmias. In any case, it is an important clue to the fact that the user has had rhythm problems in the past and thus can direct the paramedic to a worthwhile area of questioning.

FURTHER READING
Caroline NL. *Emergency Care in the Streets* (4th ed.). Boston: Little, Brown, 1991, Drug Handbook.

A 24-year-old woman is complaining of numbness around her mouth, dizziness, and cramps in the extremities. You notice that she is breathing very deeply 30 times per minute. You can thus assume that her arterial carbon dioxide level (arterial PCO_2) is

a. Lower than normal
b. Higher than normal

If this is the case, her arterial pH is

a. Lower than normal
b. Higher than normal

Thus, she is probably developing a respiratory

a. Acidosis
b. Alkalosis

A33

Our young lady is showing classic symptoms of the hyperventilation syndrome: She has unexplained tachypnea and hyperpnea, and she complains of numbness around her mouth, dizziness, and cramping in the extremities. (What other symptoms are also sometimes part of this picture?)

When a person breathes with a normal tidal volume (about 500 ml) and a normal respiratory rate (about 12–16/min), the resulting minute volume is usually just sufficient to keep the arterial PCO_2 at a normal level (around 40 mm Hg). When the minute volume increases without a corresponding increase in CO_2 production by the body, an excess of CO_2 is blown off and the arterial PCO_2 tends to fall. Thus, in the case of our patient—whose minute volume is probably several times normal, owing to increases in both her respiratory rate and tidal volume—the arterial PCO_2 is likely to be **LOWER THAN NORMAL** (answer **a**). As the PCO_2 falls, so does the level of hydrogen ions in the blood, and since the pH is computed as the negative logarithm of the hydrogen ion concentration, a fall in the concentration of hydrogen ions will be reflected as a rise in pH. Thus our patient's **pH** will be **HIGHER THAN NORMAL** (answer **b**). This, by definition, is an **ALKALOSIS** (answer **b**), and it is a *respiratory* alkalosis because the source of the problem lies in the respiratory mechanism.

FURTHER READING

Abbot Laboratories. *Acid-base balance* (pamphlet). North Chicago: Abbot, 1974.
Caroline NL. *Emergency Care in the Streets* (4th ed.). Boston: Little, Brown, 1991, Chs. 8, 22.
Flomenbaum N. Acid-base disturbances. *Emerg Med* 16(3):59, 1984.
Kassirer JP. Serious acid-base disorders. *N Engl J Med* 291:773, 1974.
Miller WC. The ABCs of blood gases. *Emerg Med* 16(3):37, 1984.
Stein JM. Interpreting arterial blood gases. *Emerg Med* 18(1):61, 1986.

Match the following terms with the phrase that best describes each:

a. Epiglottis
b. Alveolus
c. Pulmonary artery
d. Pulmonary vein
e. Trachea

1. _____ Carries blood poor in oxygen from the right ventricle to the lungs
2. _____ Terminal air sac where oxygenation of blood takes place
3. _____ Windpipe
4. _____ Structure that flops over the entrance to the lower airway during swallowing, thus preventing aspiration of food into the lungs
5. _____ Carries oxygenated blood away from the lungs to the left atrium

A34 You were promised a book of clinical problems, and suddenly there's a question on anatomy. Not fair, you say. Granted, anatomy isn't as much fun as, say, pulling someone out of a car wreck. But if you want to get around the city, you have to learn the map. And in medicine, the map is anatomy. So let's review a bit.

1. ___c___ Carries blood poor in oxygen from the right ventricle to the lungs **(pulmonary artery)**

Remember, arteries carry blood away from the heart.

2. ___b___ Terminal air sac where oxygenation of blood takes place **(alveolus)**
3. ___e___ Windpipe **(trachea)**
4. ___a___ Structure that flops over the entrance to the lower airway during swallowing, thus preventing aspiration of food into the lung **(epiglottis)**

The epiglottis is one of the landmarks you use during endotracheal intubation when you slide the curved blade into the space behind the epiglottis (the vallecula) or the straight blade over the epiglottis. The epiglottis can also become a source of life-threatening airway obstruction when it becomes swollen, as in epiglottitis.

5. ___d___ Carries oxygenated blood away from the lungs to the left atrium **(pulmonary vein)**

FURTHER READING
Caroline NL. *Emergency Care in the Streets* (4th ed.). Boston: Little, Brown, 1991, Chs. 7, 8.

1. If a person is breathing 15 times per minute with a tidal volume of 400 ml, what is his minute volume?

2. If the above individual changes his respiratory rate to 5 per minute without changing the depth of his respirations, his minute volume will

   a. Increase
   b. Decrease

3. As that happens, his arterial carbon dioxide level (arterial PCO_2) will

   a. Increase
   b. Decrease

4. As a consequence of the above, he is likely to develop a respiratory

   a. Acidosis
   b. Alkalosis

A35

1. How do we calculate the minute volume? Recall that the minute volume, or volume of air exchanged per minute, is equal to the volume of each breath (tidal volume) times the number of breaths per minute (respiratory rate):

   MINUTE VOLUME = TIDAL VOLUME × RESPIRATORY RATE

   In our patient, the tidal volume is 400 ml and the respiratory rate is 15 per minute, hence:

   MINUTE VOLUME = 400 ml × 15/min = **6,000 ml/min**

   That is in the range of normal.

2. Now something has happened to our patient to depress his rate of respirations to 5 per minute (what might cause such a change?). His tidal volume has remained unchanged at 400 ml. Thus his minute volume is

   MINUTE VOLUME = 400 ml × 5/min = 2,000 ml

   i.e., his **minute volume** has **DECREASED** (answer **b**).

3. What will happen to our patient's arterial PCO_2 with a minute volume that is now only about 30 percent of normal? Clearly his ability to exchange the gases in his lungs with environmental air is now severely impaired, for he is moving 4 liters of air less per minute in and out of his lungs than he was before. As a consequence, CO_2 will accumulate and the level of **CO_2** in his arterial blood will **INCREASE** (answer **a**).

4. Whenever the PCO_2 increases, there is always a concomitant increase in the level of carbonic acid in the blood, and if this situation continues, the patient will develop a respiratory **ACIDOSIS** (answer **a**).

FURTHER READING
Caroline NL. *Emergency Care in the Streets* (4th ed.). Boston: Little, Brown, 1991, Chs. 8, 22.
Kettel LJ. Acute respiratory acidosis. *Hosp Med* 12:31, 1976.
Miller WC. The ABCs of blood gases. *Emerg Med* 16(3):37, 1984.
Stein JM. Interpreting arterial blood gases. *Emerg Med* 18(1):61, 1986.

Which of the following patients might be expected to have a significant degree of shunt and therefore require oxygen administration? (Note: There may be more than one correct answer.)

a. A 64-year-old man with pulmonary edema
b. A 35-year-old man who has suffered a tension pneumothorax in an automobile accident
c. A child who was struck by a car and sustained a flail chest on the right side
d. A 70-year-old woman with pneumonia
e. A 24-year-old woman resuscitated after a 10-minute submersion in seawater

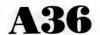

A36 Answer: ALL OF THESE PATIENTS MAY BE PRESUMED TO HAVE A SIGNIFICANT SHUNT AND NEED OXYGEN!

First, let us review the concept of shunt and look at the situation from the viewpoint of a red blood cell.

The red blood cell leaving the right side of the heart has a single mission: to paddle into the lungs, sidle up alongside an alveolus, and trade a bit of carbon dioxide for a fresh supply of oxygen. Once that mission is accomplished, the red blood cell proceeds on into the left side of the heart, from where he is pumped out into the periphery to donate his oxygen to the tissues. But suppose our red blood cell has the misfortune to snuggle up to an alveolus that has no oxygen in it—an alveolus that is, perhaps, collapsed or filled with fluid. What happens then? The poor red blood cell will not pick up any oxygen at all, and one can imagine the conversation when the red blood cell reaches the left atrium:

Left atrium: Well, where have *you* been?
Red blood cell: I've been in the left lower lobe, sir.
Left atrium: Then where's your oxygen, sonny?
Red blood cell: The alveolus I visited was out of order, sir.
Left atrium: A likely story! If you don't have any oxygen, how do I know you went through the lungs at all? Maybe you took a little shortcut, huh?
Red blood cell: No, honest, sir, I was there . . .

The red blood cell is out of luck. He will never be able to prove that he journeyed through the lungs, for he has reached the left side of the heart without oxygen, i.e., exactly as if he had been *shunted* past the lungs. And the greater the number of alveoli that are for any reason nonfunctional, the greater the volume of blood that will return to the left side of the heart without having become reoxygenated, i.e., the greater the volume of the shunt.

Now, let us return to our patients. Cases a, d, and e all have fluid in their alveoli. In the case of our 64-year-old man with pulmonary edema (answer a), the fluid is serum, which has extravasated out of the pulmonary capillaries into the alveoli because of back pressure from the failing left heart. Our 70-year-old lady with pneumonia has pus in her alveoli. Our 24-year-old near-drowning victim has her alveoli filled with seawater, which—because of its hypertonicity—draws even more water (extracellular fluid) into the alveoli with it. The net effect is the same, for blood passing by these fluid-filled alveoli will not find any oxygen there and will thus reach the left side of the heart in a desaturated (i.e., relatively unoxygenated) state.

Our trauma victims (b and c) have a somewhat different problem. Their alveoli are collapsed. In the case of the child with a flail chest (answer c), there are spotty areas of alveolar collapse (= atelectasis) because it hurts him to take a deep breath and so he does not expand all his alveoli normally on inhalation. Our patient with a tension pneumothorax (answer b) has an entire lung collapsed. In both instances, blood passing alongside the collapsed alveoli will find, instead of an air-filled sac, an empty, limp little bag, and this blood will return to the left heart without having taken on a fresh supply of oxygen—another example of shunt.

Why do these patients need oxygen? We take for granted that NOT ALL of the alveoli are nonfunctional in these patients. Granted, some of the alveoli are filled with fluid or collapsed, but others are working just fine. If we can fill the functioning alveoli with a very high concentration of oxygen, the blood passing by *those* alveoli will reach a very high PO_2. Then, when the blood that is carrying lots of oxygen reaches the left heart and mixes with the shunted blood, the net PO_2 will at least be in the normal range. The tissues, waiting in the periphery, are bound to notice the difference!

FURTHER READING
Aberman A. On understanding oxygen transport. *Emerg Med* 14(7):116, 1982.
Bourne S. Gearing up for oxygen delivery. *JEMS* 13(8):58, 1988.
Caroline NL. *Emergency Care in the Streets* (4th ed.). Boston: Little, Brown, 1991, Ch. 8.
Caroline NL. *Emergency Medical Treatment: A Text for EMT-As and EMT-Intermediates* (3rd ed.). Boston: Little, Brown, 1991, Ch. 9.
Shelly RW. Oxygen administration. *JEMS* 7(7):37, 1983.
Skorodin MS. Current oxygen prescribing practices. Problems and prospects. *JAMA* 255:3283, 1986.
Tinits P. Oxygen therapy and oxygen toxicity. *Ann Emerg Med* 12:321, 1983.
White RD. Essential drugs in emergency care. *EMT J* 1(4):51, 1977.

Indicate which of the following statements are true and which are false:

a. An oropharyngeal airway should not be used in a fully conscious patient.

TRUE   FALSE

b. If a patient is not cyanotic, one can be reasonably confident that he is adequately oxygenated.

TRUE   FALSE

c. The most common source of upper airway obstruction is a piece of meat lodged just above the vocal cords.

TRUE   FALSE

d. Confusion and agitation in a patient with chronic bronchitis may be an important sign of hypoxemia.

TRUE   FALSE

e. Every patient in respiratory distress should receive oxygen.

TRUE   FALSE

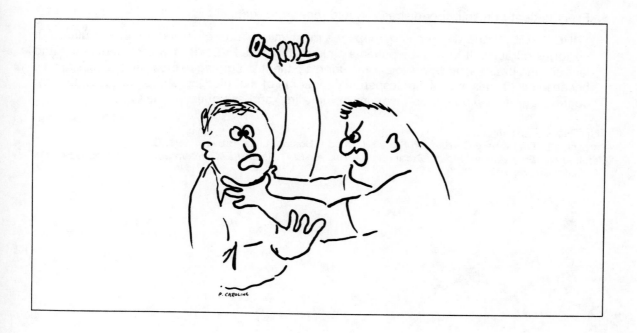

A37

It's back to the old ABCs—and in this question, a closer look at the airway and breathing—for in saving lives, that's where the money is.

a. An oropharyngeal airway should not be used in a fully conscious patient.

TRUE. If you don't believe it, just try sometime to insert an oropharyngeal airway into the throat of a conscious patient, or maybe your partner, and see what happens (make sure it's not someone with any violent tendencies). In all probability, your patient or partner will gag, cough, spit out the airway, and call you a few uncomplimentary names. Conscious patients simply do not tolerate having a rigid piece of plastic or rubber shoved into their posterior oropharynx, nor do they need such a device. Any patient who *is* sufficiently comatose to tolerate an oropharyngeal airway without gagging probably needs to have his airway protected with a cuffed endotracheal tube at the earliest possible moment.

b. If a patient is not cyanotic, one can be reasonably confident that he is adequately oxygenated.

FALSE! Granted, when cyanosis *is* present, it is a good indication of hypoxemia, but its absence is no guarantee that the patient is well oxygenated. Cyanosis becomes visible when approximately 5 gm% of the patient's hemoglobin is in the desaturated state (i.e., not carrying oxygen). Many patients, however, can reach extreme degrees of hypoxemia long before this degree of desaturation takes place, such as patients with anemia, whose hemoglobin levels are low to begin with. Moral: BLUE IS ALWAYS BLEAK, BUT PINK AIN'T ALWAYS PERFECT.

c. The most common source of upper airway obstruction is a piece of meat lodged just above the vocal cords.

FALSE! The most common source of upper airway obstruction comes supplied in every mouth and is called a tongue. In the comatose patient, the airway is very prone to become obstructed by the base of the tongue falling against the posterior oropharynx. The cure: backward tilt of the head.

d. Confusion and agitation in a patient with chronic bronchitis may be an important sign of hypoxemia.

TRUE. That big, fat, plethoric patient who is combative and giving you such a hard time may be a case of acute respiratory failure in disguise. So be nice to him and give him some oxygen, which just may calm him down a bit. But keep an eye on him, lest he calm right down into coma. He could be one of the rare patients with chronic obstructive pulmonary disease who breathes on a hypoxic drive, and if so, a few whiffs of oxygen may persuade him to stop breathing. Encourage him to cough and take deep breaths, and if necessary, assist his ventilations with a bag-valve-mask.

e. Every patient in respiratory distress should receive oxygen.

TRUE. TRUE. TRUE. Oxygen is perhaps the most valuable drug carried on an ambulance. It performs miracles: It turns blue patients pink; it abolishes PVCs; it revives stalled hearts and languishing brains. And when you come upon a patient struggling to breathe, chances are it's because his tissues are crying desperately for some of that nice, colorless, odorless gas that comes in green cylinders. So give him oxygen first, and ask questions later.

FURTHER READING
Caroline NL. *Emergency Care in the Streets* (4th ed.). Boston: Little, Brown, 1991, Ch. 8.
Caroline NL. *Emergency Medical Treatment: A Text for EMT-As and EMT-Intermediates* (3rd ed.). Boston: Little, Brown, 1991, Ch. 9.

Which of the following devices delivers the HIGHEST concentration of oxygen to the patient?

a. A Venturi mask at 4 liters per minute flow rate
b. A nonrebreathing mask at 10 liters per minute flow rate
c. A regular plastic face mask at 12 liters per minute flow rate
d. Two-pronged nasal cannulas at 6 liters per minute flow rate
e. A bag-valve-mask without oxygen reservoir at 10 liters per minute flow rate

A38

The correct answer is **b: a nonrebreathing mask at 10 liters per minute flow rate.** This device, at the oxygen flow stated, will deliver approximately 90% oxygen if fitted snugly to the patient's face. A Venturi mask at 4 liters per minute (answer a), depending on how it is designed, will deliver either 24 or 28% oxygen and is used principally for the in-hospital treatment of patients with chronic obstructive pulmonary disease. A regular plastic face mask, without a valved reservoir bag, at 12 liters per minute (answer c) cannot deliver more than 60% oxygen because at peak inhalation the patient also pulls in room air through the side holes in the mask; the room air mixes with the oxygen and decreases the net concentration inhaled. A nasal cannula set at 6 liters per minute oxygen flow (answer d) can deliver a maximum oxygen concentration of about 40%; increasing the oxygen flow will not appreciably increase the inhaled oxygen concentration but will simply lead to drying and irritation of the nasal mucosa. Finally, a bag-valve-mask device without an oxygen reservoir at 10 liters per minute oxygen flow (answer e) can deliver up to 40 to 50% oxygen.

Therefore the nonrebreathing mask is the device of choice in situations where one wishes to deliver maximal oxygen concentrations, i.e., situations in which there is a high degree of shunt (e.g., acute pulmonary edema, shock lung). The oxygen flow rate is adjusted to prevent collapse of the reservoir bag during inhalation—usually to about 10 to 12 liters per minute.

FURTHER READING

Aberman A. On understanding oxygen transport. *Emerg Med* 14(7):116, 1982.

Bourne S. Gearing up for oxygen delivery. *JEMS* 13(8):58, 1988.

Bryan CD, Taylor JP. *Manual of Respiratory Therapy.* St Louis: Mosby, 1973.

Campbell EJ et al. Subjective effects of humidification of oxygen for delivery by nasal cannula: A prospective study. *Chest* 93:289, 1988.

Caroline NL. *Emergency Care in the Streets* (4th ed.). Boston: Little, Brown, 1991, Ch. 8.

Caroline NL. *Emergency Medical Treatment: A Text for EMT-As and EMT-Intermediates* (3rd ed.). Boston: Little, Brown, 1991. Ch. 9.

Peters WR, Jolly PC. Gastric rupture from nasal oxygen catheter. *Bull Mason Clin* 26:70, 1972.

Shelly RW. Oxygen administration. *JEMS* 7(7):37, 1983.

Skorodin MS. Current oxygen prescribing practices. Problems and prospects. *JAMA* 255:3283, 1986.

Tinits P. Oxygen therapy and oxygen toxicity. *Ann Emerg Med* 12:321, 1983.

Waxman K. Oxygen delivery and resuscitation. *Ann Emerg Med* 15:1420, 1986.

White RD. Essential drugs in emergency care. *EMT J* 1(4):51, 1977.

Zagelbaum GL, Pare JAP. *Manual of Acute Respiratory Care.* Boston: Little, Brown, 1982.

Which of the following statements about endotracheal intubation is NOT true?

a. An endotracheal tube is unnecessary to protect the airway of an unconscious patient if the patient already has a nasogastric tube in place.

b. An intubation attempt should always be preceded by at least 3 minutes of ventilation with 100% oxygen.

c. An intubation attempt should not take more than 15 to 20 seconds.

d. The curved (MacIntosh) laryngoscope blade is designed to slip between the base of the tongue and the epiglottis.

e. One should always check the position of the endotracheal tube after insertion by listening for equality of breath sounds on both sides of the chest.

A39

Statement **a** is NOT true. Merely having a nasogastric tube in his stomach does not give a patient any guarantee whatsoever against aspiration. If the nasogastric tube should become blocked and fluid should accumulate in the stomach, the tube can serve as a wick along which fluid ascends into the posterior oropharynx; from there, it is only a short drop into the trachea. EVERY UNCONSCIOUS PATIENT SHOULD HAVE HIS AIRWAY PROTECTED WITH AN ENDOTRACHAEL TUBE, whether or not a nasogastric tube is being used to drain the stomach contents.

Of necessity, oxygen administration must cease during an intubation attempt, thereby subjecting the patient to a period of relative hypoxemia. For that reason, intubation attempts should be kept as brief as possible—certainly under 20 seconds (answer c)—and should be preceded by about 3 minutes of 100% oxygen administration (answer b) to bring the patient's arterial PO_2 to the highest possible level prior to interrupting oxygen therapy. That gives the patient a margin of safety to cover the 15 to 20 seconds in which he is not receiving oxygen.

The curved (MacIntosh) laryngoscope blade is designed to slide into the vallecula, the space between the base of the tongue and the epiglottis (answer d). The straight blade, on the other hand, is slid over the epiglottis and lifts the epiglottis and tongue as a unit.

Once an endotracheal tube has been inserted, one must always check to be certain that it lies in the trachea and not in the esophagus or one of the bronchi. Auscultating over both right and left lung fields provides the information one needs to make this determination (answer e). If breath sounds are not heard in either lung field, chances are the endotracheal tube is resting in the esophagus; if so, a rush of air may be audible upon auscultation over the epigastrium while ventilating through the tube. If that is the case, the endotracheal tube must be removed immediately, and the patient must be oxygenated again by bag-valve-mask before another intubation attempt is made. If while ventilating the patient breath sounds are absent or diminished on one side of the chest but well heard on the other side, the endotracheal tube has probably entered a bronchus; it should then be pulled back very slowly until breath sounds are heard equally well bilaterally as the patient is being ventilated.

FURTHER READING

Abarbanell NR. Esophageal placement of an endotracheal tube by paramedics. *Am J Emerg Med* 6:178, 1988.

Aijian P et al. Endotracheal intubation of pediatric patients by paramedics. *Ann Emerg Med* 18:489, 1989.

Applebaum AL, Bruce DW. *Tracheal intubation.* Philadelphia: Saunders, 1976.

Ballinger JA. Secrets of airway management. *Emergency* 20(12):47, 1988.

Bissinger U, Lenz G, Kuhn W. Unrecognized endobronchial intubation of emergency patients. *Ann Emerg Med* 18:853, 1989.

Bivins HG et al. The effect of axial traction during orotracheal intubation of the trauma victim with an unstable cervical spine. *Ann Emerg Med* 17:25, 1988.

Caroline NL. *Emergency Care in the Streets* (4th ed.). Boston: Little, Brown, 1991, Ch. 7.

DeLeo BC. Endotracheal intubation by rescue squad personnel. *Heart Lung* 6:851, 1977.

Dick T. Tubular tricks: Fool-proofing your field intubations. *JEMS* 14(5):26, 1989.

Forgues M. Airway: Step two. *Emergency* 22(3):26, 1990.

Guss DA, Posluszny M. Paramedic orotracheal intubation: A feasibility study. *Am J Emerg Med* 2:399, 1984.

Jacobs LM et al. Endotracheal intubation in the prehospital phase of emergency medical care. *JAMA* 250:2175, 1983.

Kalpokas M, Russell WJ. A simple technique for diagnosing oesophageal intubation. *Anaesth Intensive Care* 17:39, 1989.

Knopp RK. The safety of orotracheal intubation in patients with suspected cervical-spine injury (editorial). *Ann Emerg Med* 19:603, 1990.

Pepe PE, Copass MK, Joyce TH. Prehospital endotracheal intubation: Rationale for training emergency medical personnel. *Ann Emerg Med* 14:1085, 1985.

Pointer JE. Clinical characteristics of paramedics' performance of pediatric endotracheal intubation. *Am J Emerg Med* 7:364, 1989.

Rhee KJ et al. Oral intubation in the multiply injured patient: The risk of exacerbating spinal cord damage. *Ann Emerg Med* 19:511, 1990.

Salem MR, Mathrubhutham J, Bennet EJ. Difficult intubation. *N Engl J Med* 295:879, 1976.

Stanford TM. ET: A different approach. *Emergency* 20(12):34, 1988.

Stein JM. Endotracheal intubation in a hurry. *Emerg Med* 14(15):129, 1982.

Stein JM. Difficult adult intubation. *Emerg Med* 17(3):121, 1985.

Stewart RD et al. Field endotracheal intubation by paramedical personnel: Success rates and complications. *Chest* 85:341, 1984.

Whitten CE. Intubation for the primary physician (series): Common errors and how to avoid them, *Emerg Med* 21(15):91, 1989; Complications, *Emerg Med* 22(7):89, 1990; Difficult intubations: Tricks to remember, *Emerg Med* 22(1):85, 1990; Endotracheal anatomy, *Emerg Med* 21(8):171, 1989; Equipment for airway management, *Emerg Med* 21(12):91, 1989; Oral intubation in adults, *Emerg Med* 21(14):81, 1989; Preintubation evaluation—predicting the difficult airway, *Emerg Med* 21(10):107, 1989; Tests for tube placement, *Emerg Med* 21(17):93, 1989.

Which of the following statements about suctioning through an endotracheal tube is NOT true?

a. Suctioning through an endotracheal tube should never be carried out for more than 10 seconds at a time.

b. At least 3 minutes of oxygenation with 100% oxygen should precede every suctioning attempt.

c. The suction catheter should be used to suction out the mouth and nasopharynx before it is inserted into the endotracheal tube.

d. Every patient who is being suctioned should be monitored, since dangerous cardiac dysrhythmias may occur during the suctioning procedure.

e. Endotracheal suctioning may cause severe bronchospasm.

A40
Answer **c** is emphatically NOT true. The suction catheter should touch nothing in the patient's mouth or nasopharynx before it is inserted into the trachea, and suctioning through an endotracheal tube should be carried out with full sterile precautions (mask, sterile gloves, etc.) in order to minimize the risk of transferring bacteria from the patient's mouth or the operator's hands to the patient's lower respiratory tract. Only *after* endotracheal suctioning is complete may one use the suction catheter to sweep out secretions from the patient's mouth.

Tracheal suctioning not only vacuums out secretions; it also effectively pulls oxygen out of the respiratory tract. For that reason, a patient should be preoxygenated with 100% oxygen for at least 3 minutes before every suctioning attempt (answer b) so that he can tolerate a short period of alveolar hypoxia. For the same reason, any given suctioning attempt should not be continued for more than 10 seconds (answer a); after that time, the suction catheter should be withdrawn and the patient reoxygenated before another foray into his trachea with the suction catheter.

There are several potential complications of endotracheal suctioning, among them bronchospasm (answer e) and cardiac dysrhythmias (answer d); because of the danger of the latter, any patient who is undergoing tracheal suctioning should be monitored throughout the procedure. At the first sign of any untoward reaction, be it bronchospasm or a dysrhythmia, suctioning should be discontinued immediately and the patient reoxygenated with 100% oxygen.

FURTHER READING

Barnes CA et al. Minimizing hypoxemia due to endotracheal suctioning: A review of the literature. *Heart Lung* 15:164, 1986.

Bushnell SS. *Respiratory Intensive Care Nursing.* Boston: Little, Brown, 1973, Ch. 12.

Caroline NL. *Emergency Care in the Streets* (4th ed.). Boston: Little, Brown, 1991, Ch. 7.

Caroline NL. *Emergency Medical Treatment: A Textbook for EMT-As and EMT-Intermediates* (3rd ed.). Boston: Little, Brown, 1991, Ch. 9.

Dahlgren BE et al. Appropriate suction device in rescue medicine. *Ann Emerg Med* 16:1362, 1987.

Reigel B et al. A review and critique of the literature on preoxygenation for endotracheal suctioning. *Heart Lung* 14:507, 1985.

White PF et al. A randomized study of drugs for preventing increases in intracranial pressure during endotracheal suctioning. *Anesthesiology* 57:242, 1982.

Winston SJ, Gravelyn TR, Sitrin RG. Prevention of bradycardic responses to endotracheal suctioning by prior administration of nebulized atropine. *Crit Care Med* 15:1009, 1987.

A LOT TO SWALLOW **Q41**

Indicate which of the following statements about the esophageal obturator airway (EOA) are true and which are false.

a. Once the EOA is in place in the esophagus, there is no longer any need to maintain backward tilt of the patient's head because the EOA keeps the airway open.

TRUE FALSE

b. The EOA should be used only in unconscious patients.

TRUE FALSE

c. The EOA should not be used in children under 16 years of age.

TRUE FALSE

d. The EOA should never be removed from an unconscious patient until an endotracheal tube has been inserted, secured, and the cuff of the endotracheal tube inflated.

TRUE FALSE

e. The EOA permits better ventilation with higher tidal volumes than one can achieve with a standard mask.

TRUE FALSE

A41

a. Once the EOA is in place in the esophagus, there is no longer any need to maintain backward tilt of the patient's head because the EOA keeps the airway open.

FALSE! The EOA is no better nor worse than any other face mask. It does NOT keep an airway open; only the rescuer can keep an airway open, by maintaining backward tilt of the patient's head or by the triple airway maneuver. The only thing an EOA *does* accomplish that an ordinary mask cannot is to lessen the risk of regurgitation of stomach contents. In all other respects, it is simply an ordinary face mask and should be used as such, with due regard for airway maintenance by manual techniques.

b. The EOA should be used only in unconscious patients.

TRUE! No conscious patient is going to permit you to shove that enormous, long tube down his throat anyway, for he will cough, gag, retch, and perhaps hit you if you try it.

c. The EOA should not be used in children under 16 years of age.

TRUE. Before the age of 16, the esophagus in some children may not have reached a size sufficient to admit the EOA safely. So when you're treating kids, leave the EOA at home.

d. The EOA should never be removed from an unconscious patient until an endotracheal tube has been inserted, secured, and the cuff of the endotracheal tube inflated.

TRUE. Removal of an EOA from an unconscious patient almost invariably brings *massive* regurgitation in its wake. If the patient's airway has not been protected meanwhile with a cuffed endotracheal tube, the entire contents of the stomach may rapidly find their way into the respiratory tree, and that is not considered good medical practice. So before you pull that EOA out, whip an endotracheal tube in. Check the position of the endotracheal tube by auscultating both lungs fields (do NOT assume that just because there is already a tube in the esophagus, your endotracheal tube is in the right place; it may be sitting very comfortably beside the EOA in the esophagus); then secure the endotracheal tube well and hold it in place while you deflate the cuff on the EOA and *slowly* pull the EOA out. Make sure you have a good, strong suction handy, for you may have a considerable mess on your hands.

e. The EOA permits better ventilation with higher tidal volumes than one can achieve with a standard mask.

FALSE! The EOA is just a plain, old mask. Ventilation through it is no more or less effective than through any other mask. Granted, with the use of the EOA, less of the bag volume is transmitted to the stomach (and therefore, one might argue, more is transmitted to the lungs), but in a given breath—and that's what we are talking about when we talk about tidal volume—the difference is negligible. In the last analysis, the tidal volume is determined by the squeeze you put on the bag.

FURTHER READING

Auerbach PS, Geehr EC. Inadequate oxygenation and ventilation using the esophageal obturator gastric tube airway in the prehospital setting. *JAMA* 250:3067, 1983.

Bass R, Allison E, Hunt R. The esophageal obturator airway: A reassessment of use by paramedics. *Ann Emerg Med* 11:358, 1982.

Carlson WJ, Hunter SW, Bonnabeau RC. Esophageal perforation with obturator airway. *Emerg Med Serv* 9(5):74, 1980.

Don Michael T. Mouth-to-lung airway for cardiac resuscitation. *Lancet* 2:1329, 1968.

Donen N et al. The esophageal obturator airway: An appraisal. *Canad Anaesth Soc J* 30:194, 1983.

Garvin JM. The esophageal obturator airway—an improved model. *Emerg Med Serv* 8(4):48, 1979.

Geehr EC, Bogetz MS, Auerbach PS. Prehospital tracheal intubation versus esophageal gastric tube airway use: A prospective study. *Am J Emerg Med* 3:381, 1985.

Gertler JP et al. Esophageal obturator airway: Obturator or obtundator? *J Trauma* 25:424, 1985.

Goldenburg IF et al. Morbidity and mortality of patients prospectively randomized to receive the esophageal gastric tube airway (EGTA) or the endotracheal tube (ET) (Abstract). *Circulation* 70(suppl):57, 1984.

Gordon AS. The tongue-jaw lift for EOA and EGTA. *Emergency* 13(6):40, 1981.

Greenbaum DM, Poggi J, Grace WM. Esophageal obstruction during oxygen administration: A new method for use in resuscitation. *Chest* 65:188, 1974.

Grigsby JW, Rottman SJ. Prehospital airway management: Esophageal obturator airway or endotracheal intubation? *Topics in Emergency Medicine* 1:25, 1981.

Hammargren Y, Clinton JE, Ruiz E. A standard comparison of esophageal obturator airway and endotracheal tube in cardiac arrest. *Ann Emerg Med* 14:953, 1985.

Harrison E et al. Esophageal perforation following use of the esophageal obturator airway. *Ann Emerg Med* 9:21, 1980.

Johnson KR, Genovesi MG, Lassar KH. Esophageal obturator airway: Use and complications. *JACEP* 5:36, 1976.

Kassels SJ, Robinson WA, O'Bara KJ. Esophageal perforation associated with the esophageal obturator airway. *Crit Care Med* 8:386, 1980.

Meislin HW. The esophageal obturator airway: A study of respiratory effectiveness. *Ann Emerg Med* 9:54, 1980.

Michael TAD. Comparison of the esophageal obturator airway and endotracheal intubation in prehospital ventilation during CPR. *Chest* 87:814, 1985.

Schofferman J, Oill P, Lewis AJ. The esophageal obturator airway: A clinical evaluation. *Chest* 69:67, 1976.

Shea SR et al. Prehospital endotracheal tube airway or esophageal gastric tube airway: A critical comparison. *Ann Emerg Med* 14:102, 1985.

Smith JP et al. The esophageal obturator airway. *JAMA* 250:1081, 1982.

Smith JP et al. A field evaluation of the esophageal obturator airway. *J Trauma* 23:317, 1983.

Strate RG, Fischer RP. Midesophageal perforations by esophageal obturator airways. *J Trauma* 16:503, 1976.

Now for a little more anatomy: Trace the course that blood takes through the circulatory system, starting with the venae cavae. Arrange the following structures in the correct order:

a. Venae cavae
b. Left ventricle
c. Pulmonary artery
d. Right atrium
e. Aorta
f. Pulmonary capillaries

g. Systemic arteries
h. Left atrium
i. Pulmonary vein
j. Right ventricle
k. Systemic veins

1. __a__
2. _____
3. _____
4. _____
5. _____
6. _____

7. _____
8. _____
9. _____
10. _____
11. _____
12. __a__

Having mastered the anatomy of the cardiovascular system, you will find the physiology much easier to understand. In heart failure, for example, blood backs up behind the failing side of the heart, and a knowledge of the anatomy involved enables one to predict the associated signs and symptoms. Classify the following signs according to whether each is indicative of

a. Right heart failure
b. Left heart failure

1. _____ Foamy, blood-tinged sputum
2. _____ Jugular venous distention
3. _____ Pedal edema
4. _____ Rales
5. _____ Liver enlargement

First let's see how you did on the anatomy:

James H. Taylor

1. __a__ Venae cavae
2. __d__ Right atrium
3. __j__ Right ventricle
4. __c__ Pulmonary artery
5. __f__ Pulmonary capillaries
6. __i__ Pulmonary vein
7. __h__ Left atrium
8. __b__ Left ventricle
9. __e__ Aorta
10. __g__ Systemic arteries
11. __k__ Systemic veins
12. __a__ Venae cavae

Not bad. You have the plumbing pretty well mastered. Now let's see what happens when one of the pumps (right or left ventricle) breaks down and blood begins backing up behind it:

1. __b__ Foamy, blood-tinged sputum   **LEFT** heart failure

Blood backing up behind the left ventricle causes engorgement of the *pulmonary veins,* which in turn leads to extravasation of serum and an occasional red blood cell into the alveoli. That fluid leaking into the alveoli is coughed up as the foamy, blood-tinged sputum one sees in pulmonary edema from left heart failure.

2. __a__ Jugular venous distention   **RIGHT** heart failure

When the right pump doesn't work efficiently, on the other hand, blood backs up into the venae cavae and from there into the systemic veins. Among the most readily visible systemic veins in direct communication with the venae cavae are the external jugulars, and their engorgement with blood is easily seen on inspection of the neck.

3. __a__ Pedal edema   **RIGHT** heart failure

Once again, this is a sign that the right ventricle isn't working properly. Blood backing up into the systemic veins causes increased hydrostatic pressure within those vessels; plasma fluid thus tends to seep out of the veins into the surrounding tissues, producing edema. Dependent areas of the body, such as the feet, are relatively more affected because in those areas gravitational forces combine with hydrostatic forces to create pressure within the peripheral vessels.

4. __b__ Rales   **LEFT** heart failure

We have already discussed why there is fluid in the airways in left heart failure, and rales are simply the sound produced by the passage of air through fluid-filled airways.

5. __a__ Liver enlargement   **RIGHT** heart failure

Just as venous engorgement from right heart failure leads to seepage of fluid out of the veins into peripheral tissues, it also leads to leakage of fluids out of the veins into many tissues we cannot readily see, such as the liver. Significant swelling of the liver (hepatomegaly) may occur because of failure of the right ventricle, and liver function may be impaired as a consequence. That is important to keep in mind when administering drugs, such as lidocaine, that are detoxified in the liver, for a given dose of lidocaine may hang around in the circulation a good deal longer in a patient whose liver is not functioning properly. For the same reason, repeated doses of lidocaine or a lidocaine infusion may lead much more rapidly to toxic blood levels in a patient with liver enlargement, for the drug is not cleared from the circulation as efficiently under those circumstances.

FURTHER READING

Caroline NL. *Emergency Care in the Streets* (4th ed.). Boston: Little, Brown, 1991, Ch. 23.
Dennison DA Jr. Visual clues to cardiac diagnosis. *Emerg Med* 16(19):99, 1984.
Maydayag TM. Emergency cardiac assessment. *Emerg Med Serv* 7(5):42, 1978.
Sokolow M, McIlroy MC. *Clinical Cardiology.* Los Altos, CA: Lange, 1977. Chs. 1–3.

Match the following terms with the statement that best describes each:

a. Angina pectoris
b. Ischemia
c. Palpitations
d. Diaphoresis
e. Atherosclerosis
f. Syncope
g. Hypertension
h. Infarction
i. Anorexia
j. Tamponade

1. _____ Profuse sweating
2. _____ Acute compression of the heart caused by an accumulation of fluid or blood in the pericardial sac
3. _____ Relative deprivation of oxygen
4. _____ Fainting
5. _____ A sensation that the heart has "skipped a beat"
6. _____ Loss of appetite
7. _____ A painful or choking sensation in the chest
8. _____ High blood pressure
9. _____ A disease affecting the inner lining of certain arteries, causing narrowing of the arteries and reduction of blood flow through them
10. _____ Death of a localized area of tissue caused by the interruption of the blood supply to the area

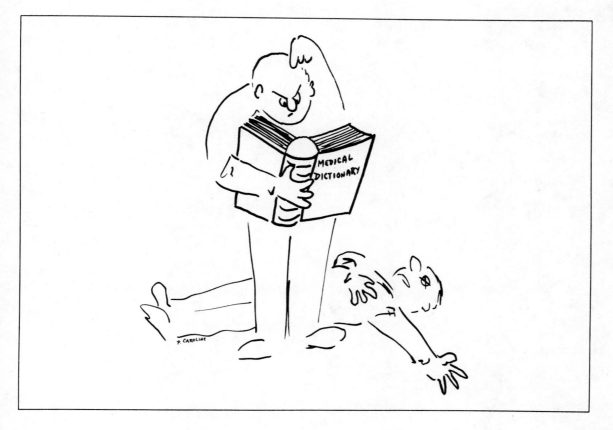

A43

There's no getting around it: If you want to talk to the natives, you have to speak their language, and doctors—like any other inhabitants of strange regions—have a language all their own. Let's see how well you did with this exercise in Medi-speak.

#		Term	Definition
1.	d	Diaphoresis	Profuse sweating
2.	j	Tamponade	Acute compression of the heart caused by an accumulation of fluid or blood in the pericardial sac
3.	b	Ischemia	Relative deprivation of oxygen
4.	f	Syncope	Fainting
5.	c	Palpitations	A sensation that the heart has "skipped a beat"
6.	i	Anorexia	Loss of appetite
7.	a	Angina pectoris	A painful or choking sensation in the chest
8.	g	Hypertension	High blood pressure
9.	e	Atherosclerosis	A disease affecting the inner lining of certain arteries, causing narrowing of the arteries and reduction of blood flow through them
10.	h	Infarction	Death of a localized area of tissue caused by the interruption of the blood supply to the area

FURTHER READING

Caroline NL. *Emergency Care in the Streets* (4th ed.). Boston: Little, Brown, 1991, Ch. 5.

Caroline NL. *Emergency Medical Treatment: A Text for EMT-As and EMT-Intermediates* (3rd ed.). Boston: Little, Brown, 1991, Ch. 3.

Frenay AC. *Understanding Medical Terminology* (6th ed.). St. Louis: Catholic Health Association, 1977.

Prendergast A. *Medical Terminology: A Text/Workbook* (2nd ed.). Reading, MA: Addison-Wesley, 1983.

Smith GL, Davis PE. *Medical Terminology: A Programmed Text* (4th ed.). New York: Wiley, 1981.

Indicate which of the following statements about acute myocardial infarction (AMI) are true and which are false.

a. Every patient suspected of AMI should have an IV lifeline inserted before he is transported to the hospital.

   TRUE   FALSE

b. If a patient's cardiac rhythm is being monitored on an ECG, there is no need to keep a finger on his pulse.

   TRUE   FALSE

c. All medications administered to patients with suspected AMI should be given intramuscularly.

   TRUE   FALSE

d. A normal ECG does not rule out the possibility that a patient is experiencing an AMI.

   TRUE   FALSE

e. If a patient with chest pain is not experiencing any difficulty breathing, there is no need to administer oxygen.

   TRUE   FALSE

f. Oxygen should be withheld from a patient with chest pain if he has a known history of chronic obstructive pulmonary disease (COPD).

   TRUE   FALSE

g. Elderly patients often suffer myocardial infarction without experiencing chest pain.

   TRUE   FALSE

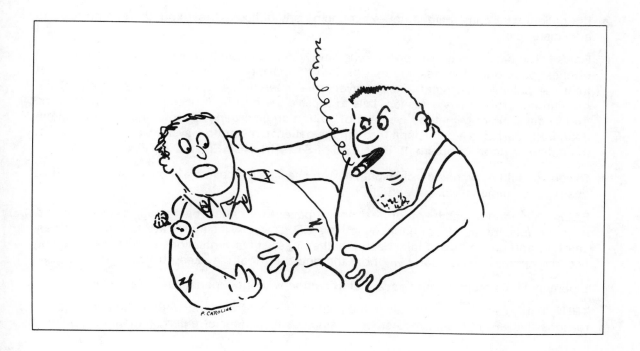

A44

a. Every patient suspected of AMI should have an IV lifeline inserted before he is transported to the hospital.

   TRUE. The whole purpose of the mobile intensive care unit is to enable early recognition and treatment of potentially life-threatening problems *before* such problems actually become life-threatening. When you see that salvo of PVCs on the monitor, that is NOT the time to start the IV, for by the time you get the IV in, the patient's heart may be fibrillating. The IV line should have been initiated at the earliest possible moment after arriving at the scene so that it is there when you need it.

b. If a patient's cardiac rhythm is being monitored on an ECG, there is no need to keep a finger on his pulse.

   FALSE! The ECG provides information only about the electric activity of the heart; it tells you nothing whatsoever about the heart's mechanical activity, i.e., the strength of cardiac contractions, or indeed whether the heart is contracting at all. The only way to get that information is to monitor the patient's pulse.

c. All medications administered to patients with suspected AMI should by given intramuscularly.

   FALSE. Intramuscular injections are to be discouraged in the field management of cardiac patients for two reasons. First, when dealing with a damaged myocardium, one cannot be certain of the efficiency of peripheral perfusion. The muscle into which you inject that dose of morphine may be very poorly perfused, and the uptake of the drug into the bloodstream will be delayed accordingly. Hours later, when perfusion improves, and after the patient has had several doses of morphine, all of the drug may suddenly be mobilized from the muscle into the circulation, and no one will understand why the patient doesn't wake up. The second reason for avoiding intramuscular injections in cardiac patients is that such injections can cause the liberation into the bloodstream of muscle enzymes, very similar to the enzymes released by a damaged myocardium. Physicians measure those enzymes in the blood in order to assess the existence and extent of myocardial damage, and extraneous enzymes from peripheral muscle can confuse the picture.

d. A normal ECG does not rule out the possibility that a patient is experiencing an AMI.

   TRUE. Electrocardiographic changes indicative of AMI may not develop for several hours after the patient begins experiencing his symptoms. For that reason, cardiologists do not rely on positive ECG findings to make their decisions regarding whether to hospitalize a patient with chest pain. If the patient has a "good story," it should be an automatic ticket of admission to the coronary care unit.

e. If a patient with chest pain is not experiencing any difficulty breathing, there is no need to administer oxygen.

   FALSE! The patient may not appear to be having difficulty breathing, but if he is complaining of chest pain, one must assume that his *heart* is having difficulty breathing, and one must treat the patient accordingly. Acute myocardial infarction occurs when a segment of the myocardium, for whatever reason, fails to receive the oxygen it needs to carry on its work. And to date, the only method we have of getting an emergency supply of oxygen to an endangered heart is to administer it through the patient's respiratory system. So whether or not the patient is short of breath, IF HE HAS CHEST PAIN, HE NEEDS OXYGEN.

f. Oxygen should be withheld from a patient with chest pain if he has a known history of chronic obstructive pulmonary disease (COPD).

   FALSE! We tried to catch you on that one. A patient with chest pain needs oxygen—no ifs, ands, or buts. If that patient happens to have COPD, you will simply have to watch him very carefully and coach him to take deep breaths or assist his ventilations should his breathing become depressed. But don't withhold the one drug that may keep his myocardium alive!

g. Elderly patients often suffer myocardial infarction without experiencing chest pain.

   TRUE. Partly because of changes in the pain threshhold that occur with aging and for other reasons that are not well understood, a significant number of elderly patients experience myocardial infarction without chest pain. Often the chief complaints are very vague and nonspecific, such as fatigue or confusion. Or the chief complaint may seem entirely unrelated to a cardiac problem, such as an accident or fall, the circumstances of which the patient cannot clearly remember. Sometimes there is no chief complaint at all, and the infarction is picked up by chance on a routine ECG. For that reason, it is always worthwhile to monitor a patient over 70 years old, regardless of his chief complaint. You may be very surprised by what the ECG shows.

FURTHER READING

Bayer AJ et al. Changing presentation of myocardial infarction with increasing old age. *J Am Ger Soc* 34:263, 1986.

Chatterjee K. Unstable angina. *Emerg Med* 15(14):271, 1983.

Chatterjee K, Rouleau JL, Parmley WW. Medical management of patients with angina. *JAMA* 252:1170, 1984.

Conti CR, Christie LG. Sorting out chest pain. *Emerg Med* 16(3):155, 1984.

Grace WJ, Chadbourne JA. The first hour in acute myocardial infarction. *Heart Lung* 3:737, 1974.

Goldberg RJ et al. Recent changes in attack and survival rates of acute myocardial infarction (1975–1981). *JAMA* 255:2774, 1986.

Hultgren HN, Giacomini JC, Miller C. Treatment of unstable angina. *JAMA* 253:2555, 1985.

Kannel WB, Abbott RD. Incidence and prognosis of unrecognized myocardial infarction: An update on the Framingham Study. *N Engl J Med* 311:1144, 1984.

Ledwich JR et al. Chest pain during myocardial infarction. *JAMA* 244:2171, 1980.

O'Doherty M et al. Five hundred patients with myocardial infarction monitored within one hour of symptoms. *Br Med J* 286:1405, 1983.

Rahimtoola SH. Unstable angina: Current status. *Mod Conc Cardiovasc Dis* 54(4):19, 1985.

Wroblewski M et al. Symptoms of myocardial infarction in old age: Clinical case retrospective and prospective studies. *Age & Aging* 15:99, 1986.

Yu PN. Prehospital care of acute myocardial infarction. *Circulation* 45:189, 1972.

1. Arrange the following components of the electric conduction system of the heart in the order in which electric impulses normally traverse them:

   a. Bundle of His
   b. Purkinje fibers
   c. SA node
   d. Atria
   e. AV node
   f. Right and left bundles

   1. _____
   2. _____
   3. _____
   4. _____
   5. _____
   6. _____

2. In the normal heart, the dominant pacemaker is usually located in

   a. The bundle of His
   b. The sinoatrial (SA) node
   c. The atrioventricular (AV) node
   d. The Purkinje fibers
   e. The posterior left bundle

A45

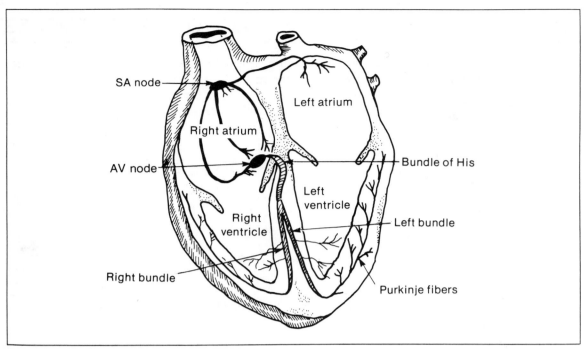

Figure 1. Electric conduction system of the heart.

1. The order in which electric impulses normally traverse the conduction tissues of the heart is as follows (Fig. 1):

    1. __c__ SA node
    2. __d__ Atria
    3. __e__ AV node
    4. __a__ Bundle of His
    5. __f__ Right and left bundles
    6. __b__ Purkinje fibers

2. The correct answer is **b**: In the normal heart, the dominant pacemaker is usually located in the **sinoatrial (SA) node**.

    Each collection of conduction tissues in the heart has its own intrinsic rate of firing. The conduction tissues with the fastest intrinsic rate—those in the SA node—normally set the pace for cardiac contractions, i.e., serve as pacemaker. If for any reason the SA node is suppressed, that part of the conduction system with the next highest intrinsic rate will take over as pacemaker, usually the AV node.

FURTHER READING

Bilitch M. *A Manual of Cardiac Arrhythmias.* Boston: Little, Brown, 1971.
Caroline NL. *Emergency Care in the Streets* (4th ed.). Boston: Little, Brown, 1991, Ch. 23.
Dubin D. *Rapid Interpretation of EKGs* (3rd ed.). Tampa: Cover, 1974.

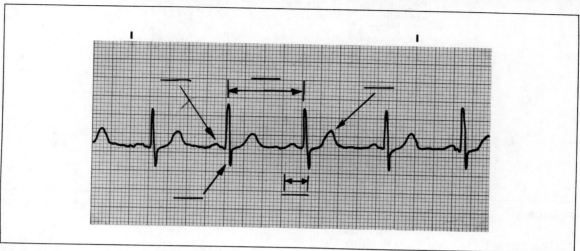

Figure 2

1. Label the following parts of the electrocardiogram in Figure 2:

   a. P wave
   b. T wave
   c. QRS complex
   d. P–R interval
   e. R–R interval

2. Each deflection or line on the ECG represents an event in the heart. Match the components of the ECG listed in part 1 above with the electric event each represents:

   1. _____ Depolarization of the ventricles
   2. _____ Repolarization of the ventricles
   3. _____ Time between two successive cardiac contractions
   4. _____ Depolarization of the atria
   5. _____ Total time it takes for an impulse to traverse the atria and AV junction

A46

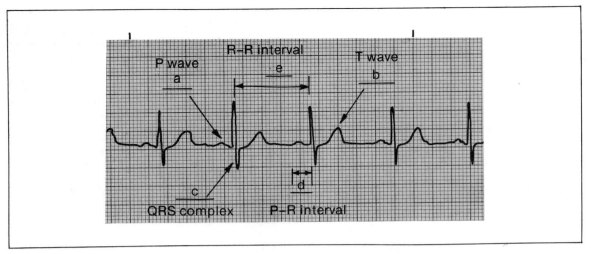

Figure 3

1. The correctly labeled ECG is shown in Figure 3.
2. The electric events of the heart as represented on the ECG are as follows:

1.	__c__	QRS complex	Depolarization of the ventricles
2.	__b__	T wave	Repolarization of the ventricles
3.	__e__	R–R interval	Time between two successive cardiac contractions
4.	__a__	P wave	Depolarization of the atria
5.	__d__	P–R interval	Total time it takes for an impulse to traverse the atria and AV junction

FURTHER READING

Bilitch M. *A Manual of Cardiac Arrhythmias.* Boston: Little, Brown, 1971.
Caroline NL. *Emergency Care in the Streets* (4th ed.). Boston: Little, Brown, 1991, Ch. 23.
Dubin D. *Rapid Interpretation of EKGs* (3rd ed.). Tampa: Cover, 1974.

Each wave and complex on the electrocardiogram corresponds to an electric event in the heart. When things have gone awry in the heart, the disturbance is often evident on the ECG, and thus it is important to understand what various ECG abnormalities signify.

1. If a P wave is absent on an ECG, one can assume

    a. There is something technically wrong with the ECG, such as a loose lead.
    b. There is damage to the Purkinje fibers in the ventricles.
    c. The pacemaker for the patient's rhythm is not in the SA node.
    d. There is complete heart block.
    e. The ventricles are not contracting.

2. A prolonged P–R interval suggests

    a. The patient is taking quinidine.
    b. There is damage to the left bundle.
    c. The atria are not contracting.
    d. There is something slowing conduction through the AV junction.
    e. There is ischemia to the heart.

A47

1. If the P wave is absent on the ECG, one can assume that **the pacemaker for the patient's rhythm is not in the SA node** (answer **c**). The normal P wave is formed when an electric impulse originating in the SA node is propagated down the atria, causing atrial depolarization. If the SA node is suppressed and the pacemaker site moves to another position in the atria, the P wave will be of a different size and configuration, reflecting the different path that the electric impulse is taking during atrial depolarization. The closer the new pacemaker site is to the AV junction, the shorter the distance between the P wave and the QRS complex, for the depolarizing impulse will reach the ventricles sooner. Indeed, if the pacemaker site is very near the AV junction, the P wave may not be seen at all, for it may be buried in the QRS complex (indicating that the atria and the ventricles were depolarized simultaneously). In low AV junctional rhythms, the P wave may even occur *after* the QRS complex, reflecting the fact that the depolarizing impulse arrived in the ventricles before it completed atrial depolarization.

    A loose lead (answer a) would cause disturbances in the ECG, but these would not be limited to the P wave; rather, one would see electric artifact or even a straight line. Damage to the Purkinje fibers in the ventricles (answer b) would appear on the ECG as irregularities (e.g., widening) of the QRS complex, for the QRS complex is the ECG representation of ventricular depolarization. In complete heart block (answer d), P waves tend to occur quite normally and regularly; the problem is that there is no consistent relationship between the P waves and the QRS complexes, for the atria and the ventricles are firing entirely independently of one another. Finally, the ECG does not provide any information, one way or the other, as to whether or how powerfully the ventricles are *contracting* (answer e); to determine that, one must palpate the patient's pulse. The ECG does indicate whether the ventricles are being *depolarized,* but this information is conveyed in the QRS complex, not the P wave.

2. A prolonged P–R interval suggests **d: There is something slowing conduction through the AV junction.**

    Recall that the P–R interval, i.e., the distance from the beginning of the P wave to the beginning of the QRS complex, represents the time it takes for an electric impulse to depolarize the atria and cross the AV junction into the ventricles. Thus a prolonged P–R interval indicates that something has slowed the conduction of the electric impulse before it could reach the ventricles, and the most common site for such a delay to occur is at the AV junction. A variety of factors, such as drugs (digitalis) and ischemia, can cause relative degrees of block at the AV junction, and when the P–R interval is delayed longer than 0.2 seconds, the dysrhythmia is termed first-degree AV block.

    Quinidine (answer a) is a drug that accelerates conduction through the AV junction; thus quinidine by itself would not be expected to cause a prolongation in the P–R interval. Damage to the left bundle (answer b) would be reflected in abnormalities in the QRS complex. Whether or not the atria are *contracting* (answer c) cannot be determined on an ECG; remember, the ECG reflects electric, not mechanical, events in the heart. If atrial *depolarization* failed to occur, one would see an absence of P waves. Finally, ischemia of the heart (answer e) is reflected on the ECG by depression of the S–T segment.

FURTHER READING
Bilitch M. *A Manual of Cardiac Arrhythmias.* Boston: Little, Brown, 1971.
Caroline NL. *Emergency Care in the Streets* (4th ed.). Boston: Little, Brown, 1991, Ch. 23.
Dubin D. *Rapid Interpretation of EKGs* (3rd ed.). Tampa: Cover, 1974.

Indicate which of the following statements about cardiac dysrhythmias are true and which are false:

a. Both very slow cardiac rhythms and very rapid cardiac rhythms may lead to decreased cardiac output.

   TRUE   FALSE

b. The administration of oxygen is sometimes all that is required to terminate PVCs.

   TRUE   FALSE

c. The vast majority of cases of cardiac arrest start out as asystole rather than ventricular fibrillation.

   TRUE   FALSE

d. Sinus arrhythmia is caused by fluctuations in vagal activity during breathing and may be entirely normal.

   TRUE   FALSE

e. The majority of patients who die from acute myocardial infarction before reaching the hospital die because of cardiogenic shock or congestive heart failure.

   TRUE   FALSE

f. In young, healthy individuals, sinus bradycardia may be a normal finding, reflecting good physical training.

   TRUE   FALSE

A48

a. Both very slow cardiac rhythms and very rapid cardiac rhythms may lead to decreased cardiac output.

TRUE. Recall the factors that determine cardiac output:

CARDIAC OUTPUT = STROKE VOLUME × HEART RATE

With very slow cardiac rhythms, i.e., bradycardias with rates below about 38 per minute, clearly the cardiac output will fall, for heart rate is a crucial component of our equation. But what about very rapid heart rates? A quick look at the equation suggests that cardiac output should *increase* as the heart rate increases. This is true, up to a point. But we have taken for granted that the stroke volume doesn't change, and that assumption is not valid at very rapid heart rates. The only time that the ventricles can fill with blood is *between heart beats* (diastole). When the heart is plodding along at about 70 per minute, or even cantering at 100 per minute, there is ample time between beats for the ventricles to refill. But a heart rate of, say, 180 beats per minute is another matter altogether; there is barely time to repolarize before the next beat, and very little blood can flow into the ventricles during this period (ventricular diastole), so there is very little blood to pump out (stroke volume). Thus, as the heart rate starts to climb above about 130 to 140 per minute, the stroke volume begins to fall, and the fall in stroke volume soon cancels out whatever benefit the increased heart rate may have accomplished in terms of increased cardiac output.

b. The administration of oxygen is sometimes all that is required to terminate PVCs.

TRUE. Premature ventricular contractions occur because an area of the ventricle has become irritable, and nothing is as likely to irritate the ventricles as local hypoxemia. Very often, therefore, a few whiffs of oxygen are all that is needed to make the ventricles happy again. When there has been significant damage to myocardial tissue, oxygen may not in itself be sufficient, and lidocaine may have to be given as well. But one always starts with oxygen at the earliest possible moment.

c. The vast majority of cases of cardiac arrest start out as asystole rather than ventricular fibrillation.

FALSE. Probably at least 90 percent cardiac arrests start out as ventricular fibrillation. By the time you see asystole, the arrest is usually relatively far advanced, and the chances for successful resuscitation are accordingly diminished.

d. Sinus arrhythmia is caused by fluctuations in vagal activity during breathing and may be entirely normal.

TRUE. Sinus arrhythmia occurs because of vagal influences during breathing, and the ECG shows a slight acceleration of heart rate during inhalation and a slight slowing during exhalation. It is an entirely normal phenomenon and is seen more commonly in children than in adults. If one is so inclined, one can calculate the respiratory rate from an ECG showing sinus arrhythmia.

e. The majority of patients who die from acute myocardial infarction before reaching the hospital die because of cardiogenic shock or congestive heart failure.

FALSE! The vast majority of patients who die from acute myocardial infarction before reaching the hospital die because of cardiac dysrhythmias that were potentially treatable!

f. In young, healthy individuals, sinus bradycardia may be a normal finding, reflecting good physical training.

TRUE. So restrain the impulse to reach for the atropine when you find a heart rate of 40 in a 20-year-old athlete. He's probably in better shape than you are.

FURTHER READING

Adelson L, Hoffman W. Sudden death from coronary disease. *JAMA:*176:129, 1961.
Adgey AAJ et al. Initiation of ventricular fibrillation outside hospital in patients with acute ischaemic heart disease. *Br Heart J* 47:55, 1982.

American Heart Association. Standards and guidelines for cardiopulmonary resuscitation (CPR) and emergency cardiac care (ECC). *JAMA* 255:2905, 1986.

Bass E. Cardiopulmonary arrest: Pathophysiology and neurologic complications. *Ann Intern Med* 103(Part 1):920, 1985.

Clinton JE et al. Cardiac arrest under age 40: Etiology and prognosis. *Ann Emerg Med* 13:1011, 1984.

Cobb LA. Cardiac arrest during sleep. *N Engl J Med* 311:1044, 1984.

Eisenberg MS et al. Out-of-hospital cardiac arrest: Significance of symptoms in patients collapsing before and after arrival of paramedics. *Am J Emerg Med* 4:116, 1986.

Goldberg AH. Cardiopulmonary arrest. *N Engl J Med* 290:381, 1974.

Liberthson RB et al. Pathophysiologic observations on prehospital ventricular fibrillation and sudden cardiac death. *Circulation* 49:790, 1974.

Schaeffer WA, Cobb LA. Recurrent ventricular fibrillation and modes of death in out-of-hospital ventricular fibrillation. *N Engl J Med* 293:259, 1975.

1. In which of the following dysrhythmias is the use of electric countershock NEVER indicated?

   a. Ventricular tachycardia
   b. Asystole
   c. Atrial flutter
   d. Ventricular fibrillation
   e. Atrial fibrillation

2. For treatment of which of the following cardiac dysrhythmias should the defibrillator NOT be set for the "synchronize" mode?

   a. Atrial flutter
   b. Atrial fibrillation
   c. Ventricular tachycardia
   d. Ventricular fibrillation
   e. Supraventricular tachycardia

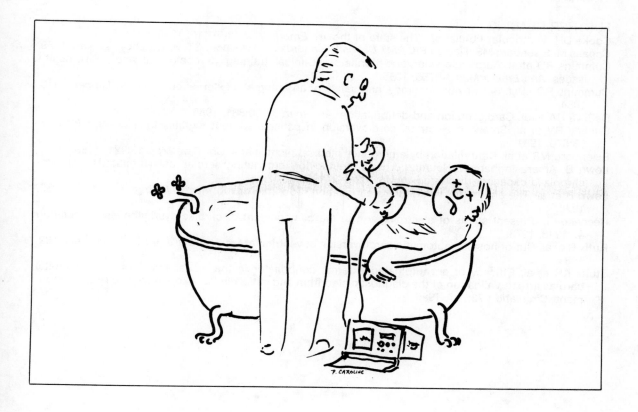

A49

1. Electric countershock is never indicated in the treatment of **asystole** (answer **b**), for it can do nothing to stimulate a heart in cardiac standstill to resume its contractions. For that, one needs epinephrine, which may stimulate the heart into a state of ventricular fibrillation—and *that* one can treat with electric countershock (answer d). Countershock is also indicated in the field treatment of ventricular tachycardia (answer a), atrial flutter (answer c), and atrial fibrillation (answer e)—when those dysrhythmias are associated with signs of poor peripheral perfusion, i.e., hypotension, cold and clammy skin, and confusion or coma.

   "So what's the big deal?" you say. "I won't do any good by shocking a patient in asystole. But I won't do any harm either." Not so. Sending 400 joules of electricity through the myocardium is NOT a harmless procedure, for countershock can itself cause myocardial damage. Like any other medical treatment, it must be reserved for those situations in which it is clearly warranted and in which its potential benefit exceeds its potential harm. Asystole is *not* one of those situations. Furthermore, defibrillation attempts in asystole may waste valuable time that could be used for constructive resuscitation procedures.

2. The defibrillator is NOT set on the "synchronize" mode for the treatment of **ventricular fibrillation** (answer **d**). The synchronize mode instructs the defibrillator to sense the peak of the R wave and then pause for a sufficient period to prevent the delivery of the electric shock on top of the next T wave, lest one precipitate ventricular fibrillation. But in ventricular fibrillation itself, there are no T waves. As a matter of fact, strictly speaking there are no R waves either. The defibrillator, however, isn't smart enough to figure that out. The defibrillator sees the positive deflections among the fibrillatory waves and assumes that these are R waves; the result is that the discharge of the defibrillator is delayed or sometimes prevented altogether.

   In all the other situations listed, the use of the synchronize mode IS indicated in order to prevent delivering the shock during the heart's vulnerable period (ventricular repolarization, as represented on the ECG by the T wave).

   If you were wide awake while reading question 2, you may have wondered what supraventricular tachycardia (answer e) is doing on the list. Is countershock the first-line treatment of choice these days for supraventricular tachycardias? In many instances, no. The problem is that it is often very difficult, even for trained cardiologists, to distinguish between some supraventricular tachycardias and some rapid ventricular tachycardias. And if the patient is showing signs of compromised peripheral perfusion—e.g., hypotension, confusion—one will often give countershock a try, even if the diagnosis of ventricular tachycardia is not 100 percent certain.

FURTHER READING

Cooke DH. Ventricular fibrillation: The state of the art. *Emerg Med* 18(5):115, 1986.

Copass M, Eisenberg MS, Damon SK. *EMT Defibrillation* (3rd ed.). Westport, CT: Emergency Training, 1989.

Cummins RO et al. Automatic external defibrillators: Clinical, training, psychological, and public health issues. *Ann Emerg Med* 14:755, 1985.

Cummins RO et al. Sensitivity, accuracy, and safety of an automatic external defibrillator. *Lancet* 2:318, 1984.

DeSilva RA et al. Cardioversion and defibrillation. *Am Heart J* 100:881, 1980.

Ditchey RV et al. Safety of electrical cardioversion in patients without digitalis toxicity. *Ann Int Med* 95:676, 1981.

Eisenberg MS et al. Defibrillation by emergency medical technicians. *Crit Care Med* 13:921, 1985.

Lown B, Amarasingham R, Neuman J. New method for terminating cardiac arrhythmias: Use of synchronized capacitor discharge. *JAMA* 182:548, 1962.

Lown B et al. The energy for ventricular defibrillation: Too little or too much? *N Engl J Med* 288:1252, 1978.

Resnekov L. Present status of electroversion in the management of cardiac dysrhythmias. *Circulation* 47:1346, 1973.

Ruffy R et al. Out-of-hospital automatic cardioversion of ventricular tachycardia. *J Am Coll Cardiol* 62:482, 1985.

Stults KR et al. Efficacy of an automated external defibrillator in the management of out-of-hospital cardiac arrest: Validation of the diagnostic algorithm and initial clinical experience in a rural environment. *Circulation* 73:701, 1986.

Which of the following statements regarding myocardial trauma are true and which are false?

a. Given the same mechanisms of injury, blunt trauma to the heart is more likely to occur to a young person than to an older person.

TRUE   FALSE

b. If a patient has sustained blunt trauma to the abdomen without evidence of chest injury, there is no need to worry about the possibility of injury to the heart.

TRUE   FALSE

c. A myocardial contusion may present with all the same signs and symptoms as an acute myocardial infarction.

TRUE   FALSE

d. A myocardial contusion may present without any signs or symptoms at all.

TRUE   FALSE

e. If a cardiac dysrhythmia occurs after trauma to the chest, it should be treated exactly as if it had occurred in the context of acute myocardial infarction.

TRUE   FALSE

A50

a. Given the same mechanisms of injury, blunt trauma to the heart is more likely to occur to a young person than to an older person.

TRUE. The thorax of a young person is more pliable than that of an older individual, for with aging, calcifications develop in the articulations of the thoracic cage, rendering it progressively more rigid. Thus the thorax of a young person is more apt to be compressed sharply against his spine on blunt impact, and the heart—lying in between—is more likely to get the squeeze.

b. If a patient has sustained blunt trauma to the abdomen without evidence of chest injury, there is no need to worry about the possibility of injury to the heart.

FALSE! Even when trauma is apparently confined to the abdomen, significant injury to the heart may occur, for the heart sits on the diaphragm, only inches from the abdominal cavity.

c. A myocardial contusion may present with all the same signs and symptoms as an acute myocardial infarction.

TRUE. Furthermore, a patient with myocardial contusion is prone to all the same complications as a patient with myocardial infarction, including dysrhythmias, myocardial rupture, and cardiogenic shock.

d. A myocardial contusion may present without any signs or symptoms at all.

Also **TRUE.** And very important. In the vast majority of cases, if you don't consider the possibility of myocardial contusion and don't check for it, you won't know it's there. Until it's too late. Maintain a high index of suspicion when managing any patient who has sustained significant trauma to his chest, and monitor his cardiac rhythm.

e. If a cardiac dysrhythmia occurs after trauma to the chest, it should be treated exactly as if it had occurred in the context of acute myocardial infarction.

TRUE. Virtually any cardiac dysrhythmia can occur after myocardial trauma, although atrial flutter and fibrillation are the most common. Whatever the dysrhythmia, it should be treated as you would treat the same dysrhythmia in a patient with acute myocardial infarction. And remember, if you're not monitoring the patient, you aren't going to detect his dysrhythmias.

FURTHER READING

Baxter BT et al. A plea for sensible management of myocardial contusion. *Am J Surg* 158:557, 1989.
Bayer MJ, Burdick D. Diagnosis of myocardial contusion in blunt chest trauma. *JACEP* 6:238, 1977.
Beresky R et al. Myocardial contusion: When does it have clinical significance? *J Trauma* 28:64, 1988.
Conn AKT. Cardiac arrest due to trauma. *Emergency* 11(12):42, 1979.
Dreifus LS. Dysrhythmias related to cardiac trauma. *Chest* 61:294, 1972.
Dubrow TJ et al. Myocardial contusion in the stable patient: What level of care is appropriate? *Surgery* 106:267, 1989.
Fabian TC et al. Myocardial contusion in blunt trauma: Clinical characteristics, means of diagnosis, and implications for patient management. *J Trauma* 28:50, 1988.
Green ED et al. Cardiac concussion following softball blow to the chest. *Ann Emerg Med* 9:155, 1980.
Guillot TS, Frame SB. Trauma Rounds. Problem: Myocardial contusion. *Emerg Med* 20(3):157, 1988.
Healey MA et al. Blunt cardiac injury: Is this diagnosis necessary? *J Trauma* 30:137, 1990.
Helling TS et al. A prospective evaluation of 68 patients suffering blunt chest trauma for evidence of cardiac injury. *J Trauma* 29:961, 1989.
Jones JW, Hewitt LW, Drapanas T. Cardiac contusion: A capricious syndrome. *Ann Surg* 181:567, 1975.
Kron IL, Cox PM. Cardiac injury after chest trauma. *Crit Care Med* 11:624, 1983.
Kunar SA et al. Myocardial contusion following nonfatal blunt chest trauma. *J Trauma* 23:327, 1983.
Miller FB, Shumate CR, Richardson JD. Myocardial contusion: When can the diagnosis be eliminated? *Arch Surg* 124:805, 1989.
Nelson RM et al. Journal club: Myocardial contusion. *Am J Emerg Med* 3:588, 1985.
Snow N, Richardson JD, Flint LM Jr. Myocardial contusion: Implications for patients with multiple traumatic injuries. *Surgery* 92:744, 1982.
Sturaitis M et al. Lack of significant long-term sequelae following traumatic myocardial contusion. *Arch Intern Med* 146:1765, 1986.
Sutherland GR et al. Frequency of myocardial injury after blunt chest trauma as evaluated by radionuclide angiography. *Chest* 84:1099, 1983.
Weisz GM, Blumenfeld Z, Barzilai A. Electrocardiographic changes in traumatized patients. *JACEP* 5:329, 1976.

Indicate whether in each of the following conditions the patient should be transported

a. Lying flat (supine or on his side)
b. Semisitting
c. Sitting straight up

1. _____ Congestive heart failure
2. _____ Hemorrhagic shock
3. _____ Stroke
4. _____ Uncomplicated myocardial infarction
5. _____ Syncope
6. _____ Severe asthmatic attack

A51

A safe position for transport of one patient may be fatal for another. By understanding the pathophysiology of various illnesses, one can make an informed decision regarding the position in which a given patient should be transported.

1. __c__ Congestive heart failure

The patient in heart failure should be transported **SITTING STRAIGHT UP** and if possible with his legs dangling, to facilitate drainage of excess volume, by gravity, out of the lungs and into the lower extremities.

2. __a__ Hemorrhagic shock

The patient in shock is transported **LYING FLAT** or with his legs and head slightly elevated. Perfusion pressures may be very low in shock and thus may not be sufficient to perfuse the brain adequately if blood has to travel uphill. The name of the game is perfuse the brain. Don't make the heart work against gravity: Lower the head to a level where blood flow can reach it most easily.

3. __a__ Stroke

Once again, we are dealing with a situation in which there has been a relative deficiency in brain perfusion, so **KEEP THE PATIENT FLAT**—unless he is hypertensive, in which case a semisitting position is often preferred.

4. __b__ Uncomplicated myocardial infarction

The less work the infarcted heart has to do, the less likelihood there is that the area of infarction will be extended. Thus we want to transport the patient in the position in which cardiac work is least, which is the **SEMISITTING POSITION.**

5. __a__ Syncope

Syncope occurs when there is a sudden interruption in adequate brain perfusion. The body, being very wise, knows that it is much harder to perfuse a brain that is towering a foot or more above the heart, so it invokes a very practical remedy: The patient falls down. Once the patient is flat on the ground, cerebral perfusion is greatly improved. Don't try to outsmart the body. If a patient has fainted and you find him flat on the ground, **KEEP HIM FLAT.** His neurons will appreciate it.

6. __c__ Severe asthmatic attack

Anyone in severe respiratory distress should be transported **SITTING STRAIGHT UP.** Indeed, the asthmatic suffering a severe attack probably won't let you position him any other way. He knows better than you what position enables him to breathe most comfortably. Respect his wishes.

FURTHER READING

Caroline NL. *Emergency Medical Treatment: A Text for EMT-As and EMT-Intermediates* (3rd ed.). Boston: Little, Brown, 1991, Ch. 37.

AMBULANCE CALLS

A 28-year-old metal worker suffered a laceration to the left upper arm when he slipped against a piece of sheet metal. You find him lying on a cot in the factory first-aid room. He is restless and anxious. His skin is cool and wet. Pulse is 140 and weak, blood pressure is 70 systolic, and respirations are 26 per minute. The remainder of the physical examination is unremarkable save for a deep laceration over the left upper arm, from which bright red blood is spurting. There is also an impressive pool of blood on the floor.

1. From this patient's clinical signs, what would you estimate his blood loss to be?

    a. Less than 5 percent of blood volume
    b. Less than 10 percent of blood volume
    c. About 15 percent of blood volume
    d. At least 40 percent of blood volume
    e. More than 70 percent of blood volume

2. What is the FIRST measure of hemorrhage control you would attempt in this case?

    a. Pressure point control
    b. Steady, direct pressure against the bleeding site
    c. Application of a tourniquet proximal to the bleeding site
    d. Application of a tourniquet distal to the bleeding site
    e. Clamping the brachial artery with a hemostat

3. Which of the following would NOT be indicated as part of this patient's management?

    a. Administer oxygen.
    b. Apply military antishock trousers.
    c. Start at least one IV line with normal saline, and run it wide open.
    d. Administer diazepam (Valium), 5 to 10 mg IV, to control the patient's restlessness.
    e. Cover the patient with a blanket.

A52

1. A pulse above 130 together with a systolic blood pressure around 70 or less in the context of hemorrhage usually implies a blood loss of **at least 40 percent of blood volume** in a young person (answer **d**). (How many units of blood would that amount to?)

2. The FIRST measure of hemorrhage control that should be attempted in our patient is **steady, direct pressure** against the bleeding site (answer **b**). In the vast majority of cases, that is the safest and most effective means of arresting hemorrhage. Pressure point control (answer a) for probable brachial artery bleeding will require pressure over the brachial plexus in the axillary area, an awkward maneuver and one that will be difficult to apply effectively or for sustained periods. A tourniquet proximal to the bleeding site (answer c) is always the *last* resort, after other measures to control bleeding have failed, for whenever one applies a tourniquet, one accepts the risk that the limb may have to be sacrificed. Tourniquets are never applied distal to the bleeding site (answer d), for their purpose is to stop arterial, not venous, bleeding. Finally, a paramedic should not be poking around in a wound with a hemostat (answer e); clamping off bleeding vessels with surgical instruments should be undertaken only by persons trained in surgical techniques and under sterile conditions.

3. The administration of diazepam (Valium) to control this patient's restlessness is emphatically NOT part of the appropriate treatment (answer **d**). The patient is restless because he is in shock, and giving medications that simply lower his blood pressure further will hardly improve the situation. What the patient needs is the restoration of his peripheral perfusion, so that peripheral tissues can again begin receiving an adequate supply of oxygen and nutrients. Thus he needs oxygen (answer a), intravenous fluids (answer c), and measures to improve his central circulation, such as the MAST (answer b). He should also be kept at a physiologic temperature to prevent chilling and shivering; thus a blanket is often necessary (answer e).

FURTHER READING

Barber JM. EMT checkpoint: Early detection of hypovolemic states. *EMT J* 2(2):72, 1978.
Bennet BR. Shock: An approach to teaching EMTs normal physiology before pathophysiology. *EMT J* 2(1):41, 1978.
Caroline NL. *Emergency Care in the Streets* (4th ed.). Boston: Little, Brown, 1991, Ch. 9.
Caroline NL. *Emergency Medical Treatment: A Text for EMT-As and EMT-Intermediates* (3rd ed.). Boston: Little, Brown, 1991, Ch. 8.
Garvin JM. Keeping shock simple. *Emerg Med Serv* 9(5):49, 1980.
Geelhoed GW. Shock and its management. *Emerg Med Serv* 5(6):42, 1976.
Shock. *Emerg Med* 12(19):47, 1980.
Wilson RF. Science and shock: A clinical perspective. *Ann Emerg Med* 14:714, 1985.

You are called to attend to a 22-year-old woman who was found unconscious in her apartment by her mother. The mother informs you that her daughter is an insulin-dependent diabetic who had been complaining over the past day or so of not feeling very well. The mother had spoken to the patient over the phone the night before, at which time the patient had mentioned that she had been vomiting. This morning, when she was unable to reach her daughter by phone, the mother became concerned and came over to her daughter's apartment to check. She found her daughter unconscious on the couch.

On physical examination, you find an unconscious woman breathing very deeply and rapidly. There is a fruity odor on her breath. The skin is warm and dry and tents slightly when pinched. Pulse is 120 and regular, blood pressure is 100/70, and respirations are 30 per minute. There is no evidence of head injury. Pupils are equal and reactive. The neck is supple, the chest is clear, the abdomen is soft, and extremities are unremarkable save for injection marks on the anterior thighs.

1. The most appropriate treatment for this patient in the field is to

   a. Administer 50% glucose, 50 ml IV.
   b. Start an IV with normal saline, and run it in rapidly.
   c. Administer regular insulin, 30 units SQ.
   d. Administer regular insulin, 15 units SQ and 15 units IV.
   e. Administer naloxone (Narcan), 0.4 mg slowly IV.

2. Which of the following statements about the emergency treatment of diabetic problems are true, and which are false?

   a. A patient with severe hypoglycemia may behave as if he were intoxicated with alcohol.

   TRUE   FALSE

   b. Polydipsia, polyuria, and polyphagia are signs of *hypo*glycemia.

   TRUE   FALSE

   c. A diabetic in coma is in danger of airway obstruction.

   TRUE   FALSE

A53

1. Our patient is showing signs of diabetic ketoacidosis: onset gradual, over 1 to 2 days; vomiting; Kussmaul's breathing; fruity odor on her breath. The most appropriate treatment is **b: Start an IV with normal saline, and run it in rapidly.** This patient is severely dehydrated—probably owing to a combination of vomiting, polyuria, hyperventilation, and inadequate intake of fluids. The most immediate danger is development of shock; it is of primary importance to start rehydrating her as rapidly as possible.

   Insulin (answers c and d) should not be given in the field unless you are many hours away from a medical facility, for optimal insulin therapy requires careful titration against measured blood sugar and ketone levels; that can be accomplished only in a hospital. Narcan (answer e) is entirely inappropriate here, for there is nothing to suggest that this patient's coma is due to an overdose of narcotic drugs. If you decided to try a bolus of 50% glucose (answer a)— because you weren't entirely sure whether this patient was comatose from hypoglycemia or hyperglycemia—that's OK. But when you failed to get a response to the glucose, you should have opened up the IV line wide.

2. Now to the true and false questions:

   a. A patient with severe hypoglycemia may behave as if he were intoxicated with alcohol.

   TRUE. When the brain cells aren't getting the glucose they need, all sorts of bizarre behavior may occur. The patient may become paranoid or combative; he may stagger as he tries to walk; his speech may be slurred. A good dose of glucose may be all that is required to turn an aggressive monster back into a charming, debonair gentleman. Try it sometime.

   b. Polydipsia, polyuria, and polyphagia are signs of *hypo*glycemia.

   FALSE. These are classic signs of *hyper*glycemia. The polydipsia (drinking massive quantities of water) occurs because the patient is dehydrated, and the thirst mechanism is therefore activated. Polyuria (excretion of large quantities of urine) occurs through osmotic diuresis because of the osmotic load a high blood sugar imposes. And polyphagia (eating excessively) reflects the fact that the body tissues are hungry; they are not benefitting from all that glucose floating around because, in the absence of insulin, the cells cannot utilize glucose properly. It is a case of hunger in the midst of plenty, on the cellular level.

   c. A diabetic in coma is in danger of airway obstruction.

   TRUE. Any patient in coma is in danger of airway obstruction, and also of regurgitation and aspiration. It's your job to prevent that.

FURTHER READING

Adler PM. Serum glucose changes after administration of 50% dextrose solution: Pre- and in-hospital calculations. *Am J Emerg Med* 4:504, 1986.

Adrogue HJ, Barrero J, Eknoyan G. Salutary effects of modest fluid replacement in the treatment of adults with diabetic ketoacidosis: Use in patients without extreme volume deficit. *JAMA* 262:2108, 1989.

Andrade A et al. Hypoglycemic hemiplegic syndrome. *Ann Emerg Med* 13:529, 1984.

Auf der Heide E. Prehospital management of diabetic emergencies. *Emerg Med Serv* 9(5):9, 1980.

Baker FJ et al. Diabetic emergencies: Hypoglycemia and ketoacidosis. *JACEP* 5:119, 1976.

Bourn S. When sugar's not sweet. *JEMS* 14(12):81, 1989.

Caroline NL. *Emergency Care in the Streets* (4th ed.). Boston: Little, Brown, 1991, Ch. 24.

Carter WP. Hypothermia: A sign of hypoglycemia. *JACEP* 5:594, 1976.

Chisholm CD, Chisholm RL. Hypoglycemia: A metabolic disorder of many faces. *JEMS* 14(6):29, 1989.

Cotton EK, Fahlberg VI. Hypoglycemia with salicylate poisoning. *Am J Dis Child* 108:171, 1964.

deCourtern-Myers G, Myers RE, Schoolfield L. Hyperglycemia enlarges infarct size in cerebrovascular occlusion in cats. *Stroke* 19:623, 1988.

Dorin RI, Crapo LM. Hypokalemic respiratory arrest in diabetic ketoacidosis. *JAMA* 257:1517, 1987.

Felig P. Diabetic ketoacidosis. *N Engl J Med* 290:1360, 1974.

Hillman K. Fluid resuscitation in diabetic emergencies—a reappraisal. *Intensive Care Med* 13:4, 1987.

Iscovith AL. Sudden cardiac death due to hypoglycemia. *Am J Emerg Med* 1:28, 1983.

Kunian L, Wasco J, Hulefeld L. Sweets for the alcoholic. *Emerg Med* 5(1):45, 1973.

Levine SN et al. Treatment of diabetic ketoacidosis. *Arch Intern Med* 141:713, 1981.

Morris LR et al. Bicarbonate therapy in severe diabetic ketoacidosis. *Ann Intern Med* 105:836, 1986.

Moss MH. Alcohol-induced hypoglycemia and coma caused by alcohol sponging. *Pediatrics* 46:445, 1970.

Rosenbloom AL. Intracerebral crises during treatment of diabetic ketoacidosis. *Diabetes Care* 13:22, 1990.

Slovis CM. Early recognition of diabetic ketoacidosis. *Emerg Med* 21(8):20, 1989.

Stapczynski JS, Haskell RJ. Duration of hypoglycemia and need for intravenous glucose following intentional overdoses of insulin. *Ann Emerg Med* 13:505, 1984.

Taigman M. Just a little sugar: Serious talk about D-50. *JEMS* 13(10):33, 1988.

You are called for a "possible OB" about 15 minutes' distance from the hospital. The patient is a 24-year-old woman in the ninth month of her second pregnancy. She states that her contractions are now less than 2 minutes apart, and she feels a strong urge to move her bowels.

You should

a. Help her to the toilet.
b. Have her cross her legs, and move her rapidly to the hospital so that delivery can take place under sterile conditions.
c. Give her 5 mg of morphine IV to ease her pain, and then move her to the hospital.
d. Set her up for delivery, since birth of the baby is imminent.

A54

The correct answer is **d: Set her up for delivery, since birth of the baby is imminent.** This is our patient's second pregnancy, and thus labor can be expected to proceed fairly rapidly. Certainly by the time contractions are less than 2 minutes apart, one can expect the baby to be making its appearance very shortly. And if we had any lingering doubts, the patient has informed us that she feels an urge to move her bowels, which is caused by the descent of the baby's head into the birth canal (the baby's head puts pressure on the rectum and thereby creates the sensation of having to move one's bowels). From that information, we can assume that the baby will make its debut at any moment, and we must quickly set the patient up for delivery at home.

Do NOT allow this patient to go to the toilet (answer a), unless you want to fish the baby out of the toilet bowl. Five mg of morphine IV (answer c) will scarcely mitigate the pain of labor, and probably by the time you've gotten the IV going and administered the morphine, the baby will have arrived anyway. No drugs that could potentially depress the baby in any way should be administered in the field to a patient in labor, and in this case, analgesic drugs are unnecessary anyway.

Under no circumstances should you have the mother cross her legs to impede delivery of the baby (answer b). When the baby decides to catapult itself into the cold, cruel world, no force on earth is going to stop it, and attempts to restrain delivery will simply jeopardize the baby's life. Nature is the timekeeper at these events, and health professionals must play according to Her watch.

FURTHER READING

Anderson B, Shapiro B. *Emergency Childbirth Handbook.* Albany, NY: Delmar, 1979.
Caroline NL. *Emergency Care in the Streets* (4th ed.). Boston: Little, Brown, 1991, Ch. 35.
Roush GM. Abdominal examination of the pregnant uterus. *EMT J* 3(2):33, 1979.
Taber B. *Manual of Gynecologic and Obstetric Emergencies.* Philadelphia: Saunders, 1979.
Williams C. Emergency childbirth. *Emerg Med Serv* 14(3):100, 1985.
Wojslawowicz JM. Emergency childbirth for emergency medical technicians. *EMT J* 1(4):66, 1977.

A 45-year-old man has sustained blunt trauma to the abdomen and is found lying supine and unconscious. Arrange the following steps of management in the correct order:

a. Start at least one IV with a large-bore needle and D5/normal saline.
b. Determine if the patient is breathing; if he is not, start artificial ventilation.
c. Apply military antishock trousers and inflate.
d. Open the patient's airway.
e. Check for fractures.
f. Determine if the patient has a pulse; if not, start external cardiac compressions.

1. _____
2. _____
3. _____
4. _____
5. _____
6. _____

A55

And now a word from our sponsor, the old ABCs:

AIRWAY
BREATHING
CIRCULATION

Remember? Hence, the steps in the management of this patient are

1. __d__ Open the patient's AIRWAY.
2. __b__ Determine if the patient is BREATHING; if he is not, start artificial ventilation.
3. __f__ Determine if the patient has a pulse (CIRCULATION); if not, start external cardiac compressions.
4. __c__ Apply military antishock trousers and inflate (CIRCULATION).
5. __a__ Start at least one IV with a large-bore needle and D5/normal saline (CIRCULATION).
6. __e__ Check for fractures (other injuries).

Perhaps you put a ahead of c, i.e., you decided to start the IV before applying the MAST garment. Strictly speaking this is not incorrect, but you are making things much harder for yourself if you do it that way. If the patient is in shock, nine times out of ten his veins will be collapsed, and you will have a very tough time finding a suitable vein for the IV. Once the MAST is inflated, however, veins have been known to start popping up like magic. So you can save a lot of time and aggravation by pumping up the MAST *before* you start the IV.

FURTHER READING
Caroline NL. *Emergency Medical Treatment: A Text for EMT-As and EMT-Intermediates* (3rd ed.). Boston: Little, Brown, 1991, Ch. 18.

A 45-year-old man calls for an ambulance because of chest pain. When you first examine him, his pulse is 72 and regular, but about 10 minutes later you note that his pulse has dropped to 38 per minute.

1. Assuming that his stroke volume did not change, what has happened to his cardiac output?

   a. Cardiac output has increased.
   b. Cardiac output has decreased.
   c. There has been no change in cardiac output.

2. Now let us assume as well that there has been no change in the patient's peripheral resistance. What, then, would we expect to happen to his blood pressure?

   a. Blood pressure would rise.
   b. Blood pressure would fall.
   c. There would be no change in blood pressure.

3. In fact, there might not be any significant change in the patient's blood pressure, because in making our assumption in question 2 above, we failed to take into account an important compensatory mechanism that the body uses to prevent the effect on blood pressure noted above. This mechanism is

   a. Vasodilation
   b. Vasoconstriction
   c. Diuresis
   d. Vagal stimulation

A56

In order to answer our questions properly, we must recall some definitions. CARDIAC OUTPUT is the amount of blood pumped out *per minute* by either ventricle; it is measured in liters per minute. STROKE VOLUME is the amount of blood pumped out by either ventricle *in a single contraction,* measured in milliliters. And HEART RATE, or pulse, is the number of cardiac contractions per minute. These terms can be related to one another in the following equation:

CARDIAC OUTPUT = STROKE VOLUME × HEART RATE

Now, let us return to our patient. When we first examined him, his heart rate was 72 per minute. For purposes of computation (and to make the math simpler), let's say his stroke volume was 100 ml. Thus his cardiac output is

CARDIAC OUTPUT = 100 ml × 72/min = 7,200 ml/min

Ten minutes later, his heart rate has fallen to 38 per minute. We have postulated that stroke volume remained unchanged, so we will use the same figure, 100 ml, for our calculations:

CARDIAC OUTPUT = 100 ml × 38/min = 3,800 ml/min

It is clear, then, that the decrease in his pulse has led to a **decrease in cardiac output** (answer **1b**). In fact, the decrease might be quite negligible, for our assumption—that stroke volume remained unchanged—was questionable. A slow heart rate permits more time between beats for the ventricles to refill; thus stroke volume increases as heart rate decreases.

In question 2, we ask what would happen to the patient's blood pressure if his cardiac output fell and there were no change in peripheral resistance (degree of constriction of the arterial system). Again, we go back to a fundamental equation:

BLOOD PRESSURE = CARDIAC OUTPUT × PERIPHERAL RESISTANCE

Since the cardiac output has fallen and the peripheral resistance has remained constant, the **blood pressure would fall** (answer **2b**).

In fact, however, the body attempts to maintain a fairly constant blood pressure, even when there are wide swings in the cardiac output, in order to maintain perfusion of the brain and other vital organs. Thus the assumption we made in question 2, that the peripheral resistance would remain unchanged, is probably not valid. For when the cardiac output falls, compensatory **vasoconstriction** (answer **3b**) occurs—i.e., peripheral resistance increases—in order to maintain the blood pressure at near normal levels. Vasoconstriction has the effect of decreasing the overall volume of the circulatory system (if you decrease the diameter of a pipe, its volume decreases; think about it) in order to accommodate a smaller cardiac output better.

Think of the circulatory system as a 7-liter rubber bag that must be kept full to maintain a certain internal pressure. The bag has a hole in the bottom, through which 7 liters of fluid escape per minute, but the bag is also being filled at the rate of 7 liters per minute (cardiac output), so it remains full. Now, what would happen if the filling rate dropped to 3.5 liters per minute, while the emptying rate remained the same? The bag would be only half full, and the pressure inside would drop. If we switched to a 3.5-liter bag, however, we could maintain the same pressure under the decreased flow conditions (decreased cardiac output). This is basically what vasoconstriction accomplishes by decreasing the volume of the arterial system.

Vasodilation (answer 3a) clearly would have the effect of switching our 7-liter bag for a 10-liter bag and would only make the situation worse. Diuresis, or the forced excretion of water (answer 3c), would decrease the volume available to the circulatory system and make it even more difficult to fill our rubber bag. Similarly, stimulation of the vagus nerve (answer 3d) would slow the heart rate even further, leading to further decreases in cardiac output. So the body wisely chooses vasoconstriction in situations where blood pressure must be maintained.

FURTHER READING

Caroline NL. *Emergency Care in the Streets* (4th ed.). Boston: Little, Brown, 1991, Ch. 23.
Caroline NL. *Emergency Medical Treatment: A Text for EMT-As and EMT-Intermediates* (3rd ed.). Boston: Little, Brown, 1991, Ch. 8.

A 50-year-old man was the driver of a car that struck another car head-on; he was thrown forward against the windshield. You find him unconscious, with obvious bruises on his forehead. His pulse is 130, weak and regular; blood pressure is 70 systolic; and respirations are 24.

1. From these findings, you can conclude that

   a. The patient has a rising intracranial pressure as a result of the injury to his head.
   b. The patient must have a source of significant blood loss elsewhere in his body.
   c. The patient has a basilar skull fracture.
   d. The patient must have had cardiac problems prior to his accident.

2. Regarding the management of the above patient, which of the following statements is NOT true?

   a. The first step in managing this patient is to establish an airway.
   b. Because he has a significant head injury, he must be assumed to have a cervical spine injury as well and should be immobilized accordingly.
   c. His state of consciousness and neurologic signs should be reassessed frequently and carefully recorded.
   d. Any blood or clear fluid seen draining from his ears should be dammed up with an occlusive dressing.

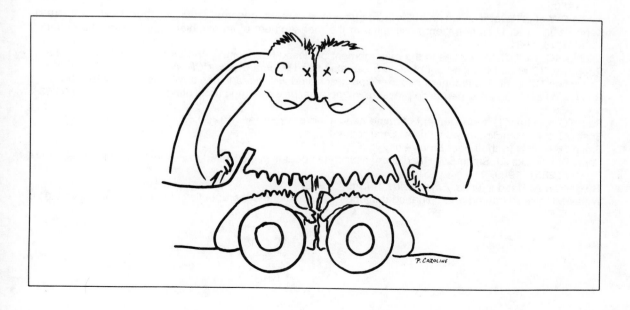

A57

The correct answer to question 1 is **b: The patient must have a source of significant blood loss elsewhere in his body.** The skull is just a little box, mainly filled with brain tissue. There is very little space for blood to accumulate within it, and certainly intracranial bleeding alone could not account for a volume of blood loss sufficient to cause hypotension and other signs of shock. When intracranial pressure does rise, in response to bleeding into the skull or edema of the brain tissues (answer 1a), the blood pressure tends to *rise,* not fall. Hypotension caused by head injury alone is a very rare finding and tends to occur in the very late stages of injury, when the patient is near death. We have no evidence from the information presented that this patient has suffered a basilar skull fracture (answer 1c), and even if he had, this would not account for his signs of shock. We also have no evidence that the patient had prior cardiac problems (answer 1d), although—given the mechanisms of injury and the likelihood of steering wheel trauma—we must consider the possibility that the patient *now* has cardiac problems, secondary to myocardial contusion. Certainly pericardial tamponade is among the possibilities that must be ruled out in trying to account for this patient's clinical picture. (What are some of the other possibilities?)

The answer to question 2 is **d**: It is definitely NOT true that any blood or clear fluid seen draining from this patient's ears should be dammed up with an occlusive dressing. Discharge from the ear may be an indication of basilar skull fracture, and damming up the flow will only increase the chances of the patient's developing high intercranial pressure. In such situations, one should *lightly* cover the ear with a sterile dressing to lessen the possibility of CNS infection.

All of the other answers in question 2 are true. The first step in managing *any* unconscious patient is always to make certain there is an adequate airway (answer 2a). It is axiomatic that *every* patient who has sustained significant trauma to the head should be assumed to have also sustained injury to the cervical spine and should be immobilized accordingly (answer 2b). Finally, frequent assessment and careful recording of the patient's neurologic status (answer 2c)—especially his state of consciousness—are among the most important aspects of management in this case.

FURTHER READING

Baxt WG et al. The impact of advanced prehospital emergency care on the mortality of severely brain-injured patients. *J Trauma* 27:365, 1987.

Bouzarth WF. Early management of acute head injury (a surgeon's viewpoint). *EMT J* 2(2):43, 1978.

Caroline NL. *Emergency Care in the Streets* (4th ed.). Boston: Little, Brown, 1991, Ch. 16.

Caroline NL. *Emergency Medical Treatment: A Text for EMT-As and EMT-Intermediates* (3rd ed.). Boston: Little, Brown, 1991, Ch. 14.

Clifton GL et al. Cardiovascular response to severe head injury. *J Neurosurg* 59:447, 1983.

Cold GE. Does acute hyperventilation provoke cerebral oligaemia in comatose patients after acute head injury? *Acta Neurochir* (Wien) 96:100, 1989.

Davidoff G et al. The spectrum of closed head injuries in facial trauma victims: Incidence and impact. *Ann Emerg Med* 17:6, 1988.

Javid M. Head injuries. *N Engl J Med* 291:890, 1974.

Jones CC, McBride MM, Hines LL. New protocols for managing the head injured patient. *Emergency* 12(7):53, 1980.

Jones PW et al. Hyperventilation in the management of cerebral oedema. *Intensive Care Med* 7:205, 1981.

Kenning JA et al. Upright patient positioning in the management of intracranial hypertension. *Surg Neurol* 15:148, 1981.

Lillehei KO, Hoff JT. Advances in the management of closed head injury. *Ann Emerg Med* 14:789, 1985.

Raphaely RC et al. Management of severe pediatric head trauma. *Pediatr Clin North Am* 27:715, 1980.

Robertson CS et al. Treatment of hypertension associated with head injury. *J Neurosurg* 59:455, 1983.

Rosner MJ et al. Cerebral perfusion pressure, intracranial pressure, and head elevation. *J Neurosurg* 65:636, 1986.

Saul TG, Ducker TB. Management of acute head injuries. *Emergency* 12(2):59, 1980.

Scali VJ et al. Handling head injuries. *Emergency* 21(11):22, 1989.

Smith S. A blow to the head. *Emergency* 22(6):16, 1990.

Sosin DM, Sacks JJ, Smith SM. Head injury-associated deaths in the United States from 1979 to 1986. *JAMA* 262:2251, 1989.

Thygerson A. Head injuries. *Emergency* 14(3):50, 1982.

Weiss MH. Head trauma and spinal cord injuries: Diagnostic and therapeutic criteria. *Crit Care Med* 2:311, 1974.

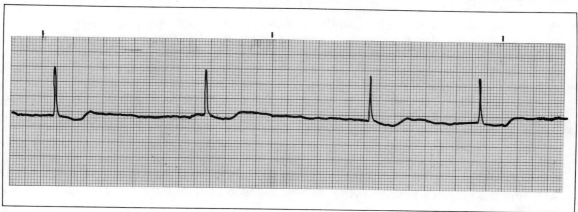

Figure 4

You are called to attend a 72-year-old man who complains that he has been "feeling poorly" lately. He states that over the past week, he seems to have lost his appetite and has been feeling quite sick to his stomach. He has had some diarrhea and in general has felt weak and tired. He has no known allergies and takes some kind of "heart pills."

On physical examination, he appears listless and somewhat confused. His vital signs are unremarkable, save for the irregularity in pulse reflected in his electrocardiogram. His pupils are equal. Neck veins are not distended. There are a few crackling rales at the bases of both lungs. The abdomen is soft and nontender; bowel sounds are slightly hyperactive. There is 1+ ankle edema.

1. Examine the electrocardiogram in Figure 4:

    a. The rhythm is _____ regular _____ irregular
    b. The rate is _____ per minute.

2. The name of this rhythm is

    a. Sinus bradycardia
    b. Junctional bradycardia
    c. Atrial fibrillation
    d. Third-degree AV block
    e. Sinus arrest

3. The patient's bradycardia is probably due to

    a. Acute myocardial infarction
    b. The effect of respirations on the vagus nerve
    c. Left heart failure
    d. Digitalis toxicity
    e. Procainamide (Pronestyl) toxicity

4. The treatment of this patient in the field is

    a. Start an IV with D5W, and add 60 mEq of potassium to the infusion.
    b. Morphine, 5 to 8 mg slowly IV.
    c. Cardioversion at 25 to 50 watt-seconds.
    d. Naloxone (Narcan), 0.4 mg IV.
    e. Supportive treatment only; notify the hospital to have a pacemaker ready.

A58

1. The patient's rhythm is **irregular.** The rate is about **40 per minute.**
2. The name of this rhythm is **atrial fibrillation** (answer **c**), with a very slow ventricular response. While the fibrillatory waves are difficult to see, the irregularly irregular rhythm is the tip-off, and the absence of P waves confirms our suspicions.
3. Our patient's bradycardia is probably due to **digitalis toxicity** (answer **d**). Certainly his history is consistent with this diagnosis, for anorexia, nausea, diarrhea, and weakness are all characteristic complaints in patients whose digitalis levels are in the toxic range. The margin between a therapeutic dose of digitalis and a toxic dose is very narrow, and for that reason, dosage of the drug is difficult to regulate. Our patient was probably prescribed digitalis for chronic heart failure (he has crackles in his lung bases and a bit of pedal edema) and chronic atrial fibrillation. But for some reason the dose he was taking was too high, and he has developed gastrointestinal and cardiac signs of toxicity.

   If you answered **a** to this question, you could be correct. One cannot discount the possibility of acute myocardial infarction (AMI), which may present in unusual ways in the elderly. The absence of chest pain, especially in an elderly patient, does not rule out the possibility of AMI, and the patient's bradyarrhythmia could be secondary to ischemic damage to the AV junction.
4. The treatment of this patient in the field is **supportive** (answer **e**). If he were showing signs of a marked decrease in peripheral perfusion (cold, clammy skin; hypotension; stupor), one might attempt to increase his cardiac rate with atropine or isoproterenol. But at the moment, he is apparently relatively stable. An IV lifeline is always a good idea—so it's there in the event his status changes—but for heaven's sake don't give him potassium (answer **a**), unless you want to stop his heart altogether. WHEN HIGH DEGREES OF AV BLOCK ARE CAUSED BY DIGITALIS TOXICITY, DO NOT GIVE POTASSIUM: It may further depress AV conduction and lead to even more dangerous dysrhythmias.

   There is no reason on earth to give this patient morphine (answer **b**), and there are a lot of reasons not to. He is not in pain. He is not in acute pulmonary edema. He does, however, have a potentially dangerous bradycardia, and morphine can only be expected to aggravate this situation. Cardioversion (answer **c**) is indicated for tachyarrhythmias, not bradyarrhythmias, and even in the former case, cardioversion is very dangerous under circumstances where the patient is fully digitalized (not to mention digitoxic!). Naloxone (Narcan) is a very specific antidote against narcotic overdose; it won't help a bit in digitalis toxicity (answer **d**).

   In the hospital, our patient will probably be monitored on the ICU for a few days, until the effects of his digitalis begin to wane. If he develops symptoms of poor cardiac output, a temporary pacemaker may be inserted to tide him over the period of digitalis toxicity, and it's a good idea for them to have a pacemaker ready in the emergency room—just in case.

FURTHER READING

Caroline NL. *Emergency Care in the Streets* (4th ed.). Boston: Little, Brown, 1991, Ch. 23.
Chung EG. Signposts to digitalis toxicity. *Drug Therapy* 1:42, 1975.
Ewy G. Digitalis therapy in the geriatric patient. *Drug Therapy* 1:36, 1972.
Moorman JR et al. The arrhythmias of digitalis intoxication. *Arch Intern Med* 145:1289, 1985.
Schwartz HS. Digitalis intoxication and poisoning. *JACEP* 6:168, 1977.
Whang R et al. Frequency of hypomagnesemia in hospitalized patients receiving digitalis. *Arch Intern Med* 145:655, 1985.

Dyspnea is a common chief complaint and may be caused by a variety of different problems for which one seeks clues in the patient's history. Match the following causes of dyspnea with the historical information that suggests each:

a. Left heart failure with pulmonary edema
b. Acute asthmatic attack
c. Pulmonary embolism
d. Decompensation of chronic bronchitis
e. Spontaneous pneumothorax

1. _____ A 55-year-old man who smokes three packs of cigarettes per day. Yesterday, he noticed that his sputum had turned green and copious, and since then he has had more and more trouble breathing.

2. _____ A 34-year-old woman reports that she had sudden onset of severe shortness of breath. She has no history of previous illness. Her only regular medications are vitamins and birth control pills.

3. _____ A 50-year-old man woke up from sleep with severe shortness of breath, which was somewhat relieved by sitting up. He has a known history of hypertension and takes digitalis at home.

4. _____ A thin, 20-year-old man developed sudden, sharp, right chest pain and dyspnea during a plane trip from Chicago to Los Angeles.

5. _____ A 20-year-old man, severely short of breath, with a history of similar attacks in the past for which he has been treated in the emergency department with a "shot" and a "breathing machine."

What would you expect the physical examination to show in each of these cases?

A59

1. __d__ There are two significant clues that our 55-year-old man is suffering from **DECOM-PENSATION OF CHRONIC BRONCHITIS:** First, his heavy smoking history makes him a prime candidate for chronic bronchitis; second, there has been a significant change in the character and volume of his sputum, which has become green (thus purulent) and more copious—telltale signs of a respiratory infection. The latter is one of the most common causes of decompensation in chronic obstructive pulmonary disease (COPD), and we know that this patient has decompensated because he himself tells us that he is having progressively more trouble breathing.

On physical examination, you would expect to find a man in obvious respiratory distress, perhaps even somewhat cyanotic. Neck veins might be distended if there is an element of right heart failure (which accompanies certain forms of COPD), and the chest can be expected to be full of noises: rales, rhonchi, wheezes. If there is accompanying right heart failure, pedal edema may be present as well.

FURTHER READING
Bates D. Chronic bronchitis and emphysema. *New Engl J Med* 278:546, 1968.
Caroline NL. *Emergency Care in the Streets* (4th ed.). Boston: Little, Brown, 1991, Ch. 22.
Caroline NL. *Emergency Medical Treatment: A Text for EMT-As and EMT-Intermediates* (3rd ed.). Boston: Little, Brown, 1991, Ch. 19.
Ersoz CJ. Prehospital support of the patient with chronic lung disease. *Emerg Med Serv* 8(3):63, 1979.
Farber SM, Wilson RHL. Chronic obstructive emphysema. *Clin Sympos* 1968.

2. __c__ The clues in the case of our 34-year-old lady are (1) the sudden onset of her symptoms and (2) the fact that she is taking birth control pills. Sudden onset could also be consistent with spontaneous pneumothorax (answer e), but the birth control pills make one highly suspicious of the possibility of **PULMONARY EMBOLISM,** for women taking birth control pills have a higher susceptibility to pulmonary embolism than do the rest of the population.

Physical examination of this woman may not reveal any abnormalities at all, save for tachypnea and tachycardia. Most often the lungs are entirely normal to auscultation in this condition, although if the lung tissue surrounding the blocked pulmonary artery has undergone infarction, one might hear a scratching sound ("friction rub") as the infarcted area of lung rubs against the parietal pleura. Usually, however, physical findings are minimal in pulmonary embolism, and a presumptive diagnosis is made largely on the basis of the patient's history. The diagnosis is confirmed by a pulmonary angiogram, a special x-ray in which dye is injected into the pulmonary arteries to try to visualize the site at which the embolus lodged.

FURTHER READING
Bell WR, Simon TL, DeMets DL. The clinical features of submassive and massive pulmonary emboli. *Am J Med* 62:355, 1977.
Cooke DH. Focusing in on pulmonary embolism. *Emerg Med* 17(9):86, 1985.
Goodall RJR et al. Clinical correlations in the diagnosis of pulmonary embolism. *Ann Surg* 191:219, 1980.
Huet Y et al. Hypoxemia in acute pulmonary embolism. *Chest* 88:829, 1985.
McGlynn TJ, Hamilton RW, Moore R. Pulmonary embolism: 1979. *JACEP* 8:532, 1979.
Park H et al. Pulmonary embolism. *Emerg Med Serv* 4(5):33, 1975.
Sabiston DC. Pathophysiology, diagnosis and management of pulmonary embolism. *Am J Surg* 138:384, 1979.
Stein PD et al. History and physical examination in acute pulmonary embolism in patients without preexisting cardiac or pulmonary disease. *Am J Cardiol* 47:218, 1981.
Sutton GC, Honey M, Gibson RV. Clinical diagnosis of acute massive pulmonary embolism. *Lancet* 1:271, 1979.
Williams MH. Pulmonary embolism. *Emerg Med* 16(4):135, 1984.

3. __a__ Our 50-year-old man who was wakened from sleep by his dyspnea is most probably suffering from **LEFT HEART FAILURE WITH PULMONARY EDEMA.** He is a good candidate for problems with the left side of his heart because he is a hypertensive, which means that his left heart has been forced for some time to work much harder than usual in order to pump blood out against a high pressure gradient. Furthermore, we suspect that he has chronic heart failure because he is taking digitalis, a medication often prescribed for heart failure. The nature of the patient's dyspnea is also significant: He tells us that he got some relief by sitting up (i.e., he had *orthopnea,* or dyspnea when lying down). Orthopnea tends to occur in conditions of cardiovascular overload because blood pools in the lungs through gravity when the

patient is supine; when he sits up or stands, the same gravitational forces enable some of the blood to leave the pulmonary vasculature and pool in the legs (this is the reason why patients in congestive heart failure should always be transported in the sitting postion).

On physical examination, this patient will undoubtedly be found sitting up and in considerable respiratory distress. His pulse will be rapid, perhaps somewhat irregular—if hypoxemia has precipitated PVCs—and his blood pressure will be elevated. Rales will be heard in the lungs, especially at the bases, and it may be possible to hear a gallop rhythm over the precordium.

FURTHER READING

Forrester JS, Staniloff HM. Heart failure. *Emerg Med* 16(4):121, 1984.
Goldberg H, Nakhjavan FK. Pathophysiology, diagnosis, and treatment of heart failure. *Hosp Med* 8(7):8, 1972.
Karas S. CHF vs. COPD. *Emergency* 10(8):49, 1978.
Robin ED, Carroll IC, Zelis R. Pulmonary edema. *N Engl J Med* 288:239, 292. 1972.
Tresch DD et al. Out-of-hospital pulmonary edema: Diagnosis and treatment. *Ann Emerg Med* 12:533, 1983.

4. ___e___ Our thin, 24-year-old man has suffered a **SPONTANEOUS PNEUMOTHORAX.** This condition occurs when a small "bleb," or area of attenuated tissue, ruptures in the lung, allowing air to escape into the pleural cavity. It is more prone to occur in young, tall, thin males who are otherwise healthy, and it may be precipitated by changes in atmospheric pressure, such as those experienced during air travel. Spontaneous pneumothorax is also seen in patients with emphysema, who may have multiple blebs in their lungs; in these patients, a spontaneous pneumothorax can be precipitated by inhaling air under positive pressure (e.g., during a treatment with a ventilator).

On physical examination, we may find our young man to be in moderate respiratory distress. If his pneumothorax is complete, there may be slight tracheal deviation to the right (toward the side of the pneumothorax). The most striking findings will be in the chest, where breath sounds will be diminished or absent on the right, and there will be hyperresonance to percussion over the right lung field.

FURTHER READING

Askins DC. Spontaneous tension pneumothorax during sexual intercourse (letter). *Ann Emerg Med* 13:303, 1984.
Cannon WB, Mark JBD, Jamplis RW. Pneumothorax: A therapeutic update. *Am J Surg* 142:26, 1981.
Caroline NL. *Emergency Medical Treatment: A Text for EMT-As and EMT-Intermediates* (3rd ed.). Boston: Little, Brown, 1991, Ch. 15
Mukherjee D et al. A simple treatment for pneumothorax. *Surg Gynecol Obstet* 156:499, 1983.
Raja OG et al. Simple aspiration of spontaneous pneumothorax. *Br J Dis Chest* 75:207, 1981.
Smith SB et al. Spontaneous pneumothorax: Special considerations. *Am Surg* 49:245, 1983.

5. ___b___ Our 20-year-old man with recurrent attacks of dyspnea is most probably suffering an **ACUTE ASTHMATIC ATTACK.** Asthma is characterized by a series of acute attacks, interspersed with periods of relatively normal respiratory function. The acute episodes may be brought on by allergy, recent respiratory infection, stress, or a variety of other factors, many of which are not well understood. Our patient has apparently visited the emergency room more than once before for this problem and was treated with aerosolized bronchodilators ("breathing machine") and aqueous epinephrine (a "shot").

On physical examination, our asthmatic is likely to be sitting up and visibly struggling to breathe. His pulse will be rapid, and his respirations somewhat shallow. Examination of the chest will reveal some hyperinflation and hyperresonance, and wheezes will be heard on exhalation. Furthermore, the expiratory phase of respiration will be abnormally prolonged. If his is a very severe attack, breath sounds may be scarcely audible at all, for with severe obstruction, the asthmatic can barely move any air in and out of his lungs.

FURTHER READING

Benatar SR. Fatal asthma. *N Engl J Med* 314:423, 1986.
Dailey RD. Asthmatic: Acute and adult. *Emerg Med* 8(4):127, 1973.
Karetzky MS. Acute asthma: The use of subcutaneous epinephrine in therapy. *Ann Allergy* 44:12, 1980.

A 26-year-old hiker became separated from his companions during a sudden snowstorm and is found a day later by a search party. He is conscious and alert and complaining of severe, burning pain in his right foot. When you remove his boots and socks in the ambulance, you notice that the right foot is pale and slightly swollen. It has a lifeless, waxy appearance, but you can indent the skin on palpation.

Which of the following is NOT part of the treatment for this injury?

a. Gradually rewarm the foot in warm water (about 41°C).
b. Give the patient hot chocolate to drink.
c. Do not permit the patient to smoke.
d. Vigorously massage the foot to restore circulation to the area.
e. Give morphine for pain.

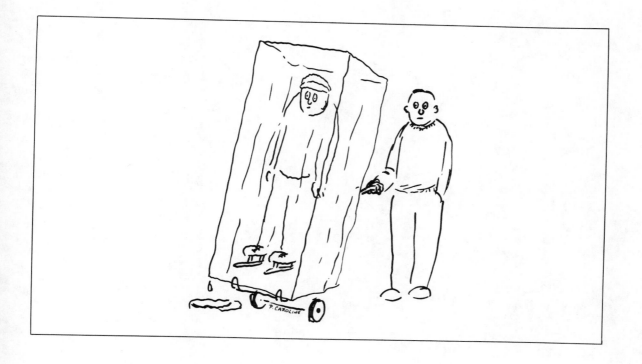

A60 Answer **d** is NOT part of the management of this patient: A frostbitten area should NEVER be massaged or rubbed, for rubbing will only aggravate the damage already sustained by the tissues. The frostbitten area requires the gentlest possible care; if it is a foot that is frostbitten, as in the present case, the patient should not be permitted to bear any weight on the injured extremity, and shoes and socks should be removed (gently!) as soon as the patient is out of the cold environment.

In a situation like this one, where the limb is not frozen solid, rewarming (answer a) is best started in the field, but only if the ambulance team has the training and equipment to do so properly. This means being able to control the temperature of a water bath within a very narrow range (between 40 and 42°C)—something that may not always be feasible under field conditions. If rewarming cannot be initiated in the field, soft, sterile gauze should be inserted gently between the patient's toes, and the foot should be wrapped in a sterile dressing. The foot may then be placed on a pillow to cushion it from sudden bumps or jars during transport. Meanwhile, the rest of the body should be kept as warm as possible.

Hot chocolate (answer b) may not assist a great deal in general warming, but does give a feeling of warmth and supply some calories. Drugs that cause peripheral vasoconstriction, such as nicotine, must be avoided; for that reason, the patient who has suffered frostbite must be forbidden to smoke (answer c).

As the frostbitten area begins to thaw out, the pain may become extremely severe, and adequate analgesia should be provided. Morphine is a good drug for this purpose, and it should be administered slowly IV at a dose of 0.1 mg per kilogram of body weight.

FURTHER READING
Bangs CC. Caught in the cold. *Emerg Med* 15(21):29, 1982.
Caroline NL. *Emergency Care in the Streets* (4th ed.). Boston: Little, Brown, 1991, Ch. 32.
Donner HJ. Out in the cold. *Emerg Med* 17(21):21, 1985.
Forgey WW. *Death by Exposure: Hypothermia.* Merrillville, IN: ICS Books, 1985.
Heggers JP et al. Experimental and clinical observations on frostbite. *Ann Emerg Med* 16:1056, 1987.
Holm PCA, Vaggaard L. Frostbite. *Plast Reconstr Surg* 54:544, 1974.
Lapp NL, Juergens LL. Frostbite. *Mayo Clin Proc* 40:932, 1965.
Lathrap TG. *Hypothermia: Killer of the Unprepared.* Portland, OR: Mazamas, 1975.
McCauley RL et al. Frostbite injuries: A rational approach based on the pathophysiology. *J Trauma* 213:143, 1983.
Mills WJ. Out in the cold. *Emerg Med* 8(1):134, 1976.
Terr AL. Environmental illness. *Arch Intern Med* 146:145, 1986.
Treatment of frostbite. *Med Lett* 18:105, 1976.
Ward M. Frostbite. *Br Med J* 1:67, 1974.
Washburn B. Frostbite. *N Engl J Med* 266:974, 1972.
Wilkerson JA (ed.). *Hypothermia, Frostbite, and Other Cold Injuries.* Seattle: Mountaineers, 1986.

The call comes in for a "sick baby," and when you arrive 5 minutes later at the apartment in question, a woman comes screaming out the door, "My baby is dead, my baby is dead." You follow her into her apartment and find an 8-month-old infant, apneic, somewhat cyanotic, and pulseless. The mother is able to tell you, between sobs, that the baby "just stopped breathing" a few minutes before you arrived.

1. You immediately begin CPR on the infant. The correct ratio of ventilations to compressions in this case is

   a. 1 to 5
   b. 1 to 15
   c. 2 to 5
   d. 2 to 15
   e. 1 to 20

2. After resuscitation has been in progress for a few minutes and the basic stabilizing measures have been taken (intubation, IV line, certain resuscitative drugs), the monitor shows coarse ventricular fibrillation. What is the correct dosage of current to defibrillate a child of this age?

   a. 5 joules
   b. 25 joules
   c. 100 joules
   d. 300 joules
   e. 400 joules

3. In the course of your resuscitation, you used the following drugs:

   a. Epinephrine
   b. Atropine
   c. Lidocaine
   d. Dopamine

   Match the drugs on the list above with the correct dosage for each:

   1. _____ 0.02 mg per kilogram IV bolus
   2. _____ 0.1 ml per kilogram of a 1:10,000 solution
   3. _____ 2–20 micrograms per kilogram per minute
   4. _____ 1 mg per kilogram IV bolus

A61

1. The correct ratio of ventilations to chest compressions when doing CPR on an infant is **1 ventilation to 5 compressions** (answer **a**), to provide about 20 ventilations and 80 to 100 compressions per minute.

2. The correct initial defibrillating dosage for an infant is about 2 joules/kg—so for an infant of 12 kg, the correct dosage would be **25 joules** (answer **b**). If defibrillation is unsuccessful at this dosage, one may try up to a maximum of 4 joules/kg; so for this 12-kg baby, this means a *maximum* of 50 joules. Larger doses are usually unnecessary and may cause considerable damage.

3. How well did you do on those pediatric dosages?

   1. **b** Atropine   0.02 mg per kilogram IV bolus
   2. **a** Epinephrine   0.1 ml per kilogram of a 1:10,000 solution
   3. **d** Dopamine   2–20 micrograms per kilogram per minute
   4. **c** Lidocaine   1 mg per kilogram IV bolus

FURTHER READING

American Heart Association. Standards and guidelines for cardiopulmonary resuscitation (CPR) and emergency cardiac care (ECC). *JAMA* 255:2905, 1986.

Atkins DL et al. Pediatric defibrillation: Importance of paddle size in determining transthoracic impedance. *Pediatrics* 82:914, 1988.

Benitz WE, Frankel LR, Stevenson DK. The pharmacology of neonatal resuscitation and cardiopulmonary intensive care. Part I: Immediate resuscitation. *West J Med* 144:704, 1986.

Brill JE. Cardiopulmonary resuscitation. *Pediatr Ann* 15:24, 1986.

Cavallaro D, Melker R. Comparison of two techniques for determining cardiac activity in infants. *Crit Care Med* 11:189, 1983.

David R. Closed chest cardiac massage in the newborn infant. *Pediatrics* 81:552, 1988.

Dierking BH. Pediatric notebook: Reviewing basic life support for children. *JEMS* 15(2):112, 1990.

Dishuk J. Cardiac care for kids. *Emergency* 21(8):29, 1989.

Eisenberg M, Bergner L, Hallstrom A. Epidemiology of cardiac arrest and resuscitation in children. *Ann Emerg Med* 12:672, 1983.

Finholt DA et al. The heart is under the lower third of the sternum: Implications for external cardiac massage. *Am J Dis Child* 140:646, 1986.

Freisen RM et al. Appraisal of pediatric cardiopulmonary resuscitation. *Can Med Assoc J* 126:1055, 1982.

Goetting MG, Paradis NA. High dose epinephrine in refractory pediatric cardiac arrest. *Crit Care Med* 17:1258, 1989.

Harris BH. The ABCs on a small scale. *Emerg Med* 17(3):24, 1985.

Holbrook PR. On opening the airway. *Emerg Med* 14(1):137, 1982.

Holbrook PR. On restarting the heart. *Emerg Med* 14(1):126, 1982.

Holbrook PR et al. Cardiovascular resuscitation drugs for children. *Crit Care Med* 8:588, 1980.

Lewis JK et al. Outcome of pediatric resuscitation. *Ann Emerg Med* 12:297, 1983.

Lubitz DS et al. A rapid method for estimating weight and resuscitation drug dosages from length in the pediatric age group. *Ann Emerg Med* 17:576, 1988.

Ludwig S, Kettrick RG, Parker M. Pediatric cardiopulmonary resuscitation: A review of 130 cases. *Clin Pediatr* 23:71, 1984.

Orlowski JP. Cardiopulmonary resuscitation in children. *Pediatr Clin North Am* 27:495, 1980.

Orlowski JP. Optimal position for external cardiac compression in infants and young children. *Ann Emerg Med* 15:667, 1986.

Phillips GWL et al. Relation of infant heart to sternum: Its significance in cardiopulmonary resuscitation. *Lancet* 1:1024, 1986.

Singer J. Cardiac arrests in children. *JACEP* 6:198, 1977.

Torphy DE, Minter MG, Thompson BM. Cardiorespiratory arrest and resuscitation of children. *Am J Dis Child* 138:1099, 1984.

Williams DR. The heartsaver-baby: A CPR course for young parents. *Can Fam Physician* 31:1005, 1985.

Zideman DA. Resuscitation of infants and children. *Br Med J* 292:1584, 1986.

Your dispatcher receives a call from a man who announces his intention to kill himself. He tells the dispatcher that he is divorced and living alone; his ex-wife and children live in another city. He sees no purpose any more in living. His father took his own life, so why shouldn't he?
Which of the following statements about this patient and his management is NOT true?

a. This patient is at high risk for successful suicide.
b. The dispatcher should keep the caller on the phone until your team can reach him.
c. When you reach the patient and interview him, you should inquire specifically whether he has made any concrete plans about how he would kill himself.
d. If the paramedic team feels that the patient is in real danger of harming himself, they may transport him against his will to the hospital.

Answer **d** is NOT true: In most localities, the only person authorized to transport anyone against his will is a law enforcement officer. If it is the opinion of the base station physician that this patient requires hospital evaluation and if the patient refuses to come along voluntarily, the police must usually be summoned—and often that can be done only after a court order has been issued. It is very important for each paramedic service to be aware of local regulations in this regard and to develop standard policies for dealing with such cases.

This patient is indeed at high risk for a successful suicide, for he has several significant risk factors: (1) he is male (the rate of successful suicide is higher among men than women), (2) he is divorced and living alone, (3) he is clearly depressed (he sees no point in living any more), and (4) he has a history of suicide in a close relative. Another factor that suggests a high risk is a history of having attempted suicide in the past, and the patient should be questioned about this in the course of the interview. One should also ask very specifically whether the patient has made any concrete plans as to how he would kill himself (answer c). Often interviewers are reluctant to broach this topic lest they "give the patient any ideas." There is usually little danger of that, and it is important to ascertain to what extent the patient has planned his demise—for the patient who has made concrete plans is generally more likely to carry them out than a patient who merely expresses a vague desire to "end it all."

It is important that someone stay on the line with the caller until your team can reach him (answer b). That will prevent him from doing anything rash in the meantime, and it will also give him an opportunity to ventilate some of his feelings. The fact that he called your dispatcher indicates that he still has some mixed feelings about killing himself; his telephone call was a plea for help and for caring human contact. This contact should not be interrupted once begun.

FURTHER READING

Bassuk EL, Fox SS, Prendergast KJ. *Behavioral Emergencies: A Field Guide for EMTs and Paramedics.* Boston: Little, Brown, 1983, Ch. 8.

Caroline NL. *Emergency Care in the Streets* (4th ed.). Boston: Little, Brown, 1991, Ch. 38.

Centers for Disease Control. Premature mortality due to suicide and homicide—United States, 1984. *MMWR* 36(32,33), 1987.

Jenike MA. Depressed in the ER. *Emerg Med* 16(6):102, 1984.

Leisner K. Trauma: Accident or attempted suicide? *Emerg Med Serv* 18(5):30, 1989.

Minoletti A et al. Suicidal behavior in the emergency room: 2. Treatment and disposition. *Can Fam Physician* 31:1668, 1985.

Motto JA et al. Development of a clinical instrument to estimate suicide risk. *Am J Psych* 142:680, 1985.

Murphy GE. Suicide and attempted suicide. *Hosp Pract* 12(11):73, 1977.

Pallis DJ et al. Estimating suicide risk among attempted suicides: I. The development of new clinical scales. *Br J Psych* 141:37, 1982.

Patterson WM et al. Evaluation of suicidal patients: The SAD PERSONS scale. *Psychosomatics* 24:343, 1983.

Perez E et al. Suicidal behavior in the emergency room: 1. Assessment of risk. *Can Fam Physician* 31:1663, 1985.

Rotheram MJ. Evaluation of imminent danger for suicide among youth. *J Orthospsychiatr* 57:102, 1987.

Roy A. Risk factors for suicide in psychiatric patients. *Arch Gen Psychiatry* 39:1089, 1982.

Rund DA. Assessment of suicide risk. *Emerg Med Serv* 18(5):27, 1989.

Ruple JA. Honing skills for suicide intervention. *JEMS* 15(1):149, 1990.

Solomon J. The suicide scenario: Rewriting the final act. *Emerg Med* 21(4):75, 1989.

Wheezes may occur in both asthma and acute pulmonary edema, but it is critically important to be able to distinguish between those two conditions because the treatment for one is considerably different from the treatment for the other.

Often the history and physical examination will provide sufficient information to permit a reasonably clear differentiation between the patient suffering from an acute asthmatic attack and the patient suffering from acute pulmonary edema. Indicate which of the following pieces of information would lead you to suspect

a. Acute asthmatic attack
b. Acute pulmonary edema

1. _____ Patient takes digitalis at home.
2. _____ Patient uses a Medihaler at home.
3. _____ Patient takes chlorothiazide (Diuril) at home.
4. _____ Patient has a known history of hypertension.
5. _____ Patient has noted a recent, rapid gain in weight.
6. _____ Patient has a known history of severe allergies.
7. _____ Patient's chest appears hyperinflated.
8. _____ A gallop rhythm is heard over the precordium.

As noted above, the treatment for the acute asthmatic attack is considerably different from the treatment for acute pulmonary edema. Indicate whether each of the following treatments is

a. Used only for asthma
b. Used only for acute pulmonary edema
c. Used for both asthma and acute pulmonary edema

1. _____ Epinephrine 1:1,000, 0.3 to 0.5 ml SQ
2. _____ Furosemide (Lasix), 40 to 80 mg IV
3. _____ Morphine, 5 to 10 mg titrated IV
4. _____ Oxygen
5. _____ Intravenous fluids at 100 to 200 ml per hour
6. _____ Aminophylline, 250 to 500 mg IV over at least 15 to 30 minutes

A63

First, let us look at the history and physical findings in our two patients:

1. __b__
2. __a__
3. __b__
4. __b__
5. __b__
6. __a__
7. __a__
8. __b__

The asthmatic patient often has an allergic history and takes bronchodilator medication (such as that dispensed by a Medihaler) at home. During the acute attack, he has relatively more obstruction to exhalation than to inhalation, the result being trapping of air in the lungs with consequent hyperinflation of the chest. The patient who is prone to develop acute pulmonary edema often has a history of high blood pressure, and indeed his high blood pressure may be at least one of the causes of his cardiac problems, for in chronic hypertension the left ventricle has to work much harder to pump blood out against a heavy afterload. Under those circumstances, the left heart may eventually fail, leading to acute pulmonary edema. Patients with chronic heart failure are frequently prescribed digitalis (to increase the rate and force of cardiac contractions) and diuretics, such as chlorothiazide, to counter their tendency toward water retention. When water retention does occur, the patient will often note a fairly sudden, rapid gain in weight. The physical examination of a patient in congestive heart failure will sometimes reveal a gallop rhythm (dum da-da, dum da-da, dum da-da . . .).

The differences between the treatment of these two conditions are considerable: What's good for the asthmatic may kill the patient in congestive heart failure, and vice versa.

1. __a__
2. __b__
3. __b__
4. __c__
5. __a__
6. __c__

EPINEPHRINE is a first-line drug in the treatment of acute asthmatic attack. Giving a shot of epinephrine to a patient in left heart failure is like making him run around the block three times, then up four flights of steps, followed by a double-somersault and five push-ups. Do you think he'll make it?

LASIX is a first-line drug in the treatment of pulmonary edema and left heart failure; it is one of several measures that are aimed at getting rid of the excess fluid volume in which the patient is literally drowning. The asthmatic does not have a problem of fluid overload; quite the contrary, he is apt to be significantly dehydrated, and a dose of Lasix is the last thing he needs under the circumstances. What he does need is a good dose of INTRAVENOUS FLUIDS, to help loosen up his secretions so he can cough them out. Remember: KEEP THE CARDIAC DRY; HYDRATE THE ASTHMATIC

Now, MORPHINE. Morphine is a wonderful drug for the patient in congestive heart failure, for by promoting peripheral pooling of blood, it decreases venous return to the heart and thereby takes a considerable volume load off the weary myocardium. In addition, its sedative effects help to allay the considerable terror associated with acute pulmonary edema. In asthma, morphine is a killer, for it adds the narcotic effect of an opiate to that of the carbon dioxide accumulating in the patient's blood. MORPHINE IS FORBIDDEN IN THE ACUTE ASTHMATIC ATTACK!

OXYGEN is always indicated for any patient in respiratory distress, and thus it is an appropriate treatment for both our asthmatic and our patient in acute pulmonary edema. Likewise, AMINOPHYLLINE is useful as a bronchodilator in both conditions; however, it should be used with extreme caution in the presence of myocardial infarction or cardiac dysrhythmias caused by hypoxemia, for aminophylline can have a significant irritant effect on the myocardium.

FURTHER READING
Acute Pulmonary Edema

Abrams J. Vasodilator therapy for chronic congestive heart failure. *JAMA* 254:3070, 1985.
Cohn JN, Fanciosa JA. Vasodilator therapy of cardiac failure. *N Engl J Med* 279:27, 254, 1977.

Forrester JS, Staniloff HM. Heart failure. *Emerg Med* 16(4):121, 1984.

Francis GS et al. Acute vasoconstrictor response to intravenous furosemide in patients with chronic congestive heart failure. *Ann Intern Med* 103:1, 1985.

Genton R, Jaffe AS. Management of congestive heart failure in patients with acute myocardial infarction. *JAMA* 256:2556, 1986.

Goldberg H, Nakhjavan FK. Pathophysiology, diagnosis, and treatment of heart failure. *Hosp Med* 8(7):8, 1972.

Hoffman JR, Reynolds S. Comparison of nitroglycerin, morphine and furosemide in treatment of presumed pre-hospital pulmonary edema. *Chest* 92:586, 1987.

Karas S. CHF vs. COPD. *Emergency* 10(8):49, 1978.

Levy DB, Pollard T. Failure of the heart. *Emergency* 20(12):22, 1988.

Marantz PR et al. Clinical diagnosis of congestive heart failure in patients with acute dyspnea. *Chest* 97:776, 1990.

Markiewicz W et al. Sublingual isosorbide dinitrate in severe congestive failure. *Cardiology* 67:172, 1981.

McKee PA et al. The natural history of congestive heart failure: The Framingham study. *N Engl J Med* 285:1441, 1971.

Parmley WM. To rescue a failing heart. *Emerg Med* 15(5):179, 1983.

Ramirez A, Abelmann WH. Cardiac decompensation. *N Engl J Med* 290:499, 1974.

Rasanen J et al. Continuous positive airway pressure by face mask in acute cardiogenic pulmonary edema. *Am J Cardiol* 55:296, 1985.

Roberts R. Inotropic therapy for cardiac failure associated with acute myocardial infarction. *Chest* 93 (1, Suppl):22S, 1988.

Robin ED, Carroll IC, Zelis R. Pulmonary edema. *N Engl J Med* 288:239, 292, 1972.

Tresch DD et al. Out-of-hospital pulmonary edema: Diagnosis and treatment. *Ann Emerg Med* 12:533, 1983.

Vaisanen IT, Rasanen J. Continuous positive airway pressure and supplemental oxygen in the treatment of cardiogenic pulmonary edema. *Chest* 92:481, 1987.

Wulf-Dirk B, Schupp D. Effect of sublingual nitroglycerin in emergency treatment of severe pulmonary edema. *Am J Cardiol* 41:931, 1978.

Asthma

Aberman A. Managing asthmatics. *Emerg Med* 18(8):26, 1986.

Appel D et al. Comparative effect of epinephrine and aminophylline in the treatment of asthma. *Lung* 159:243, 1981.

Bailskus M, Niersbach C. Matters of life and breath. *Emergency* 21(4):12, 1989.

Benatar SR. Fatal asthma. *N Engl J Med* 314:423, 1986.

Ben-Zvi Z et al. An evaluation of repeated injections of epinephrine for the initial treatment of acute asthma. *Am Rev Respir Dis* 127:101, 1983.

Brenner BE. Bronchial asthma in adults: Presentation to the emergency department. I. Pathogenesis, clinical manifestations, diagnostic evaluation, and differential diagnosis. *Am J Emerg Med* 1:50, 1983.

Carden DL et al. Vital signs including pulsus paradoxus in the assessment of acute bronchial asthma. *Ann Emerg Med* 12:80, 1983.

Cydulka R et al. The use of epinephrine in the treatment of older adult asthmatics. *Ann Emerg Med* 17:322, 1988.

Daily RD. Asthmatic: Acute and adult. *Emerg Med* 8(4):127, 1973.

Emerman CL et al. Ventricular arrhythmias during treatment for acute asthma. *Ann Emerg Med* 15:699, 1986.

Franklin WF. Treatment of severe asthma. *N Engl J Med* 290:1469, 1974.

Grandstetter RD et al. Optimal dosing of epinephrine in acute asthma. *Am J Hosp Pharm* 37:1326, 1980.

Groth ML, Hurewitz AM. Pharmacologic management of acute asthma. *Emerg Med* 21(7):23, 1989.

Johnson AJ. Circumstances of death from asthma. *Br Med J* 288:1870, 1984.

Josephson GW et al. Cardiac dysrhythmias during the treatment of acute asthma. *Chest* 78:429, 1980.

Karetzky MS. Acute asthma: The use of subcutaneous epinephrine in therapy. *Ann Allergy* 44:12, 1980.

Kavuru MS, Ahmad M. Ambulatory management of acute asthma. *Emerg Med* 20(21):111, 1988.

Kelly HW et al. Should we stop using theophylline for the treatment of the hospitalized patient with status asthmaticus? *Ann Pharmacother* 23:995, 1989.

Littenberg B. Aminophylline treatment in severe, acute asthma. *JAMA* 259:1678, 1988.

Pliss LB et al. Aerosol vs. injected epinephrine in acute asthma. *Ann Emerg Med* 10:353, 1981.

Rothstein RJ. Intravenous theophylline therapy in asthma: A clinical update. *Ann Emerg Med* 9:327, 1980.

Schneider SM et al. High-dose methylprednisolone as initial therapy in patients with acute bronchospasm. *Asthma* 25:189, 1988.

Stadnyk AM, Grossman RF. Management of life-threatening asthma. *Emerg Med* 19(15):103, 1987.

Stewart MF et al. Risk of giving intravenous aminophylline to acutely ill patients receiving maintenance treatment with theophylline. *Br Med J* 288:450, 1984.

You are called for a patient who "took too much stuff" (= took an overdose of heroin), and en route to the scene, you review briefly in your mind what you have learned about heroin overdose.

1. Which of the following is NOT part of the clinical picture of heroin overdose?

   a. Low blood pressure
   b. Cold, clammy skin
   c. Constricted pupils
   d. Deep, rapid respirations
   e. Coma

   When you arrive at the scene, a shabby apartment building, you find a man who appears to be in his late 20s comatose on the floor with a group of his friends around him. The patient does not respond to voice or painful stimuli. His pulse is 70 and regular, blood pressure is 100/70, and respirations are 6 per minute and shallow. Pupils are pinpoint. The neck is supple, the chest is clear, and the abdomen is soft. There are numerous needle tracks on both arms. While your partner begins assisting the patient's ventilations, you prepare some naloxone (Narcan).

2. The proper dosage and method of administration of this drug is

   a. 0.8 mg by rapid IV bolus
   b. 0.8 mg diluted in 9 ml of intravenous solution, slowly IV—titrated until the patient's respirations return to normal.
   c. 8 mg rapid IV bolus
   d. 8 mg diluted in 9 ml of intravenous solution, slowly IV—titrated until the patient's respirations return to normal
   e. 0.8 mg rapid IV bolus, repeated as many times as necessary until the patient is fully awake and alert

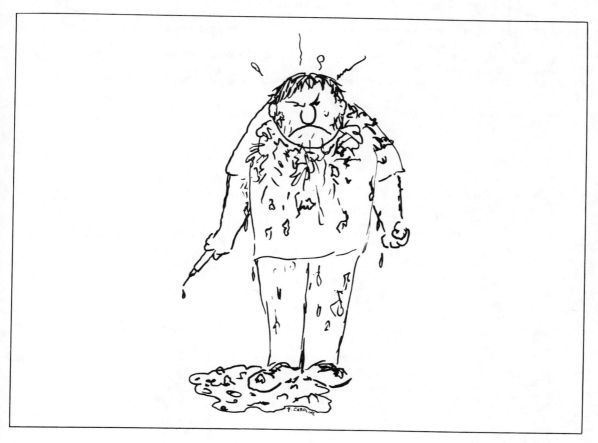

A64

The correct answer to part 1 is **d:** Deep, rapid respirations are NOT part of the clinical picture of a patient with heroin overdose. To the contrary, heroin—like all narcotics—is a respiratory depressant, and patients suffering from a heroin overdose commonly manifest very slow and shallow respirations or even outright apnea. Hypotension, pupillary constriction, clammy skin, and coma are all commonly seen in heroin overdose.

The proper dosage and method of administration of Narcan is answer **2b: 0.8 mg diluted in 9 ml of intravenous solution, SLOWLY IV—titrated until the patient's respirations return to normal.** Narcan, when administered very rapidly as a bolus, may precipitate very dramatic projectile vomiting; one needs to be standing in front of the patient only once when that happens to remember never to inject Narcan rapidly again. The dose of Narcan is titrated in the field according to the patient's *respirations*, not his state of consciousness; the goal of field treatment is to restore the patient's respirations to a normal rate and depth, NOT to waken the patient fully. The reason is a practical one. A heroin user may not be entirely appreciative of a paramedic who abolishes what was probably a rather expensive "fix." Unless you want a brawl in the back of the ambulance, it's better to let the victim of heroin overdose remain a little sleepy until you get to the hospital. Just keep titrating in your dilute solution, a few milliliters at a time, to the degree necessary to keep the patient breathing normally. Let him do his waking up in the emergency room.

FURTHER READING

Andress RA. Sudden death following naloxone administration. *Anesth Analg* 59:782, 1980.

Bradberry JC et al. Continuous infusion of naloxone in the treatment of narcotic overdose. *Drug Intell Clin Pharm* 15:945, 1981.

Cuss FM et al. Cardiac arrest after reversal of effects of opiates with naloxone. *Br Med J* 288:363, 1984.

Goldfrank LR. The several uses of naloxone. *Emerg Med* 16(10):105, 1984.

Handal KA, Schauben JL, Salamone FR. Naloxone. *Ann Emerg Med* 12:438, 1983.

Kunkel DB. Narcotic antagonist update. *Emerg Med* 19(5):97, 1987.

Levy DB. Naloxone: Negating narcotics. *Emergency* 22(7):16, 1990.

Levy DB. Naloxone: Use in shock. *Emergency* 22(8):14, 1990.

Lewis JM et al. Continuous naloxone infusion in pediatric narcotic overdose. *Am J Dis Child* 138:944, 1984.

Martin WR. Naloxone. *Ann Intern Med* 85:765, 1976.

McFeely EJ. Naloxone: A narcotic antagonist. *Emerg Med Serv* 14(10):70, 1985.

Moore RA et al. Naloxone: Underdosage after narcotic poisoning. *Am J Dis Child* 134:156, 1980.

Neal JM. Complications of naloxone. *Ann Emerg Med* 17:765, 1988.

Pallasch TJ, Gill CJ. Naloxone-associated morbidity and mortality. *Oral Surg* 52:602, 1981.

Prough DS et al. Acute pulmonary edema in healthy teenagers following conservative doses of intravenous naloxone. *Anesthesiology* 60:485, 1984.

Tandberg D, Abercrombie D. Treatment of heroin overdose with endotracheal naloxone. *Ann Emerg Med* 11:443, 1982.

Yealy DM et al. The safety of prehospital naloxone administration by paramedics. *Ann Emerg Med* 19:902, 1990.

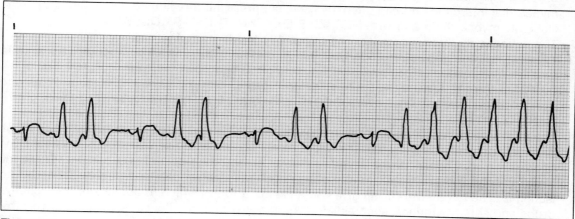

Figure 5

You have been called to a very elegant suburban home to attend a "man with chest pain." The patient is a 42-year-old executive, who complains of 1 hour of "heavy" retrosternal pain, which began while he was watching the stock market report on television. He also complains of weakness and dizziness and says that he "feels like I am going to die." On physical examination, he is pale, apprehensive, and diaphoretic. The pulse is difficult to palpate, but feels irregular, and respirations appear increased.

1. What is the FIRST thing you should do upon reaching this patient?

    a. Start an IV line with D5W.
    b. Apply monitoring electrodes.
    c. Administer oxygen.
    d. Take a detailed history and do a thorough physical examination.

2. Examine the patient's rhythm strip in Figure 5:

    a. The rhythm is _____ regular _____ irregular
    b. The rate is _____ per minute

3. The patient's rhythm is

    a. Sinus, with frequent PACs
    b. Sinus, with runs of ventricular tachycardia
    c. Supraventricular tachycardia
    d. Second-degree AV block
    e. Ventricular bigeminy

4. Which of the following would NOT be part of the treatment of this patient?

    a. Administer oxygen.
    b. Start an IV line with D5W.
    c. Administer lidocaine, 100 mg slowly IV followed by 2 to 3 mg per minute by infusion.
    d. Administer morphine, 5 to 10 mg by slow IV titration.
    e. Administer atropine 0.7 to 1.0 mg IV.

A65

1. The first action you should take upon reaching *any* middle-aged or older patient complaining of chest pain is to **administer oxygen** (answer **c**)—even before you complete your history and physical examination. Oxygen is the single most important drug in the treatment of acute myocardial infarction and can often, by itself, suppress life-threatening dysrhythmias. Do the ischemic myocardium a favor: FIRST GIVE OXYGEN, THEN ASK QUESTIONS.
2. The patient's rhythm is **irregular**. The rate is **130 to 140 per minute.**
3. The rhythm strip shows an underlying **sinus rhythm with runs of ventricular tachycardia** (answer **b**). If you look closely, you will find four sinus beats on the rhythm strip; the rest of the beats are almost certainly ventricular ectopic beats, with their wide QRS complexes and upside-down T waves. THIS IS A LIFE-THREATENING DYSRHYTHMIA AND DEMANDS URGENT TREATMENT.
4. The administration of atropine (answer **e**) would NOT be part of the treatment of this patient. His heart rate is already too rapid without atropine, and what we want to do is to calm the heart down, not speed it up. Oxygen (answer **a**), as noted above, is a critical part of the treatment of this dysrhythmia, for the dysrhythmia reflects myocardial irritability secondary to ischemia. The IV (answer **b**) will give you a lifeline through which to administer resuscitative drugs and antiarrhythmics, such as lidocaine (answer **c**). If the lidocaine fails to convert this patient's ventricular tachycardia, and if he begins to show signs of inadequate cardiac output (cold, clammy skin; hypotension; stupor or coma), cardioversion may be necessary.

    One could argue about giving this patient morphine (answer **d**) if he is already manifesting signs of hypotension (his dizziness and barely palpable pulse suggest that cardiac output is at least partially compromised). He does deserve analgesia, but perhaps nitrous oxide/oxygen would be a better choice than morphine if his ventricular tachycardia does not rapidly convert to sinus rhythm.

FURTHER READING

American Heart Association. Standards and guidelines for cardiopulmonary resuscitation (CPR) and emergency cardiac care (ECC). *JAMA* 255:2905, 1986.

Baerman JM et al. Differentiation of ventricular tachycardia from supraventricular tachycardia with aberration: Value of the clinical history. *Ann Emerg Med* 16:40, 1987.

Campbell RWF. Treatment and prophylaxis of ventricular arrhythmias in acute myocardial infarction. *Am J Cardiol* 52:55C, 1983.

Caroline NL. *Emergency Care in the Streets* (4th ed.). Boston: Little, Brown, 1991, Ch. 23.

DeSouza N et al. Evaluation of warning arrhythmias before paroxysmal ventricular tachycardia during acute myocardial infarction in man. *Circulation* 60:814, 1979.

Frank MJ. Restoring ventricular rhythm. *Emerg Med* 15(2):51, 1983.

Levitt MA. Supraventricular tachycardia with aberrant conduction versus ventricular tachycardia: Differentiation and diagnosis. *Am J Emerg Med* 6:273, 1988.

Morady F et al. Clinical symptoms in patients with sustained ventricular tachycardia. *West J Med* 142:341, 1985.

Northover BJ. Ventricular tachycardia during the first 72 hours after acute myocardial infarction. *Cardiology* 69:149, 1982.

Pennington JE, Taylor J, Lown B. Chest thump for reverting ventricular tachycardia. *New Engl J Med* 283:1192, 1970.

Sabetti K. Distinguishing between ectopic ventricular activity and aberrant ventricular conduction of supraventricular impulses. *Heart Lung* 8:949, 1979.

Tye K et al. R on T or R on P phenomenon? Relation to the genesis of ventricular tachycardia. *Am J Cardiol* 44:632, 1979.

A 50-year-old man sustained trauma to the chest in an automobile accident when he was thrown forward against the steering wheel. Your paramedic team finds him lying unconscious beside the car with an open chest wound. Arrange the following steps of management in their correct sequence:

a. Check for pulse; if absent, begin external cardiac compressions.
b. Close the open chest wound.
c. Establish an airway.
d. Control major bleeding.
e. Examine extremities for fractures.
f. Determine whether the patient is breathing; if not, start artificial ventilation.
g. Establish an IV line.

1. _____
2. _____
3. _____
4. _____
5. _____
6. _____
7. _____

A66

1. __c__ ESTABLISH AN AIRWAY.
2. __b__ CLOSE THE OPEN CHEST WOUND.
3. __f__ DETERMINE WHETHER THE PATIENT IS BREATHING; IF NOT, START ARTIFICIAL VENTILATION.
4. __a__ CHECK FOR PULSE; IF ABSENT, BEGIN EXTERNAL CARDIAC COMPRESSIONS.
5. __d__ CONTROL MAJOR BLEEDING.
6. __g__ ESTABLISH AN IV LINE.
7. __e__ EXAMINE EXTREMITIES FOR FRACTURES.

Yes, we're back to the old ABCs again. They are simply too important to ignore. The key to answering this question correctly is figuring out what constitutes part of A (airway management), what belongs in category B (breathing), and what is involved in category C (circulation).

A, the airway, comes first. On that we all agree. There might be some argument about where to place the open chest wound in this list: On the one hand, one could argue that an open chest wound interferes with efficient ventilation, so it should be part of B (breathing) and should come after the initiation of artifical ventilation. This is a reasonable argument, and if you put answer f ahead of answer b, you needn't mark it wrong. The reason for classifying an open chest wound under A (airway), however, is that—depending on the size of the hole in the chest—an open chest wound may in itself become an "airway" of sorts. That is to say, if the hole in the chest is larger than the space between the vocal cords, air will preferentially flow into the chest through the chest wound during inhalation rather than into the lungs through the larynx and trachea. In any case, the point to remember is that a hole in the chest wall can interfere with ventilation and must be sealed if effective breathing is to occur.

Now we come to C (circulation), and the first thing we must determine is whether there *is* any circulation at all, i.e., determine if there is a pulse, and if there is not, begin external cardiac compressions (answer a). Then, having established a circulation, we must make certain it is not in jeopardy from major hemorrhage, i.e., we must control any significant bleeding (answer d). And, still attending to the circulation, we must then take steps to ensure adequate circulatory volume by establishing an IV line (answer g), a measure that may have to be accomplished en route to the hospital.

Only when we have finished dealing with the ABCs may we turn our attention to other matters that are not life-threatening, such as examination for and stabilization of fractures (answer e). In the present case, which falls into the load-and-go category (by virtue of impaired consciousness and an open chest wound), the *whole patient* must be splinted rapidly to a backboard for expeditious removal to the hospital.

FURTHER READING

Caroline NL. *Emergency Care in the Streets* (4th ed.). Boston: Little, Brown, 1991, Ch. 20.
Caroline NL. *Emergency Medical Treatment: A Text for EMT-As and EMT-Intermediates* (3rd ed.). Boston: Little, Brown, 1991, Chs. 15, 18.

You are dispatched at 3:00 A.M. to a call for a "man who can't breathe," and you arrive at a somewhat run-down house, where a distraught woman is waiting for you in the front yard. As she hurries you into the house, she tells you that her 58-year-old husband has for many years suffered from "lung problems," but over the past days he has "gotten much worse." He has always been a heavy smoker—three to four packs per day—and has a chronic cough, but since last week, when he caught a cold, he has been much sicker. He is coughing more, his sputum has turned green and become much more copious, and during the past two nights he has had to sit up all night in order to breathe. Even his usual medicine—Tedrol pills and some kind of suppository—haven't seemed to help.

You find the husband sitting bolt upright in a kitchen chair. He is an obese man, distinctly cyanotic, and laboring to breathe. He appears agitated and confused. His pulse is 120 per minute and slightly irregular, his respirations are 32 per minute and shallow, and his blood pressure is 100/62. You notice that there are retractions in his supraclavicular and intercostal muscles during respiration. His neck veins are distended. There are coarse rales in both lung fields, and there are diffuse wheezes, more pronounced during exhalation. His abdomen is soft and nontender. There is 2+ pitting edema of both feet.

What is the most important aspect of the immediate treatment of this patient?

a. He should rebreathe into a paper bag in order to control his hyperventilation.
b. He should not be given oxygen because he has chronic obstructive pulmonary disease, and oxygen may cause apnea.
c. He should be given oxygen in whatever concentration is necessary and monitored closely.
d. You should open all the windows in order to give him some fresh air.

A67

Ah hah! You probably answered b. You remembered hearing somewhere that many patients with chronic obstructive pulmonary disease (COPD) breathe on a hypoxic drive, and you didn't want to give the patient oxygen lest you depress his respirations.

Very clever.

The only problem is that now, 10 minutes later, your patient is dead. Why? Because he NEEDED OXYGEN. Probably a lot of oxygen. That's what he was trying to tell you by turning blue and behaving confused.

The correct answer is **c: Give him oxygen in whatever concentration is necessary and monitor him carefully.**

Let's review the situation.

First of all, this patient suffers from COPD. How do we know? From the history, we have learned that he smokes heavily, has a chronic cough, and takes bronchodilator medications—all highly suggestive. And the physical examination reveals a typical "blue bloater": fat, cyanotic, full of rales and wheezes, showing signs of right heart failure (distended neck veins, pedal edema). Furthermore, we know that he is in a stage of *acute* decompensation. His wife told us that he's been getting worse, that he had a recent respiratory infection, and that his sputum changed in color and volume. And we can observe that this patient is in acute respiratory distress: He is struggling to breathe, using accessory muscles of respiration; he is tachypneic; and it's a safe bet that he's severely hypoxemic—not only because he's blue, but also because his brain does not seem to be getting the oxygen it needs in order to think straight. In short, we have a patient with COPD who is now in acute respiratory failure, desperately ill from hypoxemia.

What is the treatment for hypoxemia?

OXYGEN!

Now, let us return to the issue of the hypoxic drive, for it is frequently a source of confusion. The breathing of normal individuals, as we know, is regulated by fluctuations in the level of carbon dioxide in the blood (PCO_2). When the PCO_2 rises, the breathing centers in the brain are stimulated, and they in turn activate the respiratory muscles to increase their activity. So respiratory rate and depth increase until the excess CO_2 is blown off. But many patients with COPD tend to retain CO_2 because they are no longer able to blow off excess CO_2 efficiently. Eventually those patients become acclimated to high CO_2 levels in their blood. When that happens, their principal stimulus to breathe may be a drop in the level of *oxygen* in the blood (PO_2). So theoretically if you give such a patient oxygen, and thereby raise the arterial PO_2, he may lose his stimulus to breathe and stop breathing altogether.

That was the conventional wisdom for many years. The evidence does not support that view, however; studies performed to date have failed to show any suppression by oxygen of the respiratory drive in a patient with COPD. But even if it *were* the case that patients with COPD operate on an hypoxic drive, would that be a reason to withhold oxygen from a patient in acute respiratory failure?

NEVER!

If you are worried about suppressing a patient's hypoxic drive, then when you do administer oxygen to a patient with COPD, watch him closely for signs of respiratory depression. If he stops breathing, breathe for him. That's what your bag-valve-mask (with oxygen reservoir) is there for.

Moral: DON'T BE STINGY WITH OXYGEN, AND DON'T TAKE YOUR EYES OFF THE PATIENT TO WHOM YOU ADMINISTER IT.

Before we go on our next call, let's take a quick look at the other, incorrect answers:

Answer a: He should rebreathe into a paper bag in order to control his hyperventilation.

Nothing could be worse for this patient. He already has an excess of CO_2 in his blood, and rebreathing his own exhaled air will simply add to that excess. And, by the way, he is NOT hyperventilating. True, he is breathing rapidly. But the term *hyperventilation* implies that someone is overbreathing to the extent that the PCO_2 has been lowered below normal levels, which is certainly not the case with our chronic CO_2 retainer. He is breathing rapidly because he is starved for oxygen, and he isn't going to find the oxygen he needs in a paper bag.

Answer d: You should open all the windows in order to give him some fresh air.

We all need fresh air, but it won't help our patient very much. Fresh air, like "room air," has an oxygen concentration of 21%, and our patient needs a considerably higher concentration of oxygen in his inhaled air than that. Opening the windows won't help, but opening the valve on the O_2 tank could help a great deal.

FURTHER READING

Aubier M et al. Central respiratory drive in acute respiratory failure of patients with chronic obstructive pulmonary disease. *Am Rev Respir Dis* 122:191, 1980.

Aubier M et al. Effects of the administration of O_2 on ventilation and blood gases in patients with chronic obstructive pulmonary disease during acute respiratory failure. *Am Rev Respir Dis* 122:747, 1980.

Baigelman W. Exacerbation of chronic obstructive pulmonary disease. *Emerg Med* 19(9):79, 1987.

Bates D. Chronic bronchitis and emphysema. *N Engl J Med* 278:546, 1968.

Campbell EJM. Management of acute respiratory failure in chronic bronchitis and emphysema. *Am Rev Respir Dis* 96:626, 1967.

Centers for Disease Control. State-specific smoking-attributable chronic obstructive pulmonary disease mortality—United States, 1986. *MMWR* 38:552, 1989.

COPD: Gasping for breath. *Emerg Med* 19(3):86, 1987.

Ersoz CJ. Prehospital support of the patient with chronic lung disease. *Emerg Med Serv* 8(3):63, 1979.

Farber SM, Wilson RHL. Chronic obstructive emphysema. *Clin Symp* 1968.

Hunt D. Common respiratory emergencies. *Emerg Med Serv* 19(1):19, 1990.

Palevsky HI, Fishman AP. Chronic cor pulmonale. *JAMA* 263:2347, 1990.

Rice KL et al. Aminophylline for acute exacerbations of chronic obstructive pulmonary disease. *Ann Intern Med* 107:305, 1987.

Sassoon, CSH, Hassell KT, Mahutte CK. Hyperoxic-induced hypercapnia in stable chronic obstructive pulmonary disease. *Am Rev Respir Dis* 135:907, 1987.

Schmidt GA, Hall JB. Acute on chronic respiratory failure. *JAMA* 261:3444, 1989.

Seidenfeld JJ et al. Intravenous aminophylline in the treatment of acute bronchospastic exacerbations of chronic obstructive pulmonary disease. *Ann Emerg Med* 13:248, 1984.

Selinger SR et al. Effects of removing oxygen from patients with chronic obstructive pulmonary disease. *Am Rev Respir Dis* 136:85, 1987.

A 67-year-old woman was crossing the street in front of the supermarket when she was struck by a speeding car. You find her lying on her back, amidst a pile of spilled groceries, conscious and moaning. During the neurologic examination, you discover that she has no sensation to pinprick from the toes up to the nipples.

1. At what spinal level has her injury probably occurred?

   a. C3
   b. C7
   c. T4
   d. T10
   e. L4

2. An injury of this sort, because of the area of the spinal cord involved, may compromise the function of part of the autonomic nervous system. As a consequence, one might expect to see

   a. Tachycardia, due to stimulation of the parasympathetic nervous system
   b. Elevation of blood pressure, due to vasoconstriction
   c. Fall in blood pressure, due to vasodilation
   d. Rise in body temperature, due to the body's inability to dissipate heat

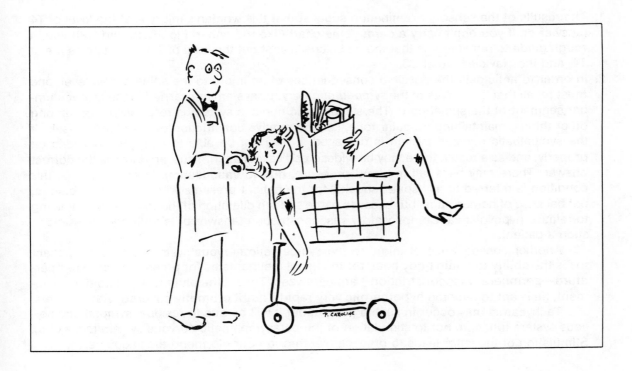

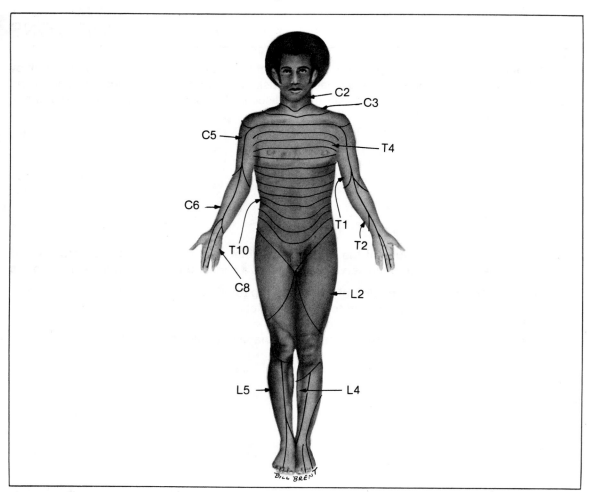

Figure 6. Distribution of spinal nerves.

1. The results of the sensory examination suggest that this woman's injury is at the level of **T4** (answer **c**). If you don't carry a dermatome chart (like the one in Fig. 6) around with you, a rough guide to remember is that the umbilicus is at about the level of T10, the nipples are at T4, and the clavicles are at C3.

2. In order to anticipate the possible consequences of an injury to the spine at this level, one must recall that the nerves of the *sympathetic* nervous system are carried in the thoracolumbar segment of the spinal cord. The sympathetic nervous system is responsible for, among other things, maintaining vascular tone, i.e., the relative constriction of the blood vessels. If the sympathetic nervous system is damaged, it may not be able to carry out that function properly, and as a result, there may be widespread vasodilation. Thus, answer **c** is the correct answer: There may be a **fall in blood pressure, due to vasodilation.** In severe cases, this condition is referred to as "spinal shock," for the patient presents with a shocklike picture, not because of hemorrhage, but because of the sudden dilatation of the vascular bed, leading to relative hypovolemia. Compensatory vasoconstriction (answer b) is no longer possible in such a patient.

   Another consequence of injury to the sympathetic nervous system is that the patient loses the ability to retain body heat, for the usual mechanisms for preserving core temperature—peripheral vasoconstriction—are paralyzed. Thus if the patient is in a cold environment, he is apt to become hypothermic very rapidly if not promptly covered with blankets.

   Tachycardia may occur in such a patient, but it will be due to residual sympathetic nervous system function, not to stimulation of the parasympathetic nervous system (answer a). Stimulation of the latter leads to bradycardia, through our old friend the vagus nerve.

FURTHER READING

Albin MS. Resuscitation of the spinal cord. *Crit Care Med* 6:270, 1978.

Anderson DK et al. Spinal cord injury and protection. *Ann Emerg Med* 14:816, 1985.

Aprahamian CA et al. Experimental cervical spine injury model: Evaluation of airway management and splinting techniques. *Ann Emerg Med* 13:584, 1984.

Aprahamian C, Thompson BM, Darin J. Recommended helmet removal techniques in a cervical spine injured patient. *J Trauma* 24:841, 1984.

Barber JM. EMT checkpoint: Spinal cord injury and neurogenic shock. *EMT J* 2(3):69, 1978.

Bayless P, Ray VG. Incidence of cervical spine injuries in association with blunt head trauma. *Am J Emerg Med* 7:139, 1989.

Bivins HG et al. The effect of axial traction during orotracheal intubation of the trauma victim with an unstable cervical spine. *Ann Emerg Med* 17:25, 1988.

Bourn S. Tell the spinal fanatics to "back off." *JEMS* 15(5):73, 1990.

Bracken MB et al. A randomized, controlled trial of methylprednisolone or naloxone in the treatment of acute spinal-cord injury. *N Engl J Med* 322:1405, 1990.

Caroline NL. *Emergency Care in the Streets* (4th ed.). Boston: Little, Brown, 1991, Ch. 16.

Caroline NL. *Emergency Medical Treatment: A Text for EMT-As and EMT-Intermediates* (3rd ed.). Boston: Little, Brown, 1991, Ch. 14.

Cline JR et al. A comparison of methods of cervical immobilization used in patient extrication and transport. *Trauma* 25:649, 1985.

Davidson JSD, Birdsell DC. Cervical spine injury in patients with facial skeletal trauma. *J Trauma* 29:1276, 1989.

Dula DJ. Trauma to the cervical spine. *JACEP* 8:504, 1979.

Grundy D et al. ABC of spinal cord injury: Early management and complications. *Br Med J* I.292:44, 1986. II.292:123, 1986.

Guthkelch AN et al. Patterns of cervical spine injury and their associated lesions. *West J Med* 147:428, 1987.

Holley J, Jorden R. Airway management in patients with unstable cervical spine fractures. *Ann Emerg Med* 18:1237, 1989.

In diving injuries . . . *Emerg Med* 14(13):139, 1982.

Jackson DW et al. Cervical spine injuries. *Clin Sports Med* 5:373, 1986.

Little NE. In case of a broken neck. *Emerg Med* 21(9):22, 1989.

O'Malley KF, Ross SE. The incidence of injury to the cervical spine in patients with craniocerebral injury. *J Trauma* 28:1476, 1988.

Reiss SJ et al. Cervical spine fractures with major associated trauma. *Neurosurgery* 18:327, 1986.

Rimel R et al. Prehospital treatment of the patient with spinal cord injuries. *EMT J* 3(4):49, 1979.

Walter J, Doris PE, Shaffer MA. Clinical presentation of patients with acute cervical spine injury. *Ann Emerg Med* 13:512, 1984.

Wolf AL. Initial management of brain- and spinal-cord injured patients. *Emerg Med Serv* 18(6):35, 1989.

You are called to see a 3-year-old child in moderate respiratory distress. His mother says that he appeared to be reasonably well during the day, but for the past two nights he has been waking up around midnight with a most alarming, high-pitched cough that sounds almost like a dog barking.

You find the child lying down in bed, looking very tired and miserable. Axillary temperature is 99.6°F (37.6°C). Respirations are stridorous, at 30 per minute, with slight retraction of the neck muscles. No wheezes or rales are heard, although it is difficult to auscultate the chest with all the barking noises going on.

Which of the following is NOT part of the field management of this patient?

a. Administer humidified oxygen.
b. Do direct laryngoscopy to make sure the airway is not obstructed by a foreign body.
c. Administer racemic epinephrine by nebulizer.
d. Transport the patient to the hospital in a supine position.

A69 Direct laryngoscopy (answer **b**) is NOT part of the field management of this patient. While the child is showing fairly classic signs of acute subglottic obstructive laryngitis (croup), there is nonetheless a small chance that the child is suffering from epiglottitis. If the latter is indeed the case, insertion of a laryngoscope or any other object into the oropharynx may be very dangerous, for it can lead to precipitous closure of the airway. There is no need whatsoever to insert a laryngoscope or any other instrument into the mouth of this child, and to do so is simply to take an unnecessary risk.

Oxygen should be administered to this child to combat hypoxemia, and it must be given in the humidified form (answer a). Dry gases will only aggravate the problem by drying out the patient's mucous membranes. The administration of racemic epinephrine (answer c) is still somewhat controversial, but many pediatricians feel it is worth a try in croup as a means of reducing the subglottic swelling that has narrowed the airway.

In general, patients in respiratory distress favor an upright position and should be so transported. In croup, however, the child often prefers to lie down, as our patient is doing, and if so, he should be transported supine (answer d).

FURTHER READING

Caroline NL. *Emergency Care in the Streets* (4th ed.). Boston: Little, Brown, 1991, Ch. 30.
Denny FW et al. Croup: An 11-year study in a pediatric practice. *Pediatrics* 71:871, 1983.
Dierking BH. Respiratory distress! *Emergency* 21(1):27, 1989.
Mauro RD et al. Differentiation of epiglottitis from laryngotracheitis in the child with stridor. *Am J Dis Child* 142:679, 1988.
Mitchell DP et al. Secondary airway support in the management of croup. *J Otolaryngol* 9:419, 1980.
Newth CJL, Levison H, Bryan AC. The respiratory status of children with croup. *J Pediatr* 81:1068, 1972.
Tintinalli J. Respiratory stridor in the young child. *JACEP* 5:195, 1976.
Zillger JJ et al. Assessment of intubation in croup and epiglottitis. *Ann Otol Rhinol Laryngol* 91:403, 1982.

Match the following types of splints with the injury for which each is most appropriately used.

a. Pillow splint
b. Air splint
c. Sling and swath
d. MAST garment
e. Backboard
f. Traction splint

1. _____ A 15-year-old halfback for the local high school football team caught his cleat in the turf as he was tackled; his right ankle is now severely swollen and tender to palpation.
2. _____ An 18-year-old swimmer dove into a shallow pool and struck his head on the bottom. Friends pulled him from the pool, and now he is lying by the side of the pool moaning and complaining of pain in his neck.
3. _____ A 34-year-old woman was struck by a car. She is lying in the road moaning. There is tenderness and instability noted on palpation of her pelvis.
4. _____ A 30-year-old man fell down several stairs. He is conscious and alert, and there is no deformity of his extremities. He complains, however, of some pain on motion of his right arm, and there is tenderness over the right clavicle.
5. _____ A 12-year-old boy slipped on a banana peel and fell onto his outstretched left hand. There is pain, deformity, and tenderness over the left forearm.
6. _____ A 16-year-old boy was struck by a car. There is marked deformity of his right thigh and tenderness to palpation over the midfemoral area on the right side.

A70

		Case	*Splint*
1.	a	Ankle sprain or fracture	Pillow splint (air splint, answer b, also OK)
2.	e	Diving injury	Backboard
3.	d	Pelvic fracture	MAST
4.	c	Clavicular fracture	Sling and swath
5.	b	Radial or Colles' fracture	Air splint
6.	f	Femoral shaft fracture	Traction splint

You get extra points if you wanted to immobilize patients 3, 4, and 6 on a backboard as well as splinting their obvious injuries. All of them sustained injuries under circumstances that might have resulted in damage to the spine, and no one would fault you for being extra cautious and using the backboard in these cases.

FURTHER READING

Anast GT. Fractures and splinting. *Emergency* 10(11):42, 1978.

Burtzloff HE. Splinting closed fractures of the extremities. *Emerg Med Serv* 10(3):70, 1981.

Canan S. Grasping objectives of long-bone splinting. *Rescue* 2(5):45, 1989.

Caroline NL. *Emergency Care in the Streets* (4th ed.). Boston: Little, Brown, 1991, Ch. 19.

Caroline NL. *Emergency Medical Treatment: A Text for EMT-As and EMT-Intermediates* (3rd ed.). Boston: Little, Brown, 1991, Ch. 17.

Connolly JF. Fracture pitfalls:
  The ankle. *Emerg Med* 16(7):49, 1984.
  The elbow. *Emerg Med* 15(11):163, 1983.
  The femur. *Emerg Med* 15(21):51, 1983.
  The forearm. *Emerg Med* 15(13):235, 1983.
  General principles. *Emerg Med* 14(17):161, 1982.
  The knee: Bone and soft tissue. *Emerg Med* 16(1):205, 1984.
  The humerus. *Emerg Med* 15(9):170, 1983.
  Metacarpals and phalanges. *Emerg Med* 15(15):201, 1983.
  Pathologic fractures. *Emerg Med* 16(11):61, 1984.
  Tibial fractures. *Emerg Med* 16(5):43, 1984.
  The wrist. *Emerg Med* 15(14):195, 1983.

Cote DJ et al. Comparison of three treatment procedures for minimizing ankle sprain swelling. *Phys Ther* 68:1072, 1988.

Evers BM, Cryer HM, Miller FB. Pelvic fracture hemorrhage: Priorities in management. *Arch Surg* 124:422, 1989.

Gustafson JE. Contraindications to the repositioning of fractured or dislocated limbs in the field. *JACEP* 5:184, 1976.

Haverson G, Iverson KV. Comparison of four ankle splint designs. *Ann Emerg Med* 16:1249, 1987.

Hedges JR, Anwar RAH. Management of ankle sprains. *Ann Emerg Med* 9:298, 1980.

Kay DB. The sprained ankle: Current therapy. *Foot Ankle* 6:22, 1985.

Lhowe D. Basics of broken bones for the nonorthopedist: 2. Primary care for nondisplaced fractures. *Emerg Med* 19(16):89, 1987.

Menkes JS. Pitfalls in orthopedic trauma:
  Part I. The upper extremity. *Emerg Med* 21(5):64, 1989.
  Part II. The lower extremity. *Emerg Med* 21(6):108, 1989.

Rayburn BK. Prehospital care of fractures and dislocations of the extremities. *EMT J* 4(2):61, 1980.

Tomford W. Basics of broken bones for the nonorthopedist: I. The fundamental principles. *Emerg Med* 19(15):25, 1987.

Thygerson AL. Finger injuries. *Emergency* 13(4):28, 13(5):82, 1981.

Thygerson AL. The sprained ankle. *Emergency* 13(2):20, 1981.

Wald DA, Ziemba TJ, Ferko JG. Upper extremity injuries. *Emergency* 21(3):25, 1989.

Winspur I, Phelps DB. Emergency care of the injured hand. Part XI: Hand dressings, splints, and casts. *Emerg Med Serv* 9(1):22, 1980.

It is 2:30 A.M. on a hot and humid summer night when a call comes in for a "woman who can't breathe." You reach the scene in about 10 minutes, a shabby row of tenements, and a neighbor hurries you to the patient's apartment. There you find a woman who appears to be in her early 20s, clad in a nightgown, and sitting bolt upright on the sofa, struggling to breathe. She is barely able to answer "yes" or "no" to your questions. On examination, you find her alert, clearly frightened, and in extreme respiratory distress. Her pulse is 120 and regular, respirations are 30 and shallow, and blood pressure is 150/80. Neck veins are not distended, and there is no tracheal deviation. The chest is somewhat hyperresonant to percussion bilaterally, and there are tight, barely audible wheezes heard in all lung fields on exhalation. There is no peripheral edema. Meanwhile, your partner returns from his reconnaissance of the medicine cabinet with a bottle of Quibron and some prednisone tablets. You conclude that this patient is probably suffering from

a. Acute pulmonary edema from left heart failure
b. Pulmonary embolism
c. Acute asthmatic attack
d. Spontaneous pneumothorax
e. A foreign body obstructing one of the bronchi

Which of the following is NOT part of the treatment of this patient?

a. Oxygen
b. Morphine
c. Intravenous fluids
d. Epinephrine

A71

This young woman is most probably suffering from an **acute asthmatic attack** (answer **c**), and a very serious one at that. The fact that she is young makes acute pulmonary edema from left heart failure (answer a) an unlikely, although possible, source of her symptoms. Pulmonary embolism (answer b) does not usually present with diffuse wheezing (there may be localized wheezing in the area of the embolism), and hyperresonance of the chest would be distinctly unusual in such a condition. Similarly, the wheezing that accompanies obstruction of a bronchus by a foreign body (answer e) is usually localized to the area of the obstruction and not heard diffusely throughout all lung fields. There is also no evidence here for pneumothorax (answer d), for breath sounds are audible throughout the chest and no difference in resonance between the left and right sides of the chest was noted on percussion. Finally, the medications culled from the medicine cabinet suggest that the patient is under treatment for asthma, for she is apparently taking Quibron (a bronchodilator) and prednisone (a steroid), both of which are often prescribed for asthmatics (the prednisone suggests that the patient suffers from a rather severe variety of asthma).

Morphine is NOT part of the treatment of a patient with an acute asthmatic attack (answer **b**), definitely and emphatically not. As an asthmatic attack progresses, the patient becomes less and less able to move an adequate tidal volume of air in and out of the lungs, and as a consequence, there is an increasing tendency toward carbon dioxide retention. As the arterial PCO_2 rises, the patient gets sleepier and sleepier because carbon dioxide is a very potent narcotic. The last thing such a patient needs is another potent narcotic—and one that depresses respirations to boot! NEVER GIVE SEDATIVES TO A PATIENT SUFFERING AN ACUTE ASTHMATIC ATTACK. If the patient is agitated, it is probably because of hypoxemia, the treatment for which is oxygen (answer a)—and for the asthmatic, make that humidified oxygen, please. Dehydration may be a significant factor in the established asthmatic attack and may lead to drying of secretions, which then form hard mucus plugs obstructing the smaller airways. For that reason, it is worthwhile to be generous with intravenous fluids (answer c) in an attempt to combat dehydration and its untoward effects on the asthmatic cycle. Finally, epinephrine (answer d) is one of the mainstays of therapy in the acute asthmatic attack, for its beta adrenergic effects promote bronchodilation. Epinephrine is given in the form of a 1:1,000 aqueous solution, 0.3 to 0.5 ml subcutaneously. The dose may be repeated after about 15 minutes.

FURTHER READING

Aberman A. Managing asthmatics. *Emerg Med* 18(8):26, 1986.
Appel D et al. Comparative effect of epinephrine and aminophylline in the treatment of asthma. *Lung* 159:243, 1981.
Bailskus M, Niersbach C. Matters of life and breath. *Emergency* 21(4):12, 1989.
Benatar SR. Fatal asthma. *N Engl J Med* 314:423, 1986.
Ben-Zvi Z et al. An evaluation of repeated injections of epinephrine for the initial treatment of acute asthma. *Am Rev Respir Dis* 127:101, 1983.
Brenner BE. Bronchial asthma in adults: Presentation to the emergency department. I. Pathogenesis, clinical manifestations, diagnostic evaluation, and differential diagnosis. *Am J Emerg Med* 1:50, 1983.
Carden DL et al. Vital signs including pulsus paradoxus in the assessment of acute bronchial asthma. *Ann Emerg Med* 12:80, 1983.
Cydulka R et al. The use of epinephrine in the treatment of older adult asthmatics. *Ann Emerg Med* 17:322, 1988.
Dailey RD. Asthmatic: Acute and adult. *Emerg Med* 8(4):127, 1973.
Emerman CL et al. Ventricular arrhythmias during treatment for acute asthma. *Ann Emerg Med* 15:699, 1986.
Franklin WF. Treatment of severe asthma. *N Engl J Med* 290:1469, 1974.
Grandstetter RD et al. Optimal dosing of epinephrine in acute asthma. *Am J Hosp Pharm* 37:1326, 1980.
Groth ML, Hurewitz AM. Pharmacologic management of acute asthma. *Emerg Med* 21(7):23, 1989.
Johnson AJ. Circumstances of death from asthma. *Br Med J* 288:1870, 1984.
Josephson GW et al. Cardiac dysrhythmias during the treatment of acute asthma. *Chest* 78:429, 1980.
Karetzky MS. Acute asthma: The use of subcutaneous epinephrine in therapy. *Ann Allergy* 44:12, 1980.
Kavuru MS, Ahmad M. Ambulatory management of acute asthma. *Emerg Med* 20(21):111, 1988.
Kelly HW et al. Should we stop using theophylline for the treatment of the hospitalized patient with status asthmaticus? *Ann Pharmacother* 23:995, 1989.
Littenberg B. Aminophylline treatment in severe, acute asthma. *JAMA* 259:1678, 1988.
Pliss LB et al. Aerosol vs. injected epinephrine in acute asthma. *Ann Emerg Med* 10:353, 1981.
Rothstein RJ. Intravenous theophylline therapy in asthma: A clinical update. *Ann Emerg Med* 9:327, 1980.
Schneider SM et al. High-dose methylprednisolone as initial therapy in patients with acute bronchospasm. *Asthma* 25:189, 1988.
Stadnyk AM, Grossman RF. Management of life-threatening asthma. *Emerg Med* 19(15):103, 1987.
Stewart MF et al. Risk of giving intravenous aminophylline to acutely ill patients receiving maintenance treatment with theophylline. *Br Med J* 288:450, 1984.

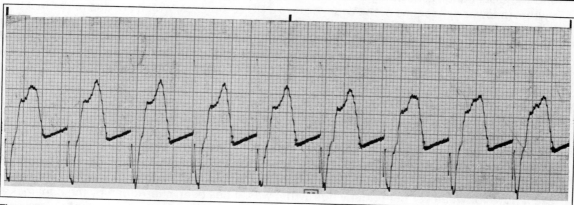

Figure 7

You are called to a downtown beauty parlor to attend to a "dizzy woman." The patient turns out to be one of the beauticians, a woman about 50, who tells you that while she was giving a permanent to one of her regular customers, she suddenly began feeling very dizzy and had to sit down. She says she is feeling better now. You take her vital signs and apply limb leads to obtain a rhythm strip.

1. Examine the rhythm strip in Figure 7:

    a. The rhythm is _____ regular _____ irregular.
    b. The rate is _____ per minute.

2. The ECG pattern is

    a. Normal sinus rhythm
    b. Junctional rhythm
    c. Pacemaker rhythm
    d. Idioventricular rhythm
    e. Second-degree AV block

3. From this rhythm strip one can conclude that

    a. The woman's dizziness was due to failure of the pacemaker to capture.
    b. The woman's dizziness was due to complete heart block.
    c. The woman had a run of supraventricular tachycardia, which remitted spontaneously prior to your arrival.
    d. The woman had been using microwave equipment.
    e. There is insufficient data to account for this woman's dizziness.

A72

1. The patient's rhythm is **regular;** the rate is approximately **90 per minute.**

2. Did you notice those little blips just before each QRS complex? Those are pacemaker spikes, and the ECG pattern shows a **pacemaker rhythm** (answer **c**). It resembles an idioventricular rhythm (answer d) because of the wide, bizarre QRS complexes, which are due to the fact that the pacemaker wire sits in the ventricle; thus the complexes that the pacemaker produces are ventricular complexes, just as if there were an ectopic focus in the ventricles. Had you placed the monitoring leads on the patient's chest instead of on her extremities, you would have noticed the bulge where the pacemaker battery was implanted beneath the skin, and it would have given the whole situation away!

3. The rhythm strip does not provide us with sufficient data to account for this patient's dizzy spell (answer **e**). We might suspect that there is something not quite right about her pacemaker, since it is firing at a rather rapid rate (most implanted pacemakers are set to fire at a rate of about 70 per minute), but certainly there is no evidence on this strip of failure of the pacemaker to capture (answer a), for each pacemaker spike is immediately followed by a QRS complex. If the patient did indeed have complete heart block in the past (answer b), we do not see it now, for whatever her underlying rhythm was, it has been overridden by the pacemaker rhythm. It is entirely possible that the patient had a run of supraventricular tachycardia prior to your arrival (answer c), but unless it recurs while she is being monitored, there is no way to prove this assumption one way or the other. As to the microwave equipment (answer d), it is true that some of the early microwave ovens that were not adequately shielded were reported to interfere with pacemaker function. Indeed, there was more than one case described of a patient keeling over while waiting for his vending machine sandwich to heat up in the microwave oven of the hospital snack bar. However, microwave technology has not yet—at least in this author's knowledge—extended to the realm of hair dryers and similar beauty parlor apparatus, so it seems unlikely that our patient had a microwave misadventure.

   In any case, with the cause of her dizziness unresolved, our beautician will certainly have to be evaluated in the hospital, where the function of her pacemaker can be thoroughly checked. An increased *or* decreased rate of firing by an implanted pacemaker may indicate a faulty pacemaker or imminent pacemaker failure.

FURTHER READING

Campo A et al. Runaway pacemaker. *Ann Emerg Med* 12:32, 1983.
Lown BL, Kosowsky B. Artificial cardiac pacemakers. *N Engl J Med* 283:907 (Part I); 971 (Part II); 1023 (Part III), 1970.
Mansour KA. Complications of cardiac pacemakers. *Ann Surg* 43:131, 1977.
Solow E, Bacharach B, Cheeng E. Runaway pacemaker. Unpredictable pacemaker failure. *Arch Intern Med* 139:1190, 1979.
Tegtmeyer CJ. Complications of cardiac pacemakers. *Am Fam Phys* 14:66, 1976.

It's a three-alarm fire in a ranch house about 10 minutes from your station. As you arrive, firemen are carrying the victims outside. The fire apparently started in the baby's room, which was tightly closed at the time. The firemen also entered the master bedroom, where they found the father unconscious in his bed and the mother leaning out the window screaming for help. In another smoky room, two other children were found fully conscious: Danny, a 10-year-old asthmatic, and his 9-year-old sister, Debby, who is not known to have any medical problems.

1. Which of these family members will be most likely to suffer significant complications from smoke inhalation? (There may be more than one correct answer.)

    a. Father
    b. Mother
    c. Baby
    d. Danny
    e. Debby

2. In examining baby, you find that he has second-degree burns about his face, and his eyelashes are singed. What urgent, life-threatening complication should you anticipate?

    a. Periorbital edema
    b. Laryngeal edema
    c. Swelling of the lips
    d. Vomiting
    e. Coughing up blood

A73

1. **Father (a), baby (c),** and **Danny (d)** are most likely to develop respiratory complications from smoke inhalation. Father was unconscious during (and perhaps as a consequence of) his exposure to smoke. Baby was in a closed space full of smoke. And Danny has a history of underlying respiratory disease. All of those situations increase the risk of suffering significant respiratory problems from smoke inhalation. Mother and Debby aren't entirely risk-free, but their prospects are considerably better, for mother had her head out the window and Debby, although exposed to more smoke, at least has no history of respiratory problems.

2. Any patient who has sustained burns to the face must be regarded as being at risk of having sustained burns to the upper airway as well, and baby is no exception. The most urgent, life-threatening complication that may arise in this situation is **laryngeal edema** (answer **b**), which can develop very quickly, closing off the upper airway within minutes. Rapid intubation by a highly skilled rescuer may forestall the need for cricothyrotomy in such a case, but intubation of an awake patient of any age is difficult, and intubation of the burned respiratory tract is not without risk. Thus whenever possible, swift transport to the hospital should be accomplished to enable definitive airway care in a safe environment.

FURTHER READING

Bascomb R, Kennedy T. Toxic gas inhalation. *Emerg Med Serv* 13(7):17, 1984.
Birky MM, Clark FB. Inhalation of toxic products from fires. *Bull NY Acad Med* 57:997, 1981.
Caroline NL. *Emergency Care in the Streets* (4th ed.). Boston: Little, Brown, 1991, Chs. 15, 22.
Cohen MA, Guzzardi LJ. Inhalation of products of combustion. *Ann Emerg Med* 12:628, 1983.
Dimick A, Wagner RG. A matter of burns and breath. *Emerg Med* 22(13):123, 1990.
DiVincenti FC, Pruitt BA Jr., Reckler JM. Inhalation injuries. *J Trauma* 11:109, 1971.
Fein A. Toxic gas inhalation. *Emerg Med* 21(7):53, 1989.
Fein A, Leff A, Hopewell PC. Pathophysiology and management of the complications resulting from fire and the inhaled products of combustion. *Crit Care Med* 8:94, 1980.
Hedges JR. Acute noxious gas exposure. *Curr Top Emerg Med* 2(10), 1978.
Heimbach DM, Waeckerle JF. Inhalation injuries. *Ann Emerg Med* 17:1316, 1988.
Injury through inspiration. *Emerg Med* 17(19):20, 1985.
Jelenko C, McKinley JC. Postburn respiratory injury. *JACEP* 5:455, 1976.
Moylan JA, Chan CK. Inhalation injury: An increasing problem. *Ann Surg* 188:24, 1978.
Robinson NB et al. Steroid therapy following isolated smoke inhalation. *J Trauma* 22:876, 1982.
Trunkey DD. Inhalation injury. *Surg Clin North Am* 8:1133, 1978.
Venus B et al. Prophylactic intubation and continuous positive airway pressure in the management of inhalation injury in burn victims. *Crit Care Med* 9:519, 1981.
Webster JR, McCabe MM, Carp M. Recognition and management of smoke inhalation. *JAMA* 201:287, 1967.
Wroblewski DA, Bower GC. The significance of facial burns in acute smoke inhalation. *Crit Care Med* 7:335, 1979.

Indicate which of the following statements about near drowning are true and which are false.

a. One of the *first* things that happens to a conscious person when he is accidentally submerged in water is the aspiration of large quantities of water into his lungs.

   TRUE   FALSE

b. When fresh water is aspirated into the lungs, it is rapidly absorbed from the lungs into the bloodstream.

   TRUE   FALSE

c. Mouth-to-mouth ventilation should be initiated immediately on the nonbreathing near-drowning victim, even before he has been removed from the water.

   TRUE   FALSE

d. A victim of near drowning is likely to have large quantities of water in his stomach and therefore is in danger of aspiration of stomach contents during resuscitation.

   TRUE   FALSE

e. Near-drowning victims tend to develop extreme metabolic acidosis.

   TRUE   FALSE

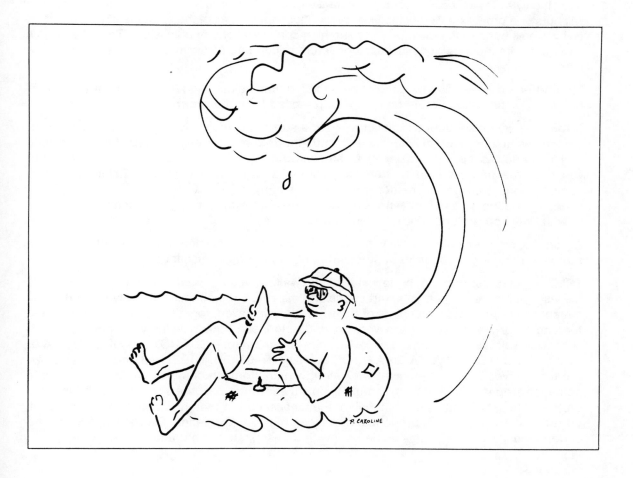

A74

a. One of the *first* things that happens to a conscious person when he is accidentally submerged in water is the aspiration of large quantities of water into his lungs.

FALSE. The aspiration of water into the lungs is a relatively *late* occurrence in the drowning process. When a person is first submerged in water, the aspiration of a very small quantity of water causes violent laryngospasm, which effectively shuts off the lower airway from further aspiration. It is only after several minutes, when the victim becomes stuporous or comatose from hypoxemia, that his laryngeal muscles relax, permitting aspiration of large quantities of water. Thus near-drowning victims who are snatched quickly from the water are likely to have dry lungs.

b. When fresh water is aspirated into the lungs, it is rapidly absorbed from the lungs into the bloodstream.

TRUE. Recall the osmotic process: Water will flow across a semipermeable membrane from a solution of lower concentration toward a solution of higher concentration. Let us regard the alveolar-capillary interface as a semipermeable membrane. The fresh water aspirated into the lungs is a solution of low solute concentration; the plasma flowing through the capillaries is a solution of higher solute concentration. Thus water will tend to flow out of the alveoli and into the capillaries.

If large quantities of fresh water are aspirated, this absorption of water into the bloodstream can have very serious consequences. Again, this is a matter of an osmotic process, but in this case we are interested in another semipermeable membrane, that surrounding the red blood cell. Ordinarily, red blood cells and the plasma in which they are suspended have roughly equivalent concentrations of solute materials, i.e., they are *isotonic,* so there is minimal flow of water either into or out of the red blood cells. But now we have a situation in which the plasma has become relatively diluted with fresh water, i.e., it has become *hypotonic* with respect to the interior of the red blood cell. What will happen? Once again, water will flow from the less concentrated solution (the plasma) into the more concentrated solution (the red blood cell). The problem is that the membrane surrounding the red blood cell can stretch only so far to accommodate an increase in volume, and at a certain point, the membrane will burst—a process called *hemolysis*. When that happens, all of the contents of the red blood cell will spill out into the plasma, including high concentrations of potassium. Thus, hemolysis can bring with it dangerous elevations of serum potassium, sometimes high enough to cause cardiac dysrhythmias.

c. Mouth-to-mouth ventilation should be initiated immediately on the nonbreathing near-drowning victim, even before he has been removed from the water.

TRUE. The victim should be rapidly turned to a supine position, his head tilted back (assuming there is no suspicion of spinal injury), and mouth-to-mouth ventilation begun immediately and continued as the victim is floated out of the water. Precious time is wasted if you wait until you have reached dry land to start oxygenating a nonbreathing patient. External cardiac compressions are another matter, for there is simply no way to accomplish closed chest cardiac massage on a patient who is bobbing up and down in an aqueous solution. That has to wait until you are both back on terra firma.

d. A victim of near drowning is likely to have large quantities of water in his stomach and therefore is in danger of aspiration of stomach contents during resuscitation.

TRUE. A person struggling in the water often swallows a great deal of water before he emits his last bubble. And when you start squeezing his chest, the chances are very good that the patient will regurgitate a few pints of the water he swallowed, together with whatever he had for lunch. For that reason, it is a very good idea to insert a nasogastric tube into the unconscious near-drowning victim at the earliest possible moment—BUT NOT BEFORE YOU HAVE PROTECTED HIS AIRWAY WITH A CUFFED ENDOTRACHEAL TUBE! Remember, a nasogastric tube serves as a very efficient wick along which stomach contents can ascend into the posterior oropharynx. And from there it is only a short hop past the vocal cords and into the bronchi. Thus, before you know it, half of that cheeseburger that the victim had for lunch will be sitting in the right main bronchus. Don't let it happen! Oxygenate the patient, and get the endotracheal tube in—or buy some time with an esophageal obturator airway (EOA).

e. Near-drowning victims tend to develop extreme metabolic acidosis.

TRUE. Indeed, this is true irrespective of whether the near-drowning victim actually experiences cardiac arrest. The reasons for this are not well understood. Certainly part of the acidosis may come from the production of large quantities of lactic acid by muscle during the patient's violent struggles in the water. In any case, victims of near drowning tend to require bicarbonate, and victims of near drowning who suffer cardiac arrest tend to require more bicarbonate than patients who suffer cardiac arrest from other causes. So give an extra ampule or two of sodium bicarbonate in these cases.

FURTHER READING

Allman FD et al. Outcome following cardiopulmonary resuscitation in severe pediatric near-drowning. *Am J Dis Child* 140:571, 1986.

Cairns FJ. Deaths from drowning. *NZ Med J* 97:65, 1984.

Colby PH. Plunging into water rescue. *JEMS* 15(7):31, 1990.

Dean JM, Kaufman ND. Prognostic indicators in pediatric near-drowning: The Glasgow coma scale. *Crit Care Med* 9:536, 1981.

Dietz PE, Baker SP. Drowning: Epidemiology and prevention. *Am J Public Health* 64:303, 1974.

Drinking and drowning (editorial). *Lancet* 2:194, 1978.

Harries MG. Drowning in man. *Crit Care Med* 9:407, 1981.

Harries MG. Clinical course of 61 serious immersion incidents. *Disaster Med* 1:263, 1983.

Hooper HA. Near drowning. *Emergency* 12(5):75, 1980.

Jacobson WK et al. Correlation of spontaneous respiration and neurologic damage in near-drowning. *Crit Care Med* 11:487, 1983.

Knopp R. Near drowning. *JACEP* 7:249, 1978.

Modell JH. Near-drowning. *Int Anesthesiol Clin* 15:107, 1977.

Modell JH. Is the Heimlich maneuver appropriate as first treatment in drowning? *Emerg Med Serv* 10(6):63, 1981.

National Safety Council. *Accident Facts, 1984.* Chicago: National Safety Council, 1984.

Nemiroff MJ. Reprieve from drowning. *Sci Am* 237:57, 1977.

Nichter MA et al. Childhood near-drowning: Is cardiopulmonary resuscitation always indicated? *Crit Care Med* 17:993, 1989.

Orlowski JP. Drowning, near-drowning, and ice-water drowning (editorial). *JAMA* 260:390, 1988.

Orlowski JP, Abulleil MM, Phillips JM. The hemodynamic and cardiovascular effects of near-drowning in hypotonic, isotonic, or hypertonic solutions. *Ann Emerg Med* 18:1044, 1989.

Ornato JP. The resuscitation of near-drowning victims. *JAMA* 256:75, 1986.

Pearn J. Secondary drowning in children. *Br Med J* 281:1103, 1980.

Pearn J. Drowning and alcohol. *Med J Aust* 141:6, 1984.

Pluekhahn V. Alcohol and accidental drowning. *Med J Aust* 141:22, 1984.

Pratt FD et al. Incidence of "secondary drowning" after saltwater submersion. *Ann Emerg Med* 15:1084, 1986.

Sarnaik AP et al. Near-drowning: Fresh, salt, and cold water immersion. *Clin Sports Med* 5:33, 1986.

Saved from a watery grave. *Emerg Med* 19(10):67, 1987.

Schuman SH et al. Risk of drowning: An iceberg phenomenon. *JACEP* 6:139, 1977.

Redding JS. Drowning and near-drowning. *Postgrad Med* 74:85, 1983.

Redmond AD et al. Resuscitation from drowning. *Arch Emerg Med* 1:113, 1984.

Stanford TM. Near-drowning. *Emergency* 21(6):30, 1989.

Thygerson AL. Drowning. *Emergency* 12(7):29, 1980.

You and your crew (two other paramedics) have arrived at a street corner where a man collapsed. Bystanders state that the patient had been walking down the street when he paused, tried to steady himself against a lamp post, and then fell to the ground. This occurred approximately 4 minutes before you arrived. No one at the scene has started CPR. You find the patient apneic and pulseless.

Indicate at what point in resuscitation each of the following should be performed:

a. Immediately upon arrival at the scene
b. Only after at least 3 to 5 minutes of adequate oxygenation
c. After the patient has been stabilized

1. _____ Intubation of the trachea
2. _____ Evacuation to the hospital
3. _____ Defibrillation
4. _____ External cardiac compressions
5. _____ Artificial ventilation
6. _____ One rescuer begins preparations to start an IV

A75 Every ambulance crew should have a well-rehearsed plan for cardiac arrest, and the order of priorities should be established according to rational principles. The moment you arrive at the scene is NOT the time to decide who does what when, for you will have your hands full simply to carry out a well-planned routine amidst the noise and confusion that often characterize the prehospital setting. So let's review a few basic principles ahead of time:

1. __b__ Intubation of the trachea

One of the most common errors in resuscitation is to attempt endotracheal intubation too early and thereby waste precious time, during which the already hypoxemic patient becomes even more hypoxemic. Our patient has been down for 4 minutes, and while we don't really know whether he has actually been apneic all that time, we have to assume the worst. What he needs right away is oxygen. The endotracheal tube can wait a few minutes until his arterial blood is fully saturated with oxygen. Then, he will be much better able to tolerate the 15 to 20 seconds without oxygen that will be required for you to get the tube in place. Meanwhile, one of your crew will have time to set up the intubation equipment and check it in an orderly fashion.

2. __c__ Evacuation to the hospital

Under most circumstances, it is preferable to get the patient stabilized to the greatest degree possible before starting transport to the hospital, for effective CPR is difficult, at best, in a moving vehicle. Certainly one wants, at least, to gain definitive control over the airway (endotracheal intubation) and get an IV line in before starting to move the patient. From there on, it will be up to the base physician to determine—taking into account the paramedics' report on conditions at the scene—what is the most appropriate moment at which to cease efforts at the scene and move on to the emergency room.

3. __b__ Defibrillation

Defibrillation is unlikely to be successful when performed on a highly hypoxic myocardium, and we must assume that our patient's myocardium has been without oxygen for about 4 minutes. Under those circumstances, immediate defibrillation is more likely to convert the rhythm to asystole than to sinus, and defibrillation is thus better postponed until the patient is better oxygenated, i.e., after a minute or two of artificial ventilation and chest compressions. Immediate defibrillation is most appropriately performed in situations of *witnessed* cardiac arrest, where the patient's level of oxygenation can be assumed to be adequate or at least marginal.

4. __a__ External cardiac compressions

External cardiac compressions should be initiated immediately upon detection of the absence of a pulse, i.e., within moments of arriving at the scene.

5. __a__ Artificial ventilation

Similarly, artificial ventilation must be started immediately upon arrival at the scene. If you neglected to take the bag-valve-mask with you when you jumped out of the ambulance, start artificial ventilation by the mouth-to-mouth method while your partner runs back to the vehicle for the equipment (you won't forget it next time . . .). And make sure he brings the oxygen back with him, for oxygen therapy should begin at the earliest possible moment as well.

6. __a__ One rescuer begins preparations to start an IV

Don't forget, there are three of you present at this case; that makes life a lot easier. While two of you are tied up with CPR, the third paramedic has the job of preparing all the equipment—the IV, the monitor, the endotracheal intubation kit. You'll want to get the IV in as rapidly as possible to provide you with a lifeline through which to administer drugs.

FURTHER READING
American Heart Association. Standards and guidelines for cardiopulmonary resuscitation (CPR) and emergency cardiac care (ECC). *JAMA* 255:2905, 1986.
CPR—it's come a long way. *Emerg Med* 17(5):77, 1985.
Fisher JM. ABC of resuscitation: Recognizing a cardiac arrest and providing basic life support. *Br Med J* 292:1002, 1986.
Luce JM et al. New developments in cardiopulmonary resuscitation. *JAMA* 244:1366, 1980.
McIntyre KM. CPR: Old problems, new techniques. *Cardiovasc Med* 10(9):16, 1985.

For each of the following situations indicate whether

a. There is ample time to get the mother to the hospital for delivery there.
b. There is NOT sufficient time to get to the hospital, and the paramedic must prepare to help deliver the baby at the scene.

1. _____ An 18-year-old woman in her third trimester is having pains 5 minutes apart. This is her first pregnancy. The hospital is 6 minutes away.
2. _____ A 24-year-old woman who is "3 weeks overdue" is having labor pains 3 minutes apart. This is her third pregnancy. The hospital is 45 minutes away.
3. _____ A 26-year-old woman in her ninth month of pregnancy is having labor pains about 2 minutes apart. She complains of a sensation of having to move her bowels. This is her fifth pregnancy. The hospital is 5 minutes away.

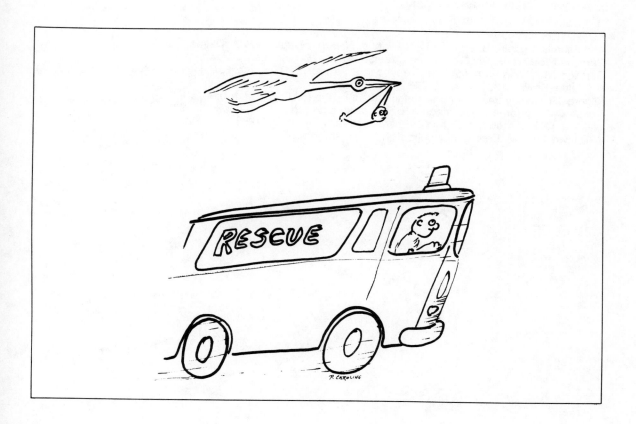

A76

In general, it is preferable for babies to be born in the hospital, where sterile conditions for delivery can more readily be provided. This is not always possible, however, for babies can be rather capricious about choosing their moment to enter the world, and the paramedic frequently faces situations in which he must decide whether there is time for a safe, unhurried transport to the hospital. Such decisions are not always easy, and where there is any doubt, the counsel of the base station physician should be sought.

1. ___a___ An 18-year-old woman in her third trimester is having pains 5 minutes apart. This is her first pregnancy. The hospital is 6 minutes away.

In this case, you can probably breathe easy. Labor during the first pregnancy is usually a leisurely affair, and if the contractions are still only 5 minutes apart, you should have lots of time—even if you get a flat tire on the way to the hospital.

2. ___b___ A 24-year-old woman who is "3 weeks overdue" is having labor pains 3 minutes apart. This is her third pregnancy. The hospital is 45 minutes away.

This is one of those tough decisions, and you'd better check with the base station physician. You might make it to the hospital, and then again, you might not. The fact that the contractions are 3 minutes apart suggests that the baby won't be coming during the next 5 to 10 minutes, but with a "multip" (a woman who has had more than two deliveries), you never can tell. If the hospital were closer, you might feel more comfortable in taking the chance, but a 45-minute ride might be pushing your luck. Thus we recommend to err on the side of caution and stay put until the baby arrives.

3. ___b___ A 26-year-old woman in her ninth month of pregnancy is having labor pains about 2 minutes apart. She complains of a sensation of having to move her bowels. This is her fifth pregnancy. The hospital is 5 minutes away.

Here the decision has been made for you, by the baby. There is virtually no doubt that you will NOT have time to get to the hospital, even a hospital 5 minutes' drive away. You'll be lucky if you have time to get set up for delivery. Remember, when the patient complains of a sensation of having to move her bowels, it means that the baby's head has descended into the birth canal, and delivery is imminent. If you want to participate, you'd better wash your hands and get your sterile duds on quickly.

FURTHER READING

Anderson B, Shapiro B. *Emergency Childbirth Handbook*. Albany, NY: Delmar, 1979.
Caroline NL. *Emergency Care in the Streets* (4th ed.). Boston: Little, Brown, 1991, Ch. 35.
Caroline NL. *Emergency Medical Treatment: A Text for EMT-As and EMT-Intermediates* (3rd ed.). Boston: Little, Brown, 1991. Chs. 32, 33.
Kilgore JR. Management of an obstetric patient by the EMT. *EMT J* 4(2):50, 1980.
Roush GM. Abdominal examination of the pregnant uterus. *EMT J* 3(2):33, 1979.
Williams C. Emergency childbirth. *Emerg Med Serv* 14(3):100, 1985.
Wojslawowicz JM. Emergency childbirth for emergency medical technicians. *EMT J* 1(4):66, 1977.

The call comes in during the early evening for a "sick baby." The patient turns out to be a 10-month-old baby who, according to mother, has been wheezing for the past 4 hours. The baby has had a "cold" for the past 3 days, with a cough and runny nose, but tonight he started to have trouble breathing. The baby has no history of allergies, and there is no family history of allergic disease.

On physical examination, you find the baby restless and cranky. Rectal temperature is 100°F (37.8°C). The respiratory rate is 64, and there are retractions of the intercostal muscles and flaring of the nostrils on inhalation. Scattered wheezes are audible throughout the chest.

Which of the following are part of the management of this child? (There may be more than one correct answer.)

a. Administer oxygen.
b. Administer epinephrine, 0.01 ml per kilogram of a 1:1,000 solution SQ.
c. Administer penicillin.
d. Administer aminophylline.
e. Transport the baby to the hospital.

A77 The correct answers are **a** and **e: Administer oxygen** and **transport the baby to the hospital.** This baby is in all probability suffering from bronchiolitis, a bronchiolar inflammation caused most often by viral infection. In many cases bronchiolitis can be managed at home, but when there is severe respiratory distress (respiratory rate above 60), signs of hypoxemia (restlessness), or dehydration, hospitalization is indicated.

Epinephrine (answer b) will have no effect on the respiratory distress of bronchiolitis, and the use of this or other bronchodilators (answer d) is therefore unwarranted. Similarly, antibiotics, such as penicillin (answer c), are of no value in uncomplicated cases, for the etiologic agent is a virus, not a bacteria, and antibiotics are ineffective against viral infections.

FURTHER READING

Caroline NL. *Emergency Care in the Streets* (4th ed.). Boston: Little, Brown, 1991, Ch. 30.

Downes J et al. Acute respiratory failure in infants with bronchiolitis. *Anesthesiology* 29:426, 1968.

Phelan P, Williams H. Sympathomimetic drugs in acute viral bronchiolitis. *Pediatrics* 44:493, 1969.

Silverman M. Bronchodilators for wheezy infants? *Arch Dis Child* 59:84, 1984.

Simpsom H et al. Acute respiratory failure in bronchiolitis in infancy: Modes of presentation and treatment. *Br Med J* 2:632, 1974.

Wohl MEB, Chernick V. Bronchiolitis: State of the art. *Am Rev Respir Dis* 118:759, 1986.

You are called to the dormitory of a local college, where a woman has been found unconscious. The patient is a 20-year-old student at the college. Her roommate informs you that the patient has been very depressed lately since a falling out with her boyfriend, and tonight when the roommate returned, she found the patient unconscious on the bed. There is an empty bottle labelled "Valium" on the bedside table.

The patient is deeply comatose, unresponsive to voice or painful stimuli. Pulse is 100 and regular, blood pressure is 90/60, and respirations are 12 per minute, with prominent snoring noises. There is no evidence of injury, and physical examination is otherwise unremarkable.

Arrange the following steps of management in the correct sequence:

a. Flush out the stomach with copious quantities of water or saline.
b. Establish an IV line.
c. Intubate the trachea.
d. Establish an airway manually.
e. Instill activated charcoal into the stomach.
f. Administer oxygen.
g. Insert a nasogastric tube.

1. _____
2. _____
3. _____
4. _____
5. _____
6. _____
7. _____

A78

1. __d__ Establish an airway manually.

Our patient's snoring respirations indicate that there is obstruction to the upper airway, probably by the base of the tongue. Backward tilt of the head may be all that is required to open the airway and permit free respirations.

2. __f__ Administer oxygen.

Since we are planning to intubate the trachea shortly, the patient will require at least 3 to 5 minutes of preoxygenation.

3. __c__ Intubate the trachea.

A patient who is deeply comatose has lost the reflexes by which one normally protects one's airway from aspiration. Thus it will be important to provide definitive airway care at the earliest possible moment, with a cuffed endotracheal tube. Then we can flush out the patient's stomach without worrying about aspiration.

4. __b__ Establish an IV line.

Diazepam (Valium), especially taken in excess, may lead to severe degrees of hypotension and eventual cardiovascular collapse. Our patient will need fluids and a route for the administration of resuscitative drugs, and we want to get the IV in before the hypotension progresses further and veins get harder to find.

5. __g__ Insert a nasogastric tube.

We waited until after we had secured the airway to insert the nasogastric tube because its insertion may lead to regurgitation and aspiration, especially if the stomach is full. Thus we wanted to make sure the airway was fully protected first. We also got our IV line in before the nasogastric tube, since an intravenous route is potentially lifesaving; a nasogastric tube is not.

6. __a__ Flush out the stomach with copious quantities of water or saline.

We don't know how long ago our patient ingested the Valium, so we cannot be sure how much of it may still be in her stomach. If there is any doubt, it's best to lavage the stomach and try to remove whatever remnants of the drug may still be there. Gastric lavage is best performed in the emergency room, but if transport times are such that lavage will be significantly delayed (i.e., more than about 20–30 minutes) by waiting until one gets to the emergency room, it may be advisable to go ahead at the scene. Consult the base station physician for orders. If you do lavage the stomach at the scene, be sure to save the fluid from the first lavage and bring it with you to the emergency room for toxicologic analysis. Just because the bottle says "Valium" does not necessarily mean that it contained Valium or that the patient didn't ingest another drug as well.

7. __e__ Instill activated charcoal into the stomach.

Once lavage of the stomach is complete, make a slurry of activated charcoal, instill it through the nasogastric tube, and clamp off the tube.

FURTHER READING

Caroline NL. *Emergency Care in the Streets* (4th ed.). Boston: Little, Brown, 1991, Ch. 27.
Caroline NL. *Emergency Medical Treatment: A Text for EMT-As and EMT-Intermediates* (3rd ed.). Boston: Little, Brown, 1991, Ch. 21.
Posner J. The comatose patient. *Emerg Med* 11:107, 1977.
Redding JS, Tabeling BB, Parham AM. Airway management in patients with central nervous system depression. *JACEP* 7:401, 1978.
Thornton WE. Sleep aids and sedatives. *JACEP* 6:408, 1977.
Wilkinson HA. Evaluation and management of the unconscious patient. *Emerg Med Serv* 75(5):24, 1978.

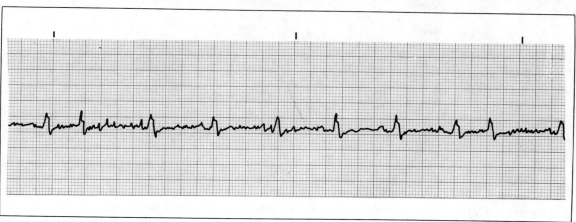

Figure 8

A 46-year-old woman was struck by a car as she was crossing the street a block from your station. Arriving at the scene, you find her lying in the street, alert and moaning. She complains of severe pain in her chest and states that "it hurts to breathe." Her pulse is strong, blood pressure is 150/80, and respirations are 20 and shallow. There is no evidence of head trauma. Pupils are equal and reactive. There is no neck vein distention. There are bruises over the right anterior chest and pain on palpation over the right fifth, sixth, seventh, and eighth ribs near the sternal border. Breath sounds are equal bilaterally, and heart sounds are well heard. The abdomen is soft and nontender. There are no deformities of the extremities; sensation and movement are intact in all extremities.

1. Examine the patient's rhythm strip in Figure 8:

   a. The rhythm is _____ regular _____ irregular.
   b. The rate is _____ per minute.

2. The patient's underlying rhythm is

   a. Sinus
   b. Atrial fibrillation
   c. Atrial flutter
   d. Junctional
   e. Idioventricular

3. Which of the following statements about this dysrhythmia is true?

   a. It is a life-threatening dysrhythmia and should be treated at once.
   b. It may reflect a contusion to the right side of the heart.
   c. It is caused by widespread ventricular irritability.
   d. It is probably due to an acute myocardial infarction.
   e. The patient will require a pacemaker.

4. The treatment for this patient's cardiac dysrhythmia is

   a. Lidocaine, 75 mg IV, followed by an infusion at 2 to 3 mg per minute
   b. Digoxin, 0.25 mg IV
   c. Procainamide (Pronestyl), 50 mg slowly IV
   d. Atropine, 0.7 to 1.0 mg IV
   e. Monitor only

A79

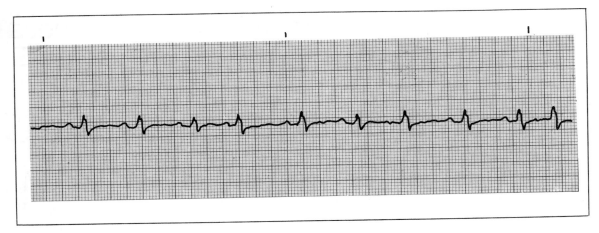

Figure 9

1. The patient's rhythm is slightly **irregular.** The rate is approximately **80 per minute.**
2. The underlying rhythm is **sinus** (answer **a**). Were you fooled by the wavy baseline into calling it atrial fibrillation (answer b)? Those are not fibrillatory waves but rather artifacts caused by a loose ECG lead. Figure 9 is another rhythm strip from the same patient taken after the leads were secured correctly, and in this strip the P waves are clearly visible. The occasional irregularities are due to premature atrial contractions (PACs), of which three are seen on the above recording. The tip-off that this rhythm was *not* atrial fibrillation was that the rhythm is *fundamentally* regular, while the hallmark of atrial fibrillation is an irregularly irregular rhythm. If you go back and look closely now at the ECG strip in Figure 8, you will be able to make out the P waves buried in the baseline artifact.
3. This patient's dysrhythmia may reflect a **contusion to the right side of the heart** (answer **b**). Right-sided chest trauma, when it produces cardiac dysrhythmias, usually produces either atrial dysrhythmias or heart block; it is thus generally less dangerous than left-sided chest trauma, which can result in ventricular dysrhythmias. Our patient's dysrhythmia is NOT life-threatening, and it reflects slight atrial, not ventricular, irritability (answers a and c respectively). There is no evidence that would lead us to believe that this patient has suffered an acute myocardial infarction (answer d); her chest pain, which is aggravated by inhalation, can be readily explained on the basis of bruised or fractured ribs. Finally, there is no need in a rhythm of this type to consider a pacemaker (answer e); there is neither heart block nor any other form of serious bradycardia present.
4. The treatment of our patient's dysrhythmia requires **monitoring only** (answer **e**). Her occasional PACs do not require any pharmacologic intervention, and none of the agents listed would be likely to abolish PACs anyway.

FURTHER READING

Bayer MJ, Burdick D. Diagnosis of myocardial contusion in blunt chest trauma. *JACEP* 6:238, 1977.
Beresky R et al. Myocardial contusion: When does it have clinical significance? *J Trauma* 28:64, 1988.
Dreifus LS. Dysrhythmias related to cardiac trauma. *Chest* 61:294, 1972.
Dubrow TJ et al. Myocardial contusion in the stable patient: What level of care is appropriate? *Surgery* 106:267, 1989.
Fabian TC et al. Myocardial contusion in blunt trauma: Clinical characteristics, means of diagnosis, and implications for patient management. *J Trauma* 28:50, 1988.
Green ED et al. Cardiac concussion following softball blow to the chest. *Ann Emerg Med* 9:155, 1980.
Guillot TS, Frame SB. Trauma rounds. Problem: Myocardial contusion. *Emerg Med* 20(3):157, 1988.
Healey MA et al. Blunt cardiac injury: Is this diagnosis necessary? *J Trauma* 30:137, 1990.
Helling TS et al. A prospective evaluation of 68 patients suffering blunt chest trauma for evidence of cardiac injury. *J Trauma* 29:961, 1989.
Jones JW, Hewitt LW, Drapanas T. Cardiac contusion: A capricious syndrome. *Ann Surg* 181:567, 1975.
Kron IL, Cox PM. Cardiac injury after chest trauma. *Crit Care Med* 11:624, 1983.
Kunar SA et al. Myocardial contusion following nonfatal blunt chest trauma. *J Trauma* 23:327, 1983.
Weisz GM, Blumenfeld Z, Barzilai A. Electrocardiographic changes in traumatized patients. *JACEP* 5:329, 1976.

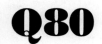

4:00 A.M. You are called to see a "child who can't breathe," and you arrive at an apartment about 20 minutes from your station, where two very distraught parents are awaiting you. They tell you that their 11-year-old son, who has a history of severe asthma, developed an attack the previous morning, and "it has just gotten worse and worse." He has been using his bronchodilator inhaler without apparent benefit.

In the bedroom you find a very ill-appearing child, sitting bolt upright in bed, struggling to breathe. He is extremely agitated and restless and does not want to sit still for your examination. There are retractions of his suprasternal muscles on inhalation. His skin is pale and dry. Pulse is 130 and regular. Respirations are 30 and shallow. The chest is full of tight wheezes and is hyper-resonant to percussion.

Which of the following is NOT part of the treatment for this child?

a. Epinephrine, to combat bronchoconstriction
b. Intravenous fluids, to combat dehydration
c. Oxygen, to combat hypoxemia
d. Sodium bicarbonate, to combat acidosis
e. Sedatives, to combat agitation

A80 The use of sedatives of any kind are absolutely contraindicated in the treatment of status asthmaticus or an acute asthmatic attack (answer **e**). Most sedative medications are also respiratory depressants, and thus they could have dangerous consequences in a patient in borderline or outright respiratory failure. Besides, our little boy is very likely, within a short time, to fall under the influence of a strong physiologic sedative: the carbon dioxide that is accumulating in his blood. He does not need further sedation. He is agitated because he has hypoxemia and is suffocating—a valid enough reason for anyone to be agitated and an indication to provide oxygen (answer c), not sedation.

Epinephrine is generally tried at least once in a severe asthmatic attack (answer a), although in this case we should not be surprised if the epinephrine is not particularly effective; the parents have told us that the child has already made considerable use of his inhaler—which probably contained epinephrine or a related drug—without benefit. Thus other bronchodilating agents, such as theophylline, may have to be tried. Intravenous fluids (answer b) will be an important part of therapy, to treat the patient's dehydration and thereby loosen up the secretions that are impacted in his airways.

By now it is a safe guess that the patient has a significant degree of acidosis. It is primarily a respiratory acidosis from carbon dioxide retention, but after more than 12 hours of struggling to breathe, there is apt to be a metabolic component to the acidosis as well, and modest bicarbonate therapy (answer d) may be indicated to try to bring the patient's pH back up into a range where bronchodilator drugs can work more effectively.

FURTHER READING

Carden DL et al. Vital signs including pulsus paradoxus in the assessment of acute bronchial asthma. *Ann Emerg Med* 12:80, 1983.

Caroline NL. *Emergency Care in the Streets* (4th ed.). Boston: Little, Brown, 1991, Ch. 30.

Fanta CH et al. Glucocorticoids in acute asthma: A critical controlled trial. *Am J Med* 74:845, 1983.

Groth ML, Hurewitz AN. Pharmacologic management of acute asthma. *Emerg Med* 21(7):23, 1989.

Harper TB et al. Techniques of administration of metered-dose aerosolized drugs in asthmatic children. *Am J Dis Child* 135:218, 1981.

Hurwitz ME et al. Clinical scoring does not accurately assess hypoxemia in pediatric asthma patients. *Ann Emerg Med* 13:1040, 1984.

Johnson AJ et al. Circumstances of death from asthma. *Br Med J* 288:1870, 1984.

Kampschulte S, Marcey J, Safar P. Simplified management of status asthmaticus in children. *Crit Care Med* 1:69, 1973.

Kattan M et al. Corticosteroids in status asthmaticus. *J Pediatr* 96:596, 1980.

Karetzky MS. Acute asthma: The use of subcutaneous epinephrine in therapy. *Ann Allergy* 44:12, 1980.

Kravis LP et al. Unexpected death in childhood asthma. *Am J Dis Child* 139:558, 1985.

Lee H et al. Aerosol bag for administration of bronchodilators to young asthmatic children. *Pediatrics* 73:230, 1984.

Leffert F. The management of acute severe asthma. *J Pediatr* 96:1, 1980.

Lulla S et al. Emergency management of asthma in children. *J Pediatr* 97:346, 1980.

Mellis CM. Important changes in the emergency management of acute asthma in children. *Med J Aust* 148:215, 1988.

Nguyen MT et al. Causes of death from asthma in children. *Ann Allergy* 55:448, 1985.

The proper use of aerosol bronchodilators (editorial). *Lancet* 1:23, 1981.

Ratto D et al. Are intravenous corticosteroids required in status asthmaticus? *JAMA* 260:527, 1988.

Reyes de la Rocha S, Brown MA. Asthma in children: Emergency management. *Ann Emerg Med* 16:79, 1987.

Silverman M. Bronchodilators for wheezy infants? *Arch Dis Child* 59:84, 1984.

Sly RM. Mortality from asthma in children 1979–1984. *Ann Allergy* 60:433, 1988.

Spiteri MA et al. Subcutaneous adrenaline versus terbutaline in the treatment of acute severe asthma. *Thorax* 43:19, 1988.

Strunk RC et al. Physiologic and psychological characteristics associated with deaths due to asthma in childhood: A case-controlled study. *JAMA* 254:1193, 1985.

Victoria MS et al. Comparison between epinephrine and terbutaline injections in the acute management of asthma. *J Asthma* 26:287, 1989.

Your patient is a 58-year-old man complaining of severe chest pain of 1 hour's duration. He describes the pain as "squeezing" and states that it radiates down his left arm. He has also felt sick to his stomach. With respect to his past medical history, the patient informs you that he has "dozens" of medical problems, for which he takes "lots of medicines," although he isn't quite sure what the medications are for. On his nightstand, you find the following:

a. Nitroglycerin
b. Methyldopa (Aldomet)
c. Furosemide (Lasix)
d. Tolbutamide (Orinase)
e. Quinidine

From this collection of medications you can already make a few assumptions about the patient's underlying medical problems. Match the above medications with the information that each suggests:

1. _____ The patient has problems of chronic fluid retention, perhaps from chronic heart failure.
2. _____ The patient has a history of cardiac dysrhythmias.
3. _____ The patient has a history of angina pectoris.
4. _____ The patient is a diabetic.
5. _____ The patient has hypertension.

On physical examination, the patient is alert, anxious, and in moderate distress. Pulse is 110 and regular, blood pressure is 180/100, and respirations are 20. As your partner is completing the physical exam, he mutters to you, "Looks like an inferior wall MI." What part of the body was your partner examining when he reached this conclusion?

a. The head
b. The neck
c. The back
d. The precordium
e. The abdomen

What did he find that led him to make his astonishing announcement?

A81

A great deal of medicine is detective work, and from the time one arrives at the scene, one is searching for clues—in the scene itself, in the patient's history, in the physical examination.

The medications a patient takes regularly may give valuable clues to his underlying medical problems. Let's see how well you did figuring out these clues in our patient's case:

1. __c__ The patient has problems of chronic fluid retention, perhaps from chronic heart failure.

   FUROSEMIDE, or other diuretic medication, is commonly prescribed to patients with chronic heart failure to counteract their tendency toward retention of excess salt and water.

2. __e__ The patient has a history of cardiac dysrhythmias.

   QUINIDINE is taken to convert certain atrial dysrhythmias, such as atrial flutter or atrial fibrillation, and also to suppress ventricular ectopic activity.

3. __a__ The patient has a history of angina pectoris.

   NITROGLYCERIN is prescribed for the pain of angina. It is usually taken under the tongue, although long-acting nitroglycerin preparations may be taken as tablets to be swallowed.

4. __d__ The patient is a diabetic.

   TOLBUTAMIDE is an oral hypoglycemic agent prescribed for stable, adult-onset diabetes.

5. __b__ The patient has hypertension.

   METHYLDOPA is an antihypertensive agent.

The physical exam too may offer surprising clues. Your partner, for example, noticed a subtle but significant finding when he was examining the patient's back (answer **c**): tenderness along the border of the left trapezius muscle. This finding is often associated with an infarction of the diaphragmatic (inferior) surface of the heart. (There was another clue that this patient might be suffering from an inferior wall infarction. Did you pick it up? The patient complained of nausea, which is more commonly associated with inferior wall infarction than with anterior infarctions. That is not a hard and fast rule, but it does serve to increase one's index of suspicion.)

FURTHER READING
Caroline NL. *Emergency Care in the Streets* (4th ed.). Boston: Little, Brown, 1991, Chs. 23, 24.

A 55-year-old man falls from the second-story window of a burning house, his sweater and trousers on fire, and lands unconscious on the lawn outside.

1. Arrange the following steps of management in the correct order:

   a. Administer oxygen.
   b. Establish an IV with normal saline solution.
   c. Cover the patient with a sterile sheet.
   d. Dress any associated wounds and immobilize any associated fractures.
   e. Establish an airway.
   f. Put out the fire.

   1. _____
   2. _____
   3. _____
   4. _____
   5. _____
   6. _____

2. Upon examining the patient, you find that he has suffered burns to the anterior and posterior surfaces of both legs, to the anterior trunk, and to the anterior and posterior surfaces of his left arm. What percent of his body was burned?

   a. 36 percent
   b. 45 percent
   c. 54 percent
   d. 63 percent
   e. 72 percent

A82

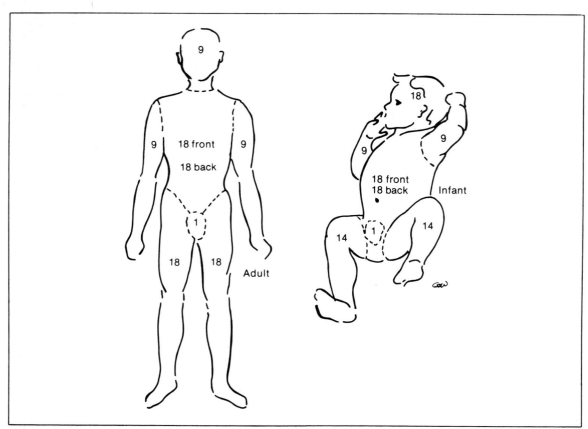

Figure 10. Rule of nines.

1. You've got the ABCs forever imprinted in your memory by now, so of course you gave primary attention to the airway. But did you remember to put out the fire first?!

1. __f__ Put out the fire!
2. __e__ Establish an airway.
3. __a__ Administer oxygen.
4. __b__ Establish an IV with normal saline solution.
5. __d__ Dress any associated wounds and immobilize any associated fractures.
6. __c__ Cover the patient with a sterile sheet.

2. If you had trouble with this question, you'd better review the rule of nines (Fig. 10).
   The correct answer is **d: 63 percent.**

right leg	= 18 percent
left leg	= 18 percent
anterior trunk	= 18 percent
left arm	= 9 percent
TOTAL	= 63 percent

FURTHER READING
Ayvazian BH, Monafo WW. Initial management of the burned patient. *Emerg Med Serv* 5(5):11, 1976.
Baxter CR, Waeckerle JF. Emergency treatment of burn injury. *Ann Emerg Med* 17:1305, 1988.
Bingham HG. Early management of the burned patient. *Emerg Med Serv* 6(5):9, 1977.
Bourn MK. Fire and smoke: Managing skin and inhalation burns. *JEMS* 14(9):62, 1989.
Dimick AR. The burn at first sight. *Emerg Med* 15(15):130, 1983.
Duda J. Burn wise. *Emergency* 21(6):44, 1989.
Edlich RF et al. Prehospital treatment of the burn patient. *EMT J* 2(3):42, 1978.
Luterman A, Talley MA. Field management of burn injuries. *Emerg Med Serv* 17(7):30, 1988.
Rodeheaver GT et al. Extinguishing the flaming burn victim. *JACEP* 8:307, 1979.
Thygerson AL. Burn treatment. *Emergency* 15(6):18, 1983.
Wachtel TL. Major burns: What to do at the scene and en route to the hospital. *Postgrad Med* 85(1):178, 1989.

It is a sunny Sunday, and you are called to a park about 5 miles outside of town to attend to a 15-year-old boy who became very ill at a family picnic. The father reports that his son was stung on the right forearm by a bee and shortly afterward began complaining of abdominal pain and difficulty in breathing. You find the boy dyspneic, with rapid, wheezing respirations. His pulse is rapid and weak. His face is swollen, and his body is covered with urticaria (hives).

1. Which of the following drugs is NOT used in the management of this type of problem?

   a. Atropine
   b. Oxygen
   c. Epinephrine
   d. Aminophylline
   e. Diphenhydramine (Benadryl)

2. In addition to pharmacologic treatment, several other measures are important in the management of this patient. Indicate which of the following is NOT appropriate in the management of our patient:

   a. Keep the patient flat, and elevate his legs.
   b. Start an IV line.
   c. Apply a tourniquet to the right arm.
   d. Give the patient ice water to drink.
   e. Remove any part of the bee's stinger that may remain in the patient's arm.

A83

1. Atropine (answer **a**) is NOT part of the treatment of this patient. As you have probably already concluded, our young man is suffering from an anaphylactic reaction. His pulse is already racing, and he hardly needs a medication to suppress the vagus nerve.

   He does most certainly need oxygen (answer b), for he is in severe respiratory distress. Epinephrine (answer c) should be given in two sites subcutaneously: 0.3 ml of a 1:1,000 solution directly into the area of the sting and the same dose subcutaneously in the other arm. The patient's bronchospasm, which is evident from his wheezing respirations, is treated with aminophylline (answer d), 5.6 mg per kilogram IV over about 20 minutes. And diphenhydramine (Benadryl, answer e) may be administered after more critical measures have been completed in order to diminish the patient's urticaria.

   Before the family takes their son home from the emergency room, they should be advised to invest in an Epi-Pen injector. If the boy is squeamish about injections, he should at least carry a Medihaler-Epi on the next picnic. Inhaled epinephrine works rapidly to reduce angioedema of the posterior pharynx and is also rapidly absorbed across the mucous membranes of the respiratory tract into the bloodstream, where it can carry out its systemic functions.

2. Answer **d** is not correct: The patient should not be given anything to drink, for stimulation of the posterior pharynx may simply aggravate existing laryngospasm. He should be kept flat (answer a), on account of his signs of hypotension, and an IV line (answer b) is needed both as a route for fluids and as a lifeline for resuscitative drugs. A tourniquet should be applied to the right arm (answer c), proximal to the bee sting, in order to isolate whatever antigen remains at the injection site from the rest of the circulation; the tourniquet should be left in place until the anaphylactic reaction is well under control. Finally, any part of the insect's stinger seen in the injection site should be removed (answer e) in order to decrease the dose of antigen still available for absorption into the patient's bloodstream.

FURTHER READING

Allergic to what he eats. *Emerg Med* 19(2):20, 1987.
Austen KF. Systemic anaphylaxis in the human being. *N Engl J Med* 291:661, 1974.
Barach EM et al. Epinephrine for treatment of anaphylactic shock. *JAMA* 251:2118, 1984.
Busse WW. Anaphylaxis: Diagnosis and management. *Emerg Med Serv* 5(2):44, 1976.
Caroline NL. *Emergency Care in the Streets* (4th ed.). Boston: Little, Brown, 1991, Ch. 26.
Casale TB, Keahey TM, Kaliner M. Exercise-induced anaphylactic syndromes. *JAMA* 255:2049, 1986.
Fischer M et al. Volume replacement in acute anaphylactoid reactions. *Intensive Care* 7:375, 1979.
Frazier CA. Food allergy emergencies. *Emerg Med Serv* 12(2):71, 1983.
Fries JH. Peanuts: Allergic and other untoward reactions. *Ann Allergy* 48:220, 1982.
Goldberg M. Systemic reactions to intravascular contrast media. *Anesthesiology* 60:46, 1984.
Hooper HA. Allergic reactions. *Emergency* 11(4):32, 1979.
Kaliner MA. Calling a halt to anaphylaxis. *Emerg Med* 21(6):51, 1989.
Kelly JF, Patterson R. Anaphylaxis: Cause, mechanisms, and treatment. *JAMA* 227:1431, 1974.
Levy DB. Anaphylaxis. *Emergency* 21(4):42, 1989.
Lucke WC, Thomas H. Anaphylaxis: Pathophysiology, clinical presentations and treatment. *J Emerg Med* 1:83, 1983.
Morrow DH, Luther RR. Anaphylaxis: Etiology and guidelines for management. *Anesth Analg* 55:493, 1976.
Perkin RM, Anas NG. Mechanisms and management of anaphylactic shock not responding to traditional therapy. *Ann Allergy* 54:202, 1985.
Raebel M. Potentiated anaphylaxis during chronic beta-blocker therapy. *Drug Intell Clin Pharm* 22:720, 1988.
Roth R. Allergic response. *Emergency* 22(6):28, 1990.
Scheffer AL. Anaphylaxis. *J Allergy Clin Immunol* 75:227, 1985.
Schwartz HJ, Sher TH. Anaphylaxis to penicillin in a frozen dinner. *Ann Allergy* 52:342, 1984.
Stark BJ, Sullivan TJ. Biphasic and protracted anaphylaxis. *J Allergy Clin Immunol* 78:76, 1986.
Vaneslow NA. Minutes to counter anaphylaxis. *Emerg Med* 20(15):121, 1988.
Yuninger JW et al. Fatal food-induced anaphylaxis. *JAMA* 260:1450, 1988.

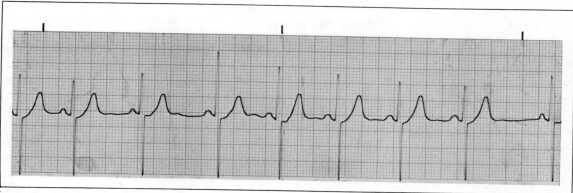

Figure 11

Your team is standing by at a four-alarm fire when you are asked to look at a firefighter who has been overcome by smoke. He is a tall, slim individual, age 26, and he appears pale and short of breath. He has a slight tachycardia. His chest is clear. After about 10 minutes he states that he is feeling better but complains of a persisting discomfort in his chest associated with respiration. You obtain the rhythm strip in Figure 11:

1. Examine the rhythm strip:

   a. The rhythm is _____ regular _____ irregular.
   b. The rate is _____ per minute.

2. This ECG pattern is

   a. Normal sinus rhythm
   b. Sinus arrhythmia
   c. Wenckebach
   d. Sinus arrest
   e. Atrial fibrillation

3. This pattern is probably due to

   a. An irritable focus in the ventricles
   b. An irritable focus in the atria
   c. The influence of respiration on the vagus nerve
   d. Damage to the sinus node
   e. Damage to the AV node

4. Which of the following statements about the management of this patient is NOT true?

   a. He should be given oxygen.
   b. He should not return to fighting the fire.
   c. He should not be permitted to smoke.
   d. He should be excused from duty and sent home to rest.
   e. He should be evaluated in the hospital.

A84

1. The patient's rhythm is **irregular.** The rate is approximately **70 per minute.**
2. The ECG pattern shown is **sinus arrhythmia** (answer **b**), i.e., the mechanism is sinus (there is a P wave prceding every QRS complex), but with slight variations in rhythm. There are no absent P waves, so there is no evidence of sinus arrest (answer d), nor are any P waves blocked as they would be in Wenckebach (answer c). In atrial fibrillation (answer e), one would not see P waves at all, but only irregular fibrillatory waves.
3. Sinus arrhythmia is usually attributable to the **stimulatory effects of respiration on the vagus nerve,** which in turn acts periodically to slow down the heart (answer **c**). It is more often seen in children or young adults than in older people and is an entirely normal finding. It does not indicate damage to any part of the conduction system (answers d, e) or myocardial irritability (answers a, b).
4. Our firefighter should NOT simply be sent home to rest (answer **d**). Significant smoke inhalation may result in relatively late complications (12–48 hours after the incident), and even though the fireman seems fine now, he could be in fulminant pulmonary edema a few hours from now. He at least deserves careful evaluation in the emergency room, and he should probably be watched overnight in the hospital (answer e.) *Any* person exposed to smoke inhalation should receive oxygen (answer a) and should not be filling his lungs with other sorts of smoke (answer c). Finally, a firefighter who has been overcome by smoke should not be permitted to return to the fray (answer b), even though his macho instincts may rebel at being restrained from rejoining his buddies on the front lines.

FURTHER READING

Bascomb R, Kennedy T. Toxic gas inhalation. *Emerg Med Serv* 13(7):17, 1984.

Birky MM, Clark FB. Inhalation of toxic products from fires. *Bull NY Acad Med* 57:997, 1981.

Cohen MA, Guzzardi LJ. Inhalation of products of combustion. *Ann Emerg Med* 12:628, 1983.

Dimick A, Wagner RG. A matter of burns and breath. *Emerg Med* 22(13):123, 1990.

DiVincenti FC, Pruitt BA Jr, Reckler JM. Inhalation injuries. *J Trauma* 11:109, 1971.

Fein A. Toxic gas inhalation. *Emerg Med* 21(7):53, 1989.

Fein A, Leff A, Hopewell PC. Pathophysiology and management of the complications resulting from fire and the inhaled products of combustion. *Crit Care Med* 8:94, 1980.

Hedges JR. Acute noxious gas exposure. *Curr Top Emerg Med* 2(10), 1978.

Heimbach DM, Waeckerle JF. Inhalation injuries. *Ann Emerg Med* 17:1316, 1988.

Injury through inspiration. *Emerg Med* 17(19):20, 1985.

Moylan JA, Chan CK. Inhalation injury: An increasing problem. *Ann Surg* 188:24, 1978.

Trunkey DD. Inhalation injury. *Surg Clin North Am* 8:1133, 1978.

Venus B et al. Prophylactic intubation and continuous positive airway pressure in the management of inhalation injury in burn victims. *Crit Care Med* 9:519, 1981.

Zarem HA, Rattenborg CC, Harmel MH. Carbon monoxide toxicity in human fire victims. *Arch Surg* 107:851, 1973.

James A. Taylor

1. A 5-year-old child was running with pencil in hand when she fell, and the pencil became impaled in her left eye. In managing this patient, you should

   a. Remove the pencil at once, patch the left eye, and transport.
   b. Remove the pencil at once, patch both eyes, and transport.
   c. Stabilize the pencil in place with a bulky dressing, patch the left eye, and transport.
   d. Stabilize the pencil in place with a bulky dressing, patch both eyes, and transport.
   e. Not waste time with dressings of any kind, but move immediately to the hospital with the patient.

2. The patient's 8-year-old brother, who was running after her and was also carrying a pencil, suffered a similar fate. But when he tripped, his pencil was jammed through his right cheek. In his case you should

   a. Stabilize the pencil in place with a bulky dressing.
   b. Suction out the mouth, and then stabilize the pencil in place with a bulky dressing.
   c. Suction out the mouth and remove the pencil; apply a dressing to the face over the entrance wound.
   d. Suction out the mouth and remove the pencil; pack the inside of the cheek with gauze, and place a dressing over the entrance wound on the face.
   e. Suction out the mouth, remove the pencil, and tape the wound shut with Steristrips.

A85

It's just as mother always said: You shouldn't run with a stick in your hand. Look what can happen.

1. In the management of our young lady with the pencil in her eye, the correct answer is **d: Stabilize the pencil in place with a bulky dressing, patch both eyes, and transport.** As a general rule, one does NOT remove impaled objects (answers a and b) but rather stabilizes them so that there will not be further motion of the impaled object that could aggravate the injury. Failure to stabilize the pencil in place (answer e) could result in its being jarred or ripped to one side during transport. Why does one patch *both* eyes and not just the injured eye (answer c)? Recall that the eyes move consensually, i.e., together. When the right eye sweeps to the right to check out the scene on that side, the left eye moves to the right as well. The object of our treatment is to keep the left eye as still as possible, so that the pencil will not be swung back and forth. Thus we patch both eyes to minimize any right-eye motion that would cause consensual movement of the left eye.

2. Big brother also has an impaled object, but his pencil is impaled in his cheek, not his eye. And the cheek is one of the rare exceptions to our general rule about not removing an impaled object. That is because the cheek is highly vascular, and massive bleeding into the mouth and airway may occur if we cannot apply adequate pressure to the wound. Thus the correct answer is **d: Suction out the mouth and remove the pencil; pack the inside of the cheek with gauze, and place a dressing over the entrance wound on the face.** Our packing and the dressing applied against it from the other side of the cheek should enable good hemorrhage control. Without the packing (answer c), bleeding would continue unchecked into the mouth. One should not attempt to close this or any other wound in the field (answer e), for field conditions do not permit adequate cleaning and debridement of a wound. Applying Steri-strips simply locks the dirt and bacteria in.

FURTHER READING
Abrahamson IA. Management of ocular foreign bodies. *Am Fam Physician* 14:81, 1976.
Caroline NL. *Emergency Care in the Streets* (4th ed.). Boston: Little, Brown, 1991, Ch. 16.
Casey TA. Examination of the eye. *Hosp Med* 7:20, 1971.
The eye emergency: 1. Basic procedures. *Emerg Med* 14(16):163, 1982.
Hale LM. Emergency eye care. *Am Fam Physician* 6:103, 1972.
Havener WH. The injured eyeball. *Emerg Med* 6(2):355, 1974.
Hoffman JR, Neuhaus RW, Baylis HI. Penetrating orbital trauma. *Am J Emerg Med* 1:22, 1983.
Karesh JW. Ocular and periocular trauma. *Emerg Med Serv* 18(6):46, 1989.
Levitsky LR. Ocular examination and contusion injuries. *Emerg Med Serv* 4(1):26, 1975.
Melamed MA. A generalist's guide to eye emergencies. *Emerg Med* 16(3):99, 1984.
Shingleton BJ. A clearer look at ocular emergencies. *Emerg Med* 21(9):52, 1989.
Soll DB, Oh KT. Industrial ocular injuries. *Am Fam Physician* 14:115, 1976.
Thygerson AL. Focus on eye injuries. *Emergency* 13(11):52, 1981.
Weinstock FJ. Blackout. *Emerg Med* 8(12):23, 1976.

A 36-year-old man suffered first- and second-degree burns over 35 percent of his body when a boiler next to which he was working exploded. Indicate which of the following statements about his management are true and which are false.

a. The second-degree burns should be covered immediately with an antibiotic ointment to prevent infection.

TRUE   FALSE

b. Any blisters forming over the second-degree burns should be ruptured with a sterile needle to prevent them from becoming infected.

TRUE   FALSE

c. Cold, sterile compresses should be applied to the burned areas to help relieve pain.

TRUE   FALSE

d. An intravenous infusion should be started, preferably in an unburned extremity, with normal saline solution.

TRUE   FALSE

e. Rings and other constricting items should be removed from burned extremities as early as possible.

TRUE   FALSE

A86

a. The second-degree burns should be covered immediately with an antibiotic ointment to prevent infection.

FALSE! Do NOT put goo on a burn! It will simply have to be scrubbed off in the emergency department, and the patient is in enough pain as it is without having to undergo a session with the scrub brush.

b. Any blisters forming over the second-degree burns should be ruptured with a sterile needle to prevent them from becoming infected.

FALSE. If your aim is to prevent infection, LEAVE THE BLISTERS ALONE. Cover them with soft, bulky, sterile dressings to protect them from being bumped or scraped. Once the blister has ruptured, all the bacteria that have been waiting in line to colonize the wound will have an easy entry. Don't give infection a helping hand; leave the blisters intact.

c. Cold, sterile compresses should be applied to the burned areas to help relieve pain.

TRUE. Pain from first- and second-degree burns can be very severe, and cold compresses often afford significant pain relief. Sterile water poured over a bulky, sterile dressing applied to the wound is suitable for this purpose. Ice packs may be applied over the sterile dressings, but be careful not to leave them in one place too long, for freezing isn't any healthier for tissues than burning is. The Water-Jel dressing is especially designed for burns and provides the desired cooling effect.

d. An intravenous infusion should be started, preferably in an unburned extremity, with normal saline solution.

TRUE. An individual with 35 percent burns can be anticipated to sustain considerable fluid losses across his damaged skin, and volume replacement should be started early with a salt-containing solution. The site for the IV will depend to a large extent upon where the burns are. It is preferable to start the IV in an unburned extremity if you have the option.

e. Rings and other constricting items should be removed from burned extremities as early as possible.

TRUE. A burned extremity can be expected to swell, and it's best to get those rings and bracelets off while you can still do it without a bolt cutter and before they begin to act as tourniquets.

FURTHER READING

Ayvazian BH, Monafo WW. Initial management of the burned patient. *Emerg Med Serv* 5(5):11, 1976.
Bingham HG. Early management of the burned patient. *Emerg Med Serv* 6(5):9, 1977.
Bloch M. Cold water for burns and scalds. *Lancet* 1:695, 1968.
Burns. *Emerg Med* 12(19):135, 1980.
Dimick AR. The burn at first sight. *Emerg Med* 15(15):130, 1983.
Gillespie RW. The burn at first sight. *Emerg Med* 16(4):141, 1984.
Edlich RF et al. Emergency department treatment, triage and transfer protocols for the burn patient. *JACEP* 7:152, 1978.
Edlich RF et al. Prehospital treatment of the burn patient. *EMT J* 2(3):42, 1978.
Gursel E, Tintinalli J. Emergency burn management. *JACEP* 7:209, 1978.
Keswani MH et al. The boiled potato peel as a burn wound dressing: A preliminary report. *Burns* 11:220, 1985.
Klippel AP, Margraf HW, Covey TH. The use of silver-zinc-allantoin powder for the prehospital treatment of burns. *JACEP* 6:184, 1977.
Lloyd JR. Comprehensive burn care. *Emerg Med Serv* 8(1):9, 8(2):16, 1979.
McKinley JC, Jelenko C, Lasseter MC. Call for help: An algorithm for burn assessment, triage and acute care. *JACEP* 5:13, 1976.
Ofeigsson OJ. First-aid treatment of scalds and burns by water cooling. *Postgrad Med* 30:4, 1961.
Raine TJ et al. Cooling the burn wound to maintain microcirculation. *J Trauma* 21:394, 1981.
Rose A. Continuous water baths for burns. *JAMA* 47:1042, 1906.
Rose HW. Initial cold water treatment for burns. *Northwest Med* 35:267, 1936.
Shulman AG. Ice water as primary treatment of burns. *JAMA* 173:1916, 1960.
Thygerson AL. Burn treatment. *Emergency* 15(6):18, 1983.

It's another one of those "possible stroke" calls, and you find yourself on the sixth floor of an office building being escorted down the hall by a harried office manager whose "whole day has been disrupted." In an office at the end of the hall, you find a 20-year-old typist complaining of numbness and tingling around her mouth and in her fingers. You notice that her hands are contorted in a flexed position.

1. She is most likely showing signs of

   a. Stroke
   b. Pulmonary embolism
   c. Hypoglycemia
   d. Hyperventilation syndrome
   e. Subdural hematoma

2. The most appropriate treatment for this patient is to

   a. Administer oxygen, and coach her to slow her breathing.
   b. Administer 50% glucose (D50) IV.
   c. Have the patient breathe into a paper bag.
   d. Administer morphine.
   e. Place the patient in a supine position, and apply the MAST garment.

3. The purpose of this treatment is

   a. To increase the level of oxygen and the level of carbon dioxide in the patient's blood.
   b. To raise the patient's blood sugar level.
   c. To muffle the patient's complaints.
   d. To enable the patient to blow off more CO_2.
   e. To bring the patient's arterial PCO_2 back up toward normal by having her rebreathe her own exhaled CO_2.

A87 Our patient is showing classic signs of the **hyperventilation syndrome** (answer **1d**), particularly the paresthesias (sensations of tingling) around the mouth and in the extremities and the carpopedal spasm (hands contorted in the flexed position). Notice that we mentioned nothing in our question about the patient's breathing; this was not to throw you off the trail but to make the point that often the hyperventilation itself may be very subtle and not immediately apparent. Indeed, when you measure the respiratory rate, it may not be dramatically above normal, for hyperventilation can also occur through hyperpnea (taking deeper breaths than normal). Remember,

MINUTE VOLUME = TIDAL VOLUME × RESPIRATORY RATE

An increase in either (or both) the tidal volume or respiratory rate can increase the minute volume, leading to a fall in arterial PCO_2.

The most appropriate treatment for this patient is to **administer oxygen and coach her to slow her breathing** (answer **2a**). We *used* to recommend having the patient breathe into a paper bag (answer 2c), but that procedure is no longer recommended in circumstances where arterial blood gases are not immediately available. For if the patient is in fact suffering from some condition other than hyperventilation syndrome—for example, an undetected pulmonary embolism—the low oxygen concentrations that will be inhaled from the paper bag after a few breaths could be lethal. Only after the patient's problem has been *proved*, in the emergency department, to be the result of hyperventilation syndrome is it appropriate to teach the patient how to lower her PCO_2 by rebreathing into a paper bag.

It is very worthwhile with such patients to demonstrate to them how their symptoms occur. Once the patient has recovered sufficiently from the acute attack and has calmed down a bit, explain to the patient that it is "overbreathing" that brings on the uncomfortable feelings he or she experiences. Have the patient breathe deeply and rapidly under your supervision until the symptoms recur, and then show the patient once again that by consciously slowing her breathing she can make the symptoms go away. Hyperventilation is often a chronic problem; a patient who understands what causes those symptoms can often learn to control the problem—and you won't get called back to the same office building for the same patient a dozen more times.

Let us look for a moment at some of the incorrect answers. First, the diagnosis: Stroke (answer 1a) would be unusual in a woman of this age, although it can occur, especially in young women taking birth control pills. However, stroke most commonly affects only one side of the body, and carpopedal spasm would be distinctly unusual. A pulmonary embolism large enough to cause symptoms (answer 1b) would be most likely to present as dyspnea, and our patient's complaint was dizziness and paresthesias. It is because we cannot rule out pulmonary embolism, however, that we've become more cautious with paper bags! She was not in any apparent respiratory distress. Hypoglycemia (answer 1c) can cause dizziness and even a whole variety of neurologic symptoms but would be unlikely to cause carpopedal spasm. As to subdural hematoma (answer 1e), there is no history of injury consistent with this diagnosis.

FURTHER READING
Blau JN et al. Unilateral somatic symptoms due to hyperventilation. *Br Med J* 286:1108, 1983.
Callaham M. Hypoxic hazards of traditional paper bag rebreathing in hyperventilation syndrome. *Am J Med* 18:622, 1989.
Caroline NL. *Emergency Care in the Streets* (4th ed.). Boston: Little, Brown, 1991, Ch. 22.
Chelmowski MK, Keelan MH. Hyperventilation and myocardial infarction. *Chest* 93:1095, 1988.
Demeter SL et al. Hyperventilation syndrome and asthma. *Am J Med* 81:989, 1986.
Grossman JE. Paper bag treatment of acute hyperventilation syndrome (letter). *JAMA* 251:2014, 1984.
Pfefer JM. Hyperventilation and the hyperventilation syndrome. *Postgrad Med* 60(Suppl 2):47, 1984.
Rice RL. Symptom patterns of the hyperventilation syndrome. *Am J Med* 8:691, 1950.
Saltzman JA, Heyman A, Sieker HO. Correlation of clinical and physiological manifestations of sustained hyperventilation. *N Engl J Med* 268:1431, 1963.
Smith CW Jr. Hyperventilation syndrome: Bridging the behavioral-organic gap. *Postgrad Med* 78(2):73, 1985.
Wheatley CE. Hyperventilation syndrome: A frequent cause of chest pain. *Chest* 68:195, 1975.
Yu PN et al. Hyperventilation syndrome. *Arch Intern Med* 103:902, 1959.

IF YOU CAN'T STAND THE HEAT, GET OUT OF THE KITCHEN

You are called one hot summer afternoon to a large bakery, where one of the employees has collapsed. As you enter the building, you estimate that the temperature near the ovens must be at least 100°F. The manager leads you to a corner of the bakery, where a somewhat heavy man, who appears to be in his middle 40s, is sitting on the floor. He is complaining of weakness and nausea and states that he began feeling ill about an hour ago. He denies any significant medical history. He has no allergies and takes no medications regularly.

The patient appears ill. His face is pale, and his skin is cold and sweaty. Pulse is 120 and weak, blood pressure is 100/80, and respirations are 20. The remainder of the physical examination is unremarkable.

Among the following possible treatments, select those that you think are appropriate for this patient.

a. Take the patient out of the bakery to a cooler location.
b. Lay the patient down, and elevate his legs.
c. Give the patient a salt-containing fluid, such as Gator-Aid, to drink.
d. Start an IV with D5W to keep the vein open.
e. Start an IV with normal saline, and run it in rapidly.
f. Administer oxygen.
g. Cool the patient down as rapidly as possible with ice baths.
h. Advise the patient not to return to work today.

A88

Our baker is suffering from heat exhaustion, a condition brought on by excessive loss of salt and water through sweating and other mechanisms. Treatment is aimed at (1) removing the precipitating causes (i.e., the exposure to heat) and (2) restoring the salt and water lost from the body. Thus, among the list presented, the appropriate measures for this patient are

a. **Take the patient out of the bakery to a cooler location.** If necessary, remove some of his clothing and sponge him down. Do NOT, however, use ice baths (answer g) in this situation, for they will simply cause the patient to become unnecessarily chilled.

b. **Lay the patient down, and elevate his legs.** Our patient's rapid pulse and relatively low blood pressure indicate that he is already symptomatic from his hypovolemia. Placing him flat will improve the circulation to his brain, and elevating his legs will increase the volume of the systemic circulation by permitting some of the blood that has pooled in his extremities to drain back into the central circulation by gravity.

e. **Start an IV with normal saline, and run it in rapidly.** As mentioned above, the central problem in heat exhaustion is a depletion of salt and water; thus salt and water are what we want to give back. A keep-open line with dextrose will not accomplish this (answer d), nor should a patient who is nauseated and hypotensive be given fluids by mouth (answer c).

f. **Administer oxygen.** The patient probably does not need oxygen, but if you chose to administer it—on the grounds that he is hypotensive and perhaps not well perfused—you certainly won't do him any harm.

h. **Advise the patient not to return to work today.** Often a liter or two of saline will make the victim of heat exhaustion "feel like a new man." The patient may announce that he feels marvelous and wants to return to work. Don't let him. He should take it easy in a cool place for the next 12 to 24 hours to give his body a chance to recover fully from the stress of a hypotensive episode. And when he does return to work, tell him he ought to make certain that he increases his intake of salt and fluids, especially for the duration of the heat wave.

FURTHER READING

Birrer RB. Heat stroke: Don't wait for the classic signs. *Emerg Med* 20(12):9, 1988.
Brill JC. Heat stroke. *Emerg Med Serv* 6(4):44, 1977.
Caroline NL. *Emergency Care in the Streets* (4th ed.). Boston: Little, Brown, 1991, Ch. 31.
Carter WA. Heat emergencies: A guide to assessment and management. *Emerg Med Serv* 9(4):29, 1980.
Clowes GHA, O'Donnell TF. Heat stroke. *N Engl J Med* 291:564, 1974.
Cummins P. Felled by the heat. *Emerg Med* 15(12):94, 1983.
Forester D. Fatal drug-induced heat stroke. *JACEP* 7:243, 1978.
Graham BS et al. Nonexertional heatstroke: Physiologic management and cooling in 14 patients. *Arch Intern Med* 146:87, 1986.
Hanson PG. Exertional heat stroke in novice runners. *JAMA* 242:154, 1979.
Hart GR et al. Epidemic classical heat stroke: Clinical characteristics and course of 28 patients. *Medicine* 61:189, 1982.
Jones TS. Morbidity and mortality associated with the July 1980 heat wave in St. Louis and Kansas City, Mo. *JAMA* 247:3327, 1982.
Kerstein MD. Heat illness in hot/humid environment. *Milit Med* 151:308, 1986.
Kilbourne EM et al. Risk factors for heatstroke. *JAMA* 247:3362, 1982.
Knochel JP. Environmental heat illness: An eclectic review. *Arch Intern Med* 133:841, 1974.
Knochel JP. Dog days and siriasis—how to kill a football player. *JAMA* 233:513, 1975.
Kunkel DB. The ills of heat. Part I: Environmental causes. *Emerg Med* 18(14):173, 1986.
Larkin JT. Treatment of heat-related illness. *JAMA* 245:570, 1981.
Parks FB, Calabro JJ. Hyperthermia: Performing when the heat is on. *JEMS* 15(8):24, 1990.
Sawka MN et al. Influence of hydration level and body fluids on exercise performance in the heat. *JAMA* 252:1165, 1984.
Slovis CM, Anderson GF, Casolaro A. Survival in a heat stroke victim with a core temperature in excess of 46.5°C. *Ann Emerg Med* 11:269, 1982.
Sprung CL. Heat stroke: Modern approach to an ancient disease. *Chest* 77:461, 1980.
Stine RJ. Heat illness. *JACEP* 8:154, 1979.
Surpure JS. Heat-related illness and the automobile. *Ann Emerg Med* 11:263, 1982.
Tintinalli JE. Heat stroke. *JACEP* 5:525, 1976.
Wettach JE, Smith DS, Stalling CE. EMS protocol for management of heat emergencies during a heat wave in an urban population. *EMT J* 5(5):328, 1981.

A 28-year-old man was thrown against the steering wheel in a two-car collision. The front end of the patient's car is crumpled, and the steering column is bent. The patient is conscious and complaining of chest pain and difficulty in breathing. His skin is pale and somewhat gray. Pulse is 120, respirations are 32 and shallow, and blood pressure is 90/60. The neck veins are slightly distended, and the trachea is deviated to the left. Breath sounds are diminished on the right, and there is hyperresonance to percussion over the right lung field.

1. The patient probably has sustained

   a. A tension pneumothorax on the right
   b. A tension pneumothorax on the left
   c. A simple pneumothorax on the right
   d. A hemothorax on the right
   e. A hemothorax on the left

2. The *first* thing to do for this patient is

   a. Start an IV with normal saline or Ringer's solution.
   b. Apply military antishock trousers.
   c. Administer oxygen.
   d. Intubate the trachea.
   e. Insert a chest tube on the left side.

A89

The correct answer to part 1 is **a**: The patient probably has **a tension pneumothorax on the right.**

Let us examine the clues in the patient's history and physical examination. To begin with, the circumstances of the injury should automatically arouse suspicion of a possible chest injury, for this patient was thrown forward with sufficient force to bend the steering column. Furthermore, the patient tells us that he is having trouble breathing, and his tachypnea and shallow ventilations attest to this. His rapid pulse and low blood pressure could be signs of significant internal bleeding, but they may also be signs of pressure in the chest cavity that is preventing adequate venous return to the heart and thereby decreasing cardiac output. At this point, we simply don't know; however, the distended neck veins certainly suggest that there is either an increase in intrapleural pressure or right heart failure, for if the patient were simply in hemorrhagic shock, we would expect his neck veins to be collapsed.

Next, we note that the trachea is deviated to the left. That narrows down the possibilities to (1) a massive hemothorax on the right, which is pushing the whole mediastinum to the left, or (2) a tension pneumothorax on the right, also pushing the whole mediastinum to the left. (In simple pneumothorax, the trachea would tend to deviate, if at all, *toward* the side of the pneumothorax; thus in simple pneumothorax on the right [answer c], the trachea would deviate to the right side, not to the left.) Auscultation of the lungs confirms that the problem is on the right side, for breath sounds on that side are diminished, but it does not help us to distinguish between our two remaining possibilities. Percussion over the chest is very helpful, however, for the right side is hyperresonant (i.e., has a more hollow sound), suggesting a cavity filled with air: a pneumothorax. If the right chest were filled with blood, we would expect it to sound dull to percussion.

The *first* thing to do for this patient is to **administer oxygen** (answer **2c**). Granted it will be important to decompress the pneumothorax with a chest tube (but *not* on the *left* side!—answer 2e), but that maneuver will take a little time; meanwhile it is important to try to overcome this patient's significant shunt and attendant hypoxemia with high concentrations of inhaled oxygen. The patient will also need an IV line (answer 2a), but that too can wait a few minutes, until you've started the oxygen. The military antishock trousers (MAST) are not called for at this time (answer 2b). The MAST is relatively contraindicated in cases of chest trauma, although it may be used when there is massive hemorrhage and adequate perfusion cannot otherwise be maintained. But at this point, we simply don't know to what extent our patient's hypotension is due to his pneumothorax, and until we decompress his chest, we cannot really evaluate this factor. The fact that the patient is conscious and alert is encouraging, for it indicates at least that his brain is still being well perfused. So we will hold off with the MAST. As to endotracheal intubation (answer 2d), in this case there is no indication for this procedure in the field; the patient is awake and fully capable of protecting his airway, and you would have quite a battle on your hands if you did try to intubate him.

FURTHER READING

Archer GJ et al. Results of simple aspiration of pneumothoraces. *Br J Chest Dis* 79:12, 1985.

Bayne CG. Pulmonary complications of the McSwain Dart. *Ann Emerg Med* 11:136, 1982.

Cannon WB, Mark JBD, Jamplis RW. Pneumothorax: A therapeutic update. *Am J Surg* 142:26, 1981.

Caroline NL. *Emergency Care in the Streets* (4th ed.). Boston: Little, Brown, 1991, Ch. 17.

Clevenger FW, Yarbrough DR, Reines HD. Resuscitative thoracotomy: The effect of field time on outcome. *J Trauma* 28:441, 1988.

Delius RE et al. Catheter aspiration for simple pneumothorax. *Arch Surg* 124:833, 1989.

Ferko JG, Singer EM. Injuries to the thorax. *Emergency* 22(4):20, 1990.

Frame SB, McSwain NE. Chest trauma. *Emergency* 21(7):22, 1989.

Guyton SW, Paull DL, Anderson RP. Introducer insertion of mini-thoracostomy tubes. *Am J Surg* 155:693, 1988.

Hansbrough JF, Chandler JE. Lung laceration following catheter insertion into the chest for pneumothorax. *Emerg Med Serv* 8(2):48, 1979.

McSwain NE Jr. A thoracostomy tube for field and emergency department use. *JACEP* 6:324, 1977.

Mukherjee D et al. A simple treatment for pneumothorax. *Surg Gynecol Obstet* 156:499, 1983.

Raja OG et al. Simple aspiration of spontaneous pneumothorax. *Br J Dis Chest* 75:207, 1981.

Semrad N. A new technique for closed thoracostomy insertion of chest tube. *Surg Gynecol Obstet* 166:171, 1988.

Smith MG. Penetrating the complexities of chest trauma. *JEMS* 14(8):50, 1989.

Vallee P et al. Sequential treatment of a simple pneumothorax. *Ann Emerg Med* 17:936, 1988.

Wayne MA, McSwain NE. Clinical evaluation of a new device for treatment of tension pneumothorax. *Ann Surg* 191:760, 1980.

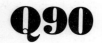
You are called about 7:00 A.M. to see one of your "regulars," a 55-year-old known alcoholic who is often brought into the emergency room because of intoxication or various injuries sustained while in that state. Today he is complaining of "pain all over." He states that for the past several hours he has felt very dizzy and has had a severe headache. He has also had intense abdominal pain, and he vomited several times during the night. Furthermore, he tells you, "everything looks blurry." He denies taking any medications or whiskey, but on close questioning he reluctantly admits that he did "take a little nip" of antifreeze last night when he found he didn't have the money to buy a more conventional beverage. He shows you the antifreeze container, and you note that the main ingredient is listed as methyl alcohol.

On physical examination, you find the patient alert and in moderate distress. Pulse is 100 and regular, blood pressure is 130/80, and respirations are 24. The pupils are dilated and barely react to light. There is no jugular venous distention. The chest is clear. Heart sounds are well heard. The abdomen is somewhat rigid and quite tender to palpation. Extremities are within normal limits, save for the usual collection of bumps and bruises.

Which of the following is NOT part of the management of this patient?

a. Start an IV.
b. Administer sodium bicarbonate, at an initial dose of 50 to 100 ml IV.
c. Give the patient a shot of Scotch (PO).
d. Administer diazepam (Valium), 5 to 10 mg slowly IV.
e. Transport the patient to the hospital for evaluation.

A90 Diazepam (Valium) is NOT part of the management of this patient (answer **d**). Methyl alcohol (methanol), like its cousin ethyl alcohol (ethanol), is likely to cause central nervous system depression, and one needn't add to that effect by administering yet another central nervous system depressant.

All of the other items listed *are* part of the appropriate management of this patient. The IV line (answer a) will be needed as a route for administration of sodium bicarbonate (answer b), which is given to combat the profound metabolic acidosis seen in cases of methanol intoxication. And, believe it or not, a shot of Scotch now and at 4-hour intervals hereafter is just what the doctor ordered (answer c). The signs and symptoms of methanol poisoning are due primarily to the accumulation of toxic products of methanol metabolism, especially formaldehyde. But the enzyme system that converts methanol to formaldehyde will preferentially use ethanol (whose metabolic products are not so toxic); thus the administration of ethanol (which is the type of alcohol in alcoholic beverages) will help to depress the metabolism of methanol and enable the latter to be excreted unchanged in the urine.

It could be argued that it is not a good idea to give anything by mouth to a patient who has been vomiting and is now complaining of abdominal pain. That is a reasonable point of view. If oral administration is considered undesirable, ethyl alcohol can also be given IV, in 5% concentration in a solution of saline or bicarbonate.

Needless to say, even though this patient is one of your "regulars," he is severely ill and needs to be evaluated in the hospital (answer e). He may require dialysis and monitoring in an intensive care unit.

FURTHER READING

Becker C. Acute methanol poisoning: "The blind drunk." *West J Med* 135:122, 1981.
Bennet IL Jr et al. Acute methyl alcohol poisoning: A review based on experiences in an outbreak of 323 cases. *Medicine* 32:431, 1953.
Ekins BR et al. Standardized treatment of severe methanol poisoning with ethanol and hemodialysis. *West J Med* 142:337, 1985.
Keyvn-Larijarni H, Tannenberg AM. Methanol intoxication. *Arch Intern Med* 134:293, 1974.
Peterson CD. Oral ethanol doses in patients with methanol poisoning. *Am J Hosp Pharm* 38:1024, 1981.
Smith ME. Inter-relations in ethanol and methanol metabolism. *J Pharmacol Exp Ther* 134:233, 1961.
Tintinalli J. Of anions, osmoles, and methanol poisoning. *JACEP* 6:417, 1977.

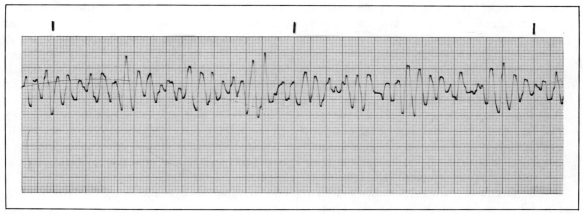

Figure 12

It's another one of those routine chest pain cases: A 45-year-old man with 1 hour of substernal pain. The patient tells you that he has never had any medical problems before. To the contrary, he has been in excellent health, and he runs 5 miles every day before breakfast. He denies any allergies, and he takes no medications regularly save for vitamin pills. On physical examination, he appears pale and apprehensive, but otherwise in no extreme distress. His pulse is 100 and regular, blood pressure is 140/88, and respirations are 16. There are no remarkable findings in the secondary survey.

You connect the patient to the monitor and see that he is in sinus rhythm with an occasional PVC. As your partner is assembling the equipment to start an IV, the patient's eyes suddenly roll back and he loses consciousness. You can no longer palpate a pulse, and the patient has ceased breathing. The monitor now shows the rhythm in Figure 12.

1. The dysrhythmia shown above is

   a. Atrial fibrillation
   b. Atrial flutter
   c. Ventricular tachycardia
   d. Ventricular fibrillation
   e. Supraventricular tachycardia

2. Your *first* action on observing this rhythm under the circumstances stated should be

   a. Administer oxygen.
   b. Immediately countershock at 200–300 joules.
   c. Start the IV, and administer 100 mg of lidocaine by bolus injection.
   d. Start the IV, and administer 50 mg of procainamide (Pronestyl) by bolus injection.
   e. Start the IV, administer 5 ml of 1:10,000 epinephrine, then countershock.

A91

1. The dysrhythmia shown is a fairly classic, coarse **ventricular fibrillation** (answer d)—entirely chaotic, lacking in true complexes, wholly irregular.

2. In the situation of *witnessed* ventricular fibrillation, the first step in treatment is **immediate countershock** (answer b), for the more quickly the shock can be delivered to a well-oxygenated patient, the more likely it is to be successful in converting the rhythm back to sinus.

    Answer a was a trick. Of course the patient should receive oxygen, but he should have been receiving it already, *before* he went into ventricular fibrillation. THE FIRST STEP OF MANAGEMENT UPON REACHING A MIDDLE-AGED OR OLDER PATIENT COMPLAINING OF CHEST PAIN IS TO ADMINISTER OXYGEN. Remember?

    Lidocaine (answer c) will be needed after you have countershocked the patient, to stabilize his rhythm—or, in the event that countershock is unsuccessful, to provide more favorable circumstances for successful conversion to sinus rhythm with the next shock. So don't put away the IV set. Just put it aside until after you've tried a 200–300 joule shock. Then get the IV in as rapidly as possible, and administer lidocaine.

    Procainamide (Pronestyl, answer d) is a second-line antiarrhythmic drug, and we will not need it unless countershock and lidocaine fail to produce a stable rhythm.

    Epinephrine (answer e) is administered as soon as possible in *unwitnessed* cardiac arrest in an attempt to create a more favorable condition for effective countershock. During the first minute or so after *witnessed* cardiac arrest, it is unlikely that the patient's endogenous adrenalin stores are yet depleted, and the situation should be optimal for successful defibrillation.

    So it wasn't just "another one of those routine chest pain cases," was it? The moral is clear: THERE IS NO SUCH THING AS A ROUTINE CASE OF CHEST PAIN.

FURTHER READING

Adgey AAJ et al. Initiation of ventricular fibrillation outside hospital in patients with acute ischaemic heart disease. *Br Heart J* 47:55, 1982.

Bilitch M. *A Manual of Cardiac Arrhythmias.* Boston: Little, Brown, 1971.

Campbell RWF. Treatment and prophylaxis of ventricular arrhythmias in acute myocardial infarction. *Am J Cardiol* 52:55C, 1983.

Caroline NL. *Emergency Care in the Streets* (4th ed.). Boston: Little, Brown, 1991, Ch. 23.

Cooke DH. Ventricular fibrillation: The state of the art. *Emerg Med* 18(5):115, 1986.

Copass M, Eisenberg MS, Damon SK. *EMT Defibrillation* (3rd ed.). Westport, CT: Emergency Training, 1989.

Cranefield PF. Ventricular fibrillation. *N Engl J Med* 289:732, 1973.

Dubin D. *Rapid Interpretation of EKGs* (3rd ed.). Tampa: Cover, 1974.

Frank MJ. Restoring ventricular rhythm. *Emerg Med* 15(2):51, 1983.

Liberthson RB et al. Pathophysiologic observations on prehospital ventricular fibrillation and sudden cardiac death. *Circulation* 49:790, 1974.

McDonald JL. Coarse ventricular fibrillation presenting as asystole or very low amplitude ventricular fibrillation. *Crit Care Med* 10:790, 1982.

Schaeffer WA, Cobb LA. Recurrent ventricular fibrillation and modes of death in out-of-hospital ventricular fibrillation. *N Engl J Med* 293:259, 1975.

Stein RA et al. The modern monitor-defibrillator: A potential source of falsely abnormal ECG recordings. *JAMA* 246:1697, 1981.

You have performed endotracheal intubation on a patient in cardiac arrest. On auscultation of the patient's chest, you cannot hear breath sounds on the left side. What has most likely happened?

a. The endotracheal tube is in the esophagus.
b. The endotracheal tube is in the right main bronchus.
c. The patient has a pneumothorax on the left as a result of the intubation attempt.
d. It is normal not to hear breath sounds on the left side because the heart muffles them.

In the above situation, you should

a. Pull back the tube very slightly, ventilate through it again, and recheck both lung fields for breath sounds.
b. Immediately deflate the cuff and remove the tube.
c. Decompress the chest with a large-gauge Intracath and flutter valve.
d. Insert the tube a few centimeters farther, and secure it in place with tape.

A92 The correct answer to the first part is **b**: The endotracheal tube has probably come to rest in the right main bronchus; thus when you ventilate through it, the right lung is ventilated, but the left lung is not, so the movement of air is heard only on the right side of the chest. If the endotracheal tube were in the esophagus (answer a)—a very common problem, but not the problem with our patient—breath sounds would be absent on BOTH sides of the chest, while the movement of air could be heard on auscultation over the epigastrium. Pneumothorax (answer c) would be an extraordinarily unusual complication of an intubation attempt; and had the patient suffered a pneumothorax *prior to* resuscitation, ventilation through a properly placed endotracheal tube would be expected to reinflate the collapsed lung—thus breath sounds would be audible on both sides of the chest. It *is* normal to hear breath sounds on the left, the presence of the heart notwithstanding (answer d). For checking the position of an endotracheal tube, it is best to listen over the apex (superior portion) of the lung on each side, where breath sounds can be expected to be equal if both lungs are being ventilated adequately.

In a situation where the endotracheal tube has been inadvertently inserted too far and comes to rest in the right main bronchus, the appropriate action to take is to **pull back the tube very slightly, ventilate through it again, and recheck both lung fields for breath sounds** (answer **a**). Do NOT, for heaven's sake, remove the tube altogether (answer b)! THE SECOND INTUBATION ATTEMPT IS ALWAYS MORE DIFFICULT THAN THE FIRST! Just keep pulling the tube back, a centimeter at a time, and rechecking its position by auscultating both lung fields. When breath sounds are heard equally well at both apexes, secure the tube in place and mark the tube at the point where it emerges from the patient's mouth (so you can determine later whether it has slipped in or out). Clearly, inserting the tube even farther (answer d) will only compound the situation. And there is no indication whatsoever that this patient has suffered a pneumothorax, so there is no need to start sticking needles in his chest (answer c).

FURTHER READING
Applebaum AL, Bruce DW. *Tracheal intubation.* Philadelphia: Saunders, 1976.
Chander S et al. Correct placement of endotracheal tubes. *NY State J Med* 79:1843, 1979.
DeLeo BC. Endotracheal intubation by rescue squad personnel. *Heart & Lung* 6:851, 1977.
Geehr EC et al. Prehospital tracheal intubation versus esophageal gastric tube airway use: A prospective study. *Am J Emerg Med* 3:381, 1985.
Guss DA, Posluszny M. Paramedic orotracheal intubation: A feasibility study. *Am J Emerg Med* 2:399, 1984.
Jacobs LM et al. Endotracheal intubation in the prehospital phase of emergency medical care. *JAMA* 250:2175, 1983.
Johnson KG et al. Esophageal perforation associated with endotracheal intubation. *Anesthesiology* 64:281, 1986.
Kacmarek RM. The art of artificial airways. *Emerg Med* 16(17):30, 1984.
Natanson C, Shelhamer J, Perrillo J. Intubation of the trachea in the critical care setting. *JAMA* 253:1160, 1985.
Pepe PE, Copass MK, Joyce TH. Prehospital endotracheal intubation: Rationale for training emergency medical personnel. *Ann Emerg Med* 14:1085, 1985.
Salem MR, Mathrubhutham J, Bennet EJ. Difficult intubation. *N Engl J Med* 295:879, 1976.
Scott DB. Endotracheal intubation: Friend or foe? *Br Med J* 292:157, 1986.
Shapiro BA. Airway access in the struggling patient. *Emerg Med* 16(7):102, 1984.
Stein JM. Difficult adult intubation. *Emerg Med* 17(3):121, 1985.
Stein JM. Endotracheal intubation in a hurry. *Emerg Med* 14(15):129, 1982.
Stein JM. Nasotracheal intubation. *Emerg Med* 16(13):183, 1984.
Stewart RD et al. Field endotracheal intubation by paramedical personnel: Success rates and complications. *Chest* 85:341, 1984.
Stewart RD et al. Effect of varied training techniques on field endotracheal intubation success rates. *Ann Emerg Med* 13:1032, 1984.
Stewart RD, Paris PM. Signs of endotracheal intubation in the field setting (letter). *Ann Emerg Med* 14:276, 1985.
Vollmer TP et al. Use of a lighted stylet for guided orotracheal intubation in the prehospital setting. *Ann Emerg Med* 14:324, 1985.
White RD, Billes BP. Endotracheal vs. esophageal intubation. *Emergency* 10(9):49, 1978.

You are called to a small farm about 10 miles from your station for a "sick man." The farm manager tells you that one of his temporary workers has been spraying insecticides for the past few days, and today he has begun complaining of abdominal cramps and diarrhea. You find the worker in considerable distress. He is pale, sweating profusely, and coughing up watery sputum. Pulse is 52 and slightly irregular, blood pressure is 150/90, and respirations are 30 and shallow. Pupils are constricted. There is no jugular venous distention. Scattered wheezes are heard throughout the chest. Bowel sounds are noisy and hyperactive. There are fine twitches in the muscles of the extremities.

Which of the following is NOT part of the management of this patient?

a. Remove the patient's clothes, and wash his skin thoroughly with soap and water.
b. Start an IV with D5W.
c. Administer morphine, 5 to 10 mg slowly IV.
d. Administer oxygen at a high concentration.
e. Administer atropine, 2 mg IM.

A93

Our farm worker is displaying classic signs of organophosphate poisoning. Organophosphates are found in many insecticides (e.g., in parathion, malathion, TEPP, HETP, OMPA) and are very potent *anticholinesterases*. That means that they interfere with the enzyme (cholinesterase) that ordinarily functions at the interface between nerve and muscle to inactivate the transmitter substance acetylcholine. The result is that acetylcholine, instead of being neutralized after it has given its message to the muscle, remains active, so there is constant stimulation of the muscles involved. The clinical picture is thus one of massive, total stimulation of the parasympathetic nervous system.

Administration of morphine (answer **c**) is definitely NOT part of the management of this patient, even though he seems to (and may, in fact) be manifesting signs of pulmonary edema. Morphine has its own parasympathetic-like effects, which will only aggravate this patient's problem.

Vigorous washing of the whole body with soap and water (answer a) is a very important part of the therapy of this patient, for organophosphate insecticides are rapidly absorbed through intact skin. The IV line (answer b) will be needed as a lifeline in the event that resuscitative drugs must be administered. High concentrations of oxygen are indicated because the patient is likely to have a high degree of shunt (answer d), owing to copious bronchial secretions. Finally, atropine (answer e) is a specific antidote for anticholinesterases, for atropine opposes the effects of acetylcholine at the neuromuscular junction. A dose of 2 mg is given IM and repeated every 10 minutes until the signs of the poisoning are controlled—which may require very high cumulative doses of atropine. An intravenous dose of 1 to 2 mg may be given at the same time as the intramuscular dose to permit a more immediate therapeutic effect.

FURTHER READING

Done AK. Autonomic toxicology primer. *Emerg Med* 15(13):134, 1983.
Done AK. Autonomics unravelled: I. Cholinergics. *Emerg Med* 15(14):287, 1983.
Done AK. Nerve gases in the war against pests. *Emerg Med* 5(5):250, 1973.
Heath DF. *Organophosphate Poisons.* Oxford: Pergamon, 1961.
Midtling JE et al. Clinical management of field worker organophosphate poisoning. *West J Med* 142:514, 1985.
The toxic effects of agriculture. *Emerg Med* 16(11):119, 1984.
Wyckoff DW et al. Diagnostic and therapeutic problems of parthion poisonings. *Ann Intern Med* 68:875, 1968.

A high school student was working in the chemistry laboratory when some hydrochloric acid splashed into his right eye.

1. The correct treatment for this emergency is

   a. Flush the eye for at least 20 minutes with water.
   b. Flush the eye for 30 to 60 seconds with water; more flushing won't do any good.
   c. Flush the eye with soap solution in order to neutralize the hydrochloric acid.
   d. Patch the eye immediately without flushing.

2. How would you modify your management of this case if the student was wearing contact lenses?

A94

The correct answer to part 1 is **a: Flush the eye for at least 20 minutes with water.** A few squirts of water delivered over 30 to 60 seconds is NOT sufficient (answer b), and the eye should NEVER be rinsed with any liquids other than water or saline (answer c). Chemical antidotes are NOT used in the eyes. Patching the eye without flushing it out (answer d) will leave the hydrochloric acid in contact with the corneal surface, allowing the chemical burn to progress. The principle of treatment is to remove the chemical from contact with the patient's eye, and that can only be accomplished by copious flushing over an adequate period of time.

If the student is wearing contact lenses, the **lenses should be removed** prior to flushing, for otherwise they will serve as a reservoir for the caustic chemical and hinder the removal of the chemical from the eye. Usually, the patient will be able to remove his contact lenses himself, but if not, you should hold his eye open and remove the contact lens with a small suction bulb designed especially for this purpose. The bulb is available from any optician and should be standard equipment aboard the ambulance.

FURTHER READING

Casey TA. Examination of the eye. *Hosp Med* 7:20, 1971.
The eye emergency:
    1. Basic procedures. *Emerg Med* 14(16):163, 1982.
    2. Burns about the eye. *Emerg Med* 14(17):232, 1982.
Hale LM. Emergency eye care. *Am Fam Physician* 6:103, 1972.
Jelenko C. Chemical burns. *Emerg Med* 5(6):33, 1973.
Luterman A, Fields C, Curreri W. Treatment of chemical burns. *Emerg Med Serv* 17(9): 36, 1988.
Melamed MA. A generalist's guide to eye emergencies. *Emerg Med* 16(3):99, 1984.
Shingleton BJ. A clearer look at ocular emergencies. *Emerg Med* 21(9):52, 1989.
Soll DB, Oh KT. Industrial ocular injuries. *Am Fam Physician* 14:115, 1976.
Thygerson AL. Focus on eye injuries. *Emergency* 13(11):52, 1981.

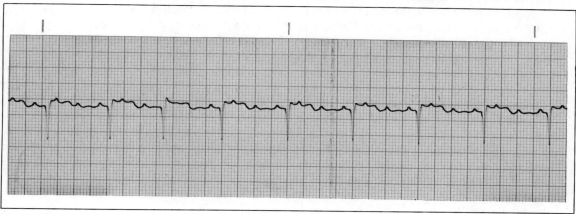

Figure 13

There's usually one on every shift, a patient whose chief complaint is "sick all over." On your shift, it is a 68-year-old woman who lives alone in a housing project on the west side of town. She is an impressively fat woman, who has a long list of complaints to communicate to you, chief among which seem to be weakness, dizziness, and a "sick feeling" all afternoon. She is apparently under treatment for several dozen maladies, including "rheumatism," rashes, "blood pressure," backaches, chronic indigestion, headaches, and constipation. She is allergic to tomatoes, strawberries, and "little white pills." On physical examination, she appears somewhat pale and apprehensive. Her pulse is strong. Blood pressure is 170/98, and respirations are 20 per minute. There are no remarkable findings on physical examination, save for a scattered, erythematous rash on the extremities. The patient's ECG tracing is shown in Figure 13.

1. Examine the patient's rhythm strip:

   a. The rhythm is _____ regular _____ irregular.
   b. The rate is _____ per minute.

2. The ECG pattern is

   a. Normal sinus rhythm
   b. Atrial flutter
   c. Second-degree block: Wenckebach
   d. Paroxysmal atrial tachycardia (PAT) with block
   e. Complete heart block

3. Which of the following statements about this patient is true?

   a. Her rhythm may be normal in older patients and is not necessarily indicative of cardiac disease.
   b. Her symptoms are probably attributable to dietary indiscretion.
   c. She may be suffering an acute myocardial infarction (AMI).
   d. She is probably simply a "crock" and does not really need to be evaluated in the hospital.

4. Which of the following is NOT part of the management of this patient?

   a. Administer oxygen.
   b. Start an IV with D5W.
   c. Administer atropine, 0.02 mg per kilogram IV.
   d. Continue monitoring the patient's cardiac rhythm.
   e. All of the above.

A95

1. The patient's rhythm is **basically regular** save for one beat (the third QRS complex shown); the rate is **approximately 75 per minute.**

2. The ECG pattern is that of **PAT with block** (answer **d**); only every third P wave is conducted through to the ventricles. Since the P–R intervals of the conducted P waves are fixed, this is not Wenckebach (answer **c**), for Wenckebach is characterized by progressive prolongation of the P–R interval until there is a dropped beat. It is not normal sinus rhythm (answer **a**), for not every P wave is followed by a QRS complex; indeed, only one out of three P waves is conducted. We do not see the sawtooth pattern characteristic of atrial flutter (answer **b**), and the fixed relationship between the P waves and fairly normal QRS complexes makes complete heart block unlikely (answer **e**).

3. The only statement on the list that is true is that our fat lady **may be suffering an acute myocardial infarction** (answer **c**). Don't write her off just because she wasn't obliging enough to give you a classic history for AMI. Remember, in older patients the classic signs and symptoms of AMI may be entirely absent, and AMI can present simply as weakness, confusion, or a general feeling of being ill.

    PAT with block is never a "normal" rhythm (answer **a**) and must be taken seriously. It is often a sign of toxicity.

    While there is every reason to believe that this patient regularly commits all sorts of dietary indiscretions (answer **b**), there are no grounds to attribute her current symptoms to this source. Fat people get sick too, indeed they are often more prone to illness than their lean contemporaries.

    A paramedic or any other health professional who uses terms such as "crock" (answer **d**) or "turkey" to refer to a patient simply displays his own immaturity and unsuitability for medical work. THE USE OF DEROGATORY TERMS TO REFER TO PATIENTS IS INEXCUSABLE! Any person who turns to a health professional for help clearly feels a need for help. It is not up to you to pass judgment on the patient's distress. Furthermore, any time one dismisses a patient's complaints as "functional" or "imaginary," one runs an enormous risk of overlooking serious medical pathology. Had you decided, for example, that our fat lady was "just another crock" who did not warrant an electrocardiogram, you might well have overlooked a possible AMI and a potentially dangerous cardiac dysrhythmia.

    The moral: DO NOT DISMISS A LONG LIST OF COMPLAINTS AS A SIGN OF TRIVIAL ILLNESS. THE PATIENT WHO IS "SICK ALL OVER" MAY BE VERY SICK INDEED.

4. Administration of atropine is NOT part of the management of this patient (answer **c**). The rate is not dangerously slow, and certainly it is not such as to compromise cardiac output. Assuming that one could abolish the block entirely with atropine (and that assumption is highly unlikely) and enable every P wave to be conducted, this patient would then have a ventricular rate of 150 (her current atrial rate—measure it and see), and that *would* compromise her cardiac output. Thus at the moment, there is no need to fool with the cardiac rhythm. The patient simply needs the standard measures for any patient with suspected myocardial infarction: oxygen (answer **a**), an IV lifeline (answer **b**), and continuous cardiac monitoring (answer **d**).

FURTHER READING

Bilitch M. *A Manual of Cardiac Arrhythmias.* Boston: Little, Brown, 1971.
Caroline NL. *Emergency Care in the Streets* (4th ed.). Boston: Little, Brown, 1991, Ch. 23.
Dubin D. *Rapid Interpretation of EKGs* (3rd ed.). Tampa: Cover, 1974.

3:15 A.M. The call comes in as a "woman with a headache." Ten minutes later you arrive at the designated address, an apartment building downtown, and are admitted to a modest flat by an anxious, sleepy man in his late 20s. He tells you that his wife, who is near the end of her last trimester of pregnancy, has been complaining of a severe headache and has become very restless.

You find the patient sitting up in bed. She appears to be in moderate distress, and you immediately notice that she has diffuse edema, even around her face. Her pulse is 80 and regular, blood pressure is 170/100, and respirations are 14. Fetal heart sounds are audible.

Which of the following is NOT part of the management of this patient?

a. Position the patient on her side in a darkened area.
b. Administer oxygen.
c. Draw up 5 to 10 mg of diazepam (Valium) in a syringe, and tape the syringe to the stretcher to have ready if seizures occur.
d. Start an IV and administer magnesium sulfate, 2 to 4 gm of a 10% solution IV.
e. Get the patient to the hospital as rapidly as possible, using full lights and sirens to expedite passage through traffic.

A96 Answer **e** is NOT part of the management of this patient. Our young woman is suffering from eclampsia, and unless you want to take care of a grand mal seizure, do not subject this lady to flashing lights and wailing sirens. Sensory stimulation should be kept to an absolute minimum: Keep the lights low while attending her at home (answer a), carry her gently and quietly to the ambulance, make her comfortable inside the ambulance, and see to it that she has a smooth, *quiet* ride to the hospital. Even with those precautions, seizures may occur. We try to minimize the possibility further by giving magnesium sulfate (answer d), but should seizure activity commence despite all our precautions, we should have diazepam (Valium) ready for immediate administration (answer c). Oxygen therapy (answer b) is undertaken mainly as a precautionary measure; in the event that seizures do occur, the preoxygenation will give mother and baby an added reserve to tide them over the drop in PO_2 that is apt to occur during seizure activity.

FURTHER READING
Caroline NL. *Emergency Care in the Streets* (3rd ed.). Boston: Little, Brown, 1987, Ch. 11.
Ferris TF. Hypertensive and pregnant. *Emerg Med* 15(7):29, 1983.
Kaunitz AM et al. Causes of maternal mortality in the United States. *Obstet Gynecol* 65:605, 1985.
Kaplan PW et al. No, magnesium sulfate should not be used in treating eclamptic seizures. *Arch Neurol* 45:1361, 1988.
The many faces of preeclampsia. *Emerg Med* 9(2):289, 1977.
Nixon RG. Third trimester obstetric complications. Part II: Eclampsia and postpartum hemorrhage. *Emerg Med Serv* 10(4):52, 1981.
Ogle ME, Sanders AB. Preeclampsia. *Ann Emerg Med* 13:368, 1984.
Pritchard JA. The use of magnesium sulfate in preeclampsia-eclampsia. *J Reprod Med* 23:107, 1979.
Pritchard JA. Standardized treatment of 154 consecutive cases of eclampsia. *Am J Obstet Gynecol* 123:543, 1975.
Sibai BM et al. Eclampsia: Observations from 67 recent cases. *Obstet Gynecol* 58:609, 1981.
Smith JC et al. An assessment of the incidence of maternal mortality in the United States. *Am J Pub Health* 74:780, 1984.
White JD. Treatment for hypertension with eclampsia. *Ann Emerg Med* 10:166, 1981.

The call is for an "unconscious man" in an apartment building not far from the university. When you arrive, his friends, who seem to have been holding some kind of a party on the premises, tell you that the patient took an overdose of "downers." The patient, a man in his early 20s, is lying unconscious on the sofa, where some of his friends are trying without success to rouse him. They show you the bottle of "yellows" (phenobarbital) that the patient apparently took.

The patient is deeply unconscious and does not respond to pinching or other noxious stimulation. His pulse is 100 and regular, blood pressure is 100/80, and respirations are 10 and shallow. Pupils are dilated and equal and react sluggishly to light. Otherwise the physical examination is unremarkable.

Which of the following is NOT part of the management of this patient?

a. Administer oxygen; assist ventilations as needed.
b. Intubate the trachea.
c. Start an IV line with normal saline solution.
d. Administer naloxone (Narcan), 0.4 mg slowly IV.
e. Administer sodium bicarbonate, 50 to 100 ml IV.

A97 The administration of naloxone (answer **d**) is NOT part of the management of this patient. Naloxone is a very specific antidote for narcotic overdose, and we have no evidence that this patient has taken narcotics. His pupils are dilated, not constricted. We have not found needle tracks on his arms. Nor have we found any medication bottles other than the bottle that had contained phenobarbital.

Oxygen and assisted ventilation (answer a) are clearly indicated, for the patient has obvious signs of respiratory depression: slow, shallow respirations. Because he is deeply comatose, his airway must be protected with a cuffed endotracheal tube as well (answer b), especially if we have any plans to insert a nasogastric tube to flush out the stomach. The IV line (answer c) will enable us to support the patient's circulation with fluids and will give us a route through which we can administer resuscitative drugs, should the need arise. Finally, sodium bicarbonate (answer e) is sometimes used in the treatment of phenobarbital overdose because it promotes the excretion of phenobarbital through the kidneys.

FURTHER READING

Berg MJ et al. Acceleration of the body clearance of phenobarbital by oral activated charcoal. *N Engl J Med* 307:642, 1982.

Costello JB et al. Treatment of massive phenobarbital overdose with dopamine diuresis. *Arch Intern Med* 14:938, 1981.

Done AK. To sleep, perchance to die. *Emerg Med* 7(9):277, 1975.

McCarron MM et al. Short-acting barbiturate overdosage: Correlation of intoxication score with serum barbiturate concentration. *JAMA* 248:55, 1982.

Pond SM et al. Randomized study of the treatment of phenobarbital overdose with repeated doses of activated charcoal. *JAMA* 251:3104, 1984.

Thornton WE. Sleep aids and sedatives. *JACEP* 6:408, 1977.

Wright N. An assessment of the unreliability of the history given by self-poisoned patients. *Clin Toxicol* 16:381, 1980.

For each of the following situations, indicate whether

a. Vomiting should be induced.
b. Vomiting should not be induced.

1. _____ A 3-year-old child who swallowed 40 aspirin tablets 10 minutes before you arrived. The child is awake and crying.
2. _____ A 40-year-old man who drank 200 ml of drain cleaner in a suicide attempt.
3. _____ A 20-year-old woman who swallowed the contents of a bottle of chlorpromazine (Thorazine) in a suicide attempt. She is confused and lapses easily into sleep.
4. _____ A 46-year-old man who ingested 60 diazepam (Valium) pills 45 minutes before you arrived. He is alert and responsive.
5. _____ A 26-year-old man who accidentally ingested about 50 ml of gasoline while siphoning the gas out of his car.
6. _____ A middle-aged philosopher named Socrates, who has just ingested a cup of hemlock.

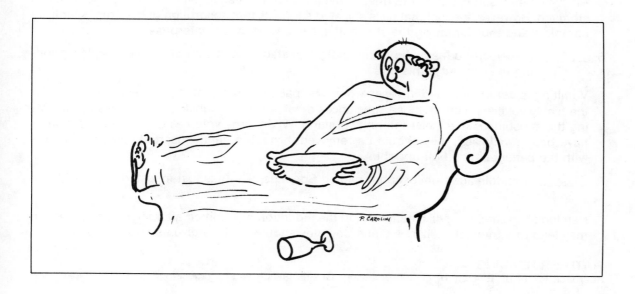

A98

The purpose of inducing vomiting after ingestion of a poison or an excess of some medication is to empty the stomach of whatever residual of the poison may remain there before the toxic substance can be absorbed into the bloodstream. However, there are certain situations in which the induction of vomiting is contraindicated because the potential dangers outweigh the potential benefits.

1. ___a___ A 3-year-old child who swallowed 40 aspirin tablets 10 minutes before you arrived. The child is awake and crying.

There is a very good chance, after only 10 minutes, that a significant amount of the aspirin is still in the child's stomach and thus can be eliminated by vomiting. Furthermore, there is nothing in the child's overall condition to preclude the induction of vomiting: He is wide awake and hence fully able to protect his airway. It probably won't be easy to persuade him to swallow the syrup of ipecac (not to mention the ugly black glop called activated charcoal that you will try to foist on him afterwards!), but it is certainly worthwhile to do so.

2. ___b___ A 40-year-old man who drank 200 ml of drain cleaner in a suicide attempt.

Vomiting should NOT be induced after the ingestion of a caustic chemical. To begin with, the chemical has already doubtless wreaked all sorts of havoc on the esophageal tissues as it made its descent into the stomach; it serves little purpose to bathe the esophagus in drain cleaner a second time in the process of bringing it all back up. Furthermore, the muscular contractions attendant upon vomiting may tear esophageal tissues if they have been seriously damaged by chemicals. Transport this patient rapidly, in a sitting position, to the hospital, where gentle nasogastric intubation may be attempted to lavage and drain the stomach.

3. ___b___ A 20-year-old woman who swallowed the contents of a bottle of chlorpromazine (Thorazine) in a suicide attempt. She is confused and lapses easily into sleep.

There are two good reasons NOT to induce vomiting in this patient. First of all, her overall condition precludes it: She is stuporous, probably on the verge of coma, and by the time your syrup of ipecac would be expected to take effect, she may be entirely unable to protect her airway against aspiration—and by then, don't forget, she'll also have a glass of water added to the contents of her stomach. In the second place, the drug she has taken happens to be an antiemetic, i.e., a medication that prevents vomiting. Thus, if you administer ipecac and then fill her stomach with water in the prescribed fashion, she may not vomit anyway; she may simply fall into coma with a full stomach and then proceed to regurgitate and aspirate the whole lot. If you want to empty her stomach, put in a nasogastric tube—but not before you have protected her airway with a cuffed endotracheal tube.

4. ___a___ A 46-year-old man who ingested 60 diazepam (Valium) pills about 45 minutes before you arrived. He is alert and responsive.

After 45 minutes, it is difficult to guess how much of the Valium still remains in the patient's stomach. However, the fact that he is still alert suggests that absorption of the drug is far from complete and thus emptying the stomach is still a worthwhile enterprise.

5. ___b___ A 26-year-old man who accidentally ingested about 50 ml of gasoline while siphoning the gas out of his car.

Vomiting is contraindicated in cases where the patient has ingested petroleum products, for the highly volatile nature of those substances creates a risk of inhaling their fumes or aspirating the substances themselves during vomiting. When large volumes of petroleum products have been swallowed, they should be removed through a gently inserted nasogastric tube, with the patient sitting bolt upright.

6 ___b___ A middle-aged philosopher named Socrates, who has just ingested a cup of hemlock.

Hemlock has strychnine-like actions, and the induction of vomiting after strychnine ingestion may lead to intractable seizures. Thus Socrates should NOT be given syrup of ipecac.

FURTHER READING
Auerback PS et al. Efficacy of gastric emptying: Gastric lavage versus emesis induced with ipecac. *Ann Emerg Med* 15:692, 1986.

Caroline NL. *Emergency Care in the Streets* (4th ed.). Boston: Little, Brown, 1991, Ch. 27.

Eason J et al. Efficacy and safety of gastrointestinal decontamination in the treatment of oral poisoning. *Pediatr Clin North Am* 26:827, 1979.

Flomenbaum NE, Hoffman R. GI evacuation: Is it still worthwhile? *Emerg Med* 22(2):80, 1990.

Freedman GE, Pasternak S, Krenzelok EP. A clinical trial using syrup of ipecac and activated charcoal concurrently. *Ann Emerg Med* 16:164, 1987.

Grande GA et al. The effect of fluid volume on syrup of ipecac emesis time. *Clin Toxicol* 25:473, 1987.

Ipecac syrup and activated charcoal for treatment of poisoning in children. *Med Lett* 21:70, 1979.

King WD. Syrup of ipecac: A drug review. *Clin Toxicol* 17:353, 1980.

Krenzelok EP et al. Preserving the emetic effect of syrup of ipecac with concurrent activated charcoal administration: A preliminary study. *Clin Toxicol* 24:159, 1986.

Krenzelok EP et al. Effectiveness of 15-ml vs 30-ml doses of syrup of ipecac in children. *Clin Pharm* 6:715, 1987.

Kulig K et al. Management of acutely poisoned patients without gastric emptying. *Ann Emerg Med* 14:562, 1985.

Levy DB. Syrup of ipecac review. *Emergency* 21(12):20, 1989.

Lipscomb JW et al. Response in children to 15-ml or 30-ml doses of ipecac syrup. *Clin Pharm* 5:234, 1986.

Mofenson HC. Benefits/risks of syrup of ipecac. *Pediatrics* 77:551, 1986.

Rumack BH. Ipecac use in the home. *Pediatrics* 75:1148, 1985.

Tandberg D, Diven BG, McLeod JW. Ipecac-induced emesis versus gastric lavage: A controlled study in normal adults. *Am J Emerg Med* 4:205, 1986.

Tenenbein M. Inefficacy of gastric emptying procedures. *J Emerg Med* 3:133, 1985.

Tenenbein M, Cohen S, Sitar DS. Efficacy of ipecac-induced emesis, orogastric lavage, and activated charcoal for acute drug overdose. *Ann Emerg Med* 16:838, 1987.

You are called to the scene of an accident, where an automobile has careened off the road into a ditch. When you arrive, the upholstery of the rear seat of the car and the brush adjacent to the car are on fire. The driver is conscious and screaming that he cannot move his legs.
  You should

a. Carefully extricate the patient from the vehicle with a short and long backboard, since he has very likely sustained an injury to his spinal cord.
b. Summon a fire company to put out the fire before you attempt to extricate the patient.
c. Administer 100% oxygen to the patient immediately, for he is probably suffering from smoke inhalation.
d. Do a thorough secondary survey before attempting to move the patient in any way.
e. Get the patient out of the vehicle and to safe ground as fast as possible, even if this may result in further damage to his spine.

A99 One of the cardinal principles of triage is that THE SALVAGE OF LIFE TAKES PRECEDENCE OVER THE SALVAGE OF LIMB. Thus answer **e** is the correct answer: **Get the patient out of the vehicle and to safe ground as fast as possible, even if this may result in further damage to his spine.** In general, we teach that any patient who may have sustained an injury to his spine should be carefully immobilized on a backboard before he is moved in any way, and under ordinary circumstances, answer a would be correct. But these are not ordinary circumstances. The patient is in a smoldering car, which may at any moment turn into an inferno of blazing gasoline. There simply isn't time to immobilize this patient on a backboard or to do the usual methodical examination (answer d). Certainly there isn't time to wait around for a fire truck to reach the scene (answer b), nor would it improve the situation to fill the automobile with a gas (oxygen, answer c) that supports combustion. In this situation, where the patient's life is at stake (and yours too, if you are caught fiddling around inside the vehicle when the gasoline tank ignites!), you must simply accept the risk that moving the patient may aggravate his spine injury. Get him and yourself to a safe place as rapidly as possible.

FURTHER READING

Caroline NL. *Emergency Care in the Streets* (4th ed.). Boston: Little, Brown, 1991, Ch. 20.
Caroline NL. *Emergency Medical Treatment: A Text for EMT-As and EMT-Intermediates* (3rd ed.). Boston: Little, Brown, 1991. Ch. 18.
Champion HR et al. Assessment of injury severity: The triage index. *Crit Care Med* 8:201, 1980.
Champion HR. Field triage of trauma patients (editorial). *Ann Emerg Med* 11:160, 1982.

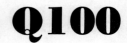
A 34-year-old factory worker was driving home after a hurricane and found the road ahead of him blocked by debris. He got out of his car and began clearing branches from the road. In the course of reaching for a branch, he inadvertently grabbed hold of a downed electric wire and collapsed immediately.

Which of the following statements about electric burns are true and which are false?

a. A current of only 0.1 ampere passing through the heart may cause ventricular fibrillation.

   TRUE   FALSE

b. Alternating current (AC) causes tetanic muscle spasms, which may cause the victim to "freeze" to the current source.

   TRUE   FALSE

c. If a patient who has suffered an electric burn shows little damage to the skin, there is unlikely to be significant injury to tissues inside the body.

   TRUE   FALSE

d. The victim of an electric burn usually has two visible injuries, an entrance burn and an exit burn.

   TRUE   FALSE

e. The *first* step in treating the victim of an electric burn is to determine whether his airway is open.

   TRUE   FALSE

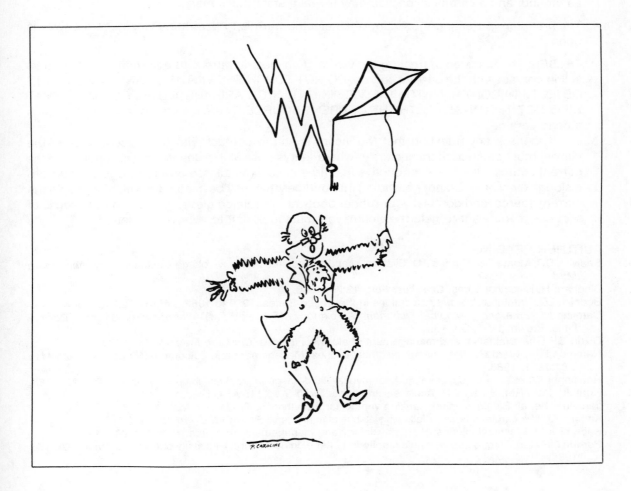

A100

a. A current of only 0.1 ampere passing through the heart may cause ventricular fibrillation.

TRUE. Even small currents, if delivered directly to the heart, may put the heart into fibrillation. Patients sustaining electric burns in which the direction of current flow is across the chest—e.g., an entrance burn on the right hand and an exit burn on the left leg—are particularly at risk of developing this complication. Needless to say, the more powerful the current source, the greater the risk of cardiac arrest, regardless of the path of current flow.

b. Alternating current (AC) causes tetanic muscle spasms, which may cause the victim to "freeze" to the current source.

TRUE. The child who has picked up the frayed end of an electric cord, for example, may clutch the cord with enormous force as the current goes through his hand and sends the hand muscles into spasm. Violent tetanic contractions may occur in all muscle groups, sometimes with sufficient force to fracture long bones.

c. If a patient who has suffered an electric burn shows little damage to the skin, there is unlikely to be significant injury to tissues inside the body.

FALSE! Electric burns may produce devastating damage to internal tissues with scarcely any injury visible on the surface of the body. For that reason, every electric burn must be considered critical until proved otherwise.

d. The victim of an electric burn usually has two visible injuries, an entrance burn and an exit burn.

TRUE, although you may have to hunt very carefully to find them. The entrance burn will usually be more obvious and may show a bull's-eye appearance, with a central, charred zone of third-degree burn, a middle zone of gray, dry tissue, and an outer, red zone. The location of the exit burn will be determined by the route through which the current left the body, i.e., what part of the body served as a ground. Usually, but not invariably, it is one of the feet that served as ground, and a careful inspection may reveal a small black mark.

e. The *first* step in treating the victim of an electric burn is to determine whether his airway is open.

FALSE!!! The first step in treating the victim of an electric burn is to determine whether he is still in contact with the current source. DO NOT TOUCH THE VICTIM OR ANY CONDUCTING OBJECTS IN CONTACT WITH THE VICTIM UNTIL YOU ARE ABSOLUTELY CERTAIN THAT HE IS NOT IN CONTACT WITH THE CURRENT SOURCE. There is nothing more useless than a dead paramedic.

If there is any question that the victim is still in contact with the current source, the current must be shut off immediately (where that is possible) or the victim dislodged from the current source. Use a nonconductive instrument, such as a lasso or a long wooden stick, to dislodge the victim. Do not go wading into puddles that may be in contact with him or with the current source, and don't let your rubber boots and insulated gloves give you a false sense of security. If you want to help the victim, you must look first to your own safety.

FURTHER READING

Beswick DR, Morse SD, Barnes AU. Bilateral scapular fractures from low-voltage electrical injury. *Ann Emerg Med* 11:676, 1982.

Bingham H. Electrical burns. *Clin Plast Surg* 13:75, 1986.

Budnick LD. Bathtub-related electrocutions in the United States, 1979 to 1982. *JAMA* 252:918, 1984.

Caroline NL. *Emergency Medical Treatment: A Text for EMT-As and EMT-Intermediates* (3rd ed.). Boston: Little, Brown, 1991, Ch. 13.

Dixon GF. The evaluation and management of electrical injuries. *Crit Care Med* 11:384, 1983.

Hammond JS, Ward G. High-voltage electrical injuries: Management and outcome of 60 cases. *South Med J* 81:1351, 1988.

Housinger TA et al. A prospective study of myocardial damage in electrical injuries. *J Trauma* 25:122, 1985.

Hunt JL, Sato RM, Baxter CR. Acute electric burns. *Arch Surg* 115:434, 1980.

Jensen PJ et al. Electrical injury causing ventricular arrhythmias. *Br Heart J* 57:279, 1987.

Kinney TJ. Myocardial infarction following electrical injury. *Ann Emerg Med* 11:622, 1982.

Kobernick M. Electrical injuries: Pathophysiology and management. *Ann Emerg Med* 11:633, 1982.

Purdue GF et al. Electrocardiographic monitoring after electrical injury: Necessity or luxury. *J Trauma* 26:166, 1986.

Reichl M et al. Electrical injuries due to railway high tension cables. *Burns* 11:423, 1985.

Salisbury R. High-voltage electrical injuries. *Emerg Med* 21(13):86, 1989.

Seward PN. Electrical injuries: Trauma with a difference. *Emerg Med* 19(9):66, 1987.

Solem L, Fischer RP, Strate RG. The natural history of electric injury. *J Trauma* 17:487, 1977.

Wilkinson C, Wood M. High voltage electric injury. *Am J Surg* 136:693, 1978.

Yang JY et al. Electrical burn with visceral injury. *Burns* 11:207, 1985.

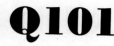

You are called to attend to a 28-year-old woman who has had several seizures in the past hour. When you arrive at the scene, you find the woman lying on the floor, groggy and disoriented. Her husband states that she had a seizure about 5 minutes ago. As you are examining her, you notice that her eyes suddenly deviate to the left, and a moment later she is once again having a grand mal convulsion.

1. Continuous seizures, or status epilepticus, are a dire medical emergency. When death occurs from seizures, it is usually due to

   a. Head injury
   b. Fracture of the long bones
   c. Dehydration and hypovolemia
   d. Stroke
   e. Hypoxemia

2. For that reason, one of the most crucial lifesaving measures in treating a patient with repeated seizures is to

   a. Place a pillow under the patient's head.
   b. Apply tight restraints to prevent the patient from moving.
   c. Infuse large volumes of normal saline solution.
   d. Administer diazepam (Valium).
   e. Maintain an open airway and administer oxygen.

3. Upon calling to the base hospital for orders, you are instructed to administer 5 to 10 mg of diazepam slowly IV. What potential complication of that treatment should you anticipate?

   a. Ventricular dysrhythmias
   b. Hypoglycemia
   c. Hypotension
   d. Vomiting
   e. Pupillary constriction

A101

1. You were entirely correct to regard this patient's repeated seizures as a dire medical emergency, for this woman may indeed die very soon if she does not receive adequate treatment. When death does occur from status epilepticus, it is usually due to **hypoxemia** (answer **e**). While fractures of the long bones (answer b), modest degrees of dehydration (answer c), and even head injury (answer a) may occur from continuous seizures, they are rarely the cause of death. And in general, it is more likely that stroke will cause seizures than vice versa (answer d).

2. Since this patient is at risk of dying from hypoxemia, clearly the most crucial therapeutic measure is to **maintain an open airway and administer oxygen** (answer **e**). A pillow under the patient's head (answer a) is apt to flex the head forward and lead to upper airway obstruction. Tight restraints (answer b) are apt to cause more problems than they prevent, for the patient may injure herself in the course of jerking violently against the restraints. It is better simply to clear the area around the patient of any furniture or other items on which she might injure herself, rather than try to restrain the patient herself. Position yourself at the patient's vertex, where you will be able to maintain her airway and suction any vomitus or secretions.

   Large volumes of normal saline solution (answer c) probably won't do this patient any harm, but they won't do that much good at this stage either. Besides, you are going to have quite a job on your hands trying to start an IV on a patient who is flailing all over the floor. If you do get the line in, much more important than giving a volume load is the administration of 50% glucose. There is, to begin with, always the possibility that this patient's seizures were caused by hypoglycemia. But even if hypoglycemia was not the cause of her condition, it may by now be the result; violent muscular contractions burn up a lot of glucose, and the brain's demand for glucose probably increases as well during seizure activity. So when you do get the IV line established (and very well secured!), consider a bolus of D50.

   Diazepam (answer d) may help to terminate the seizures, but it won't do a thing for this patient's hypoxemia, and it is hypoxemia—not the seizures per se—that is going to kill her. So *first* make certain that she has an open airway and is breathing a high concentration of inhaled oxygen. The diazepam can wait a few minutes.

3. OK, you've established an airway, administered oxygen, gotten the IV going, and now you have an order to administer diazepam. What untoward side effect might occur as a consequence of giving this drug?

   The correct answer is **c: hypotension,** which is a frequent side effect of diazepam administration. For that reason, diazepam is always given slowly, 2 to 3 mg at a time, and the blood pressure is monitored closely after each dose. At the first sign that the blood pressure is dropping, diazepam should be discontinued and no further doses given.

   There is another potential adverse effect of diazepam. Can you remember it? (See Question 15.)

FURTHER READING

Barber JM. EMT checkpoint: Seizures. *EMT J* 2(1):75, 1978.
Bell HE, Bertino JS. Constant diazepam infusion in the treatment of continuous seizure activity. *Drug Intell Clin Pharmacol* 18:965, 1984.
Bernat JL. Getting a handle on an adult's first seizure. *Emerg Med* 21(1):20, 1989.
Cloyd JC, Gumnit RJ, McLain W Jr. Status epilepticus: The role of intravenous phenytoin. *JAMA* 244:1479, 1980.
Curry HB. Fits and faints: Causes and cures. *Emerg Med* 14(3):70, 1982.
Delgado-Escueta AV et al. Management of status epilepticus. *N Engl J Med* 306:1337, 1982.
Drawbaugh RE, Deibler CG, Eitel DR. Prehospital administration of rectal diazepam in pediatric status epilepticus. *Prehosp Disaster Med* 5(2):155, 1990.
Finelli PF, Cardi JK. Seizures as a cause of fracture. *Neurology* 39:858, 1989.
Gress D. Stopping seizures. *Emerg Med* 22(1):22, 1990.
Leppik IE. Status epilepticus. *Clin Ther* 7:272, 1985.
Nicol CF. Status epilepticus. *Emerg Med* 11:114, 1976.
Parrish GA, Skiendzielewski JJ. Bilateral posterior fracture-dislocations of the shoulder after convulsive status epilepticus. *Ann Emerg Med* 14:264, 1985.
Phenobarbital for status epilepticus. *Emerg Med* 20(18):45, 1988.
Rothner AD et al. Status epilepticus. *Pediatr Clin North Am* 27:593, 1980.
Shaner DM et al. Treatment of status epilepticus. *Neurology* 38:202, 1988.
Sonander H et al. Effects of the rectal administration of diazepam. *Br J Anaesth* 57:578, 1985.

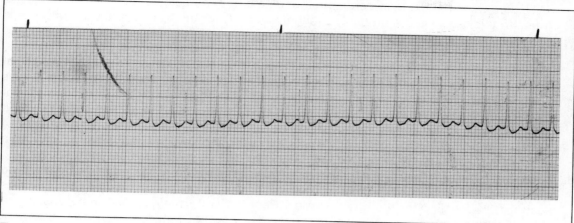

Figure 14

You are called to a large office building for a "dizzy woman." The patient is the boss's 38-year-old secretary, and you find her lying on a sofa in the boss's office, surrounded by an anxious office staff. She states that while she was typing the Annual Report, she suddenly began to feel very weak and dizzy. This has happened to her once or twice before, but it has always passed quickly before. She denies any significant illnesses, and she takes no medications regularly. On physical examination, she appears pale and anxious. The pulse is weak and very rapid. Blood pressure is 96/70, and respirations are 18 per minute. The remainder of the examination is unremarkable. The patient's rhythm strip is shown in Figure 14.

1. Examine the patient's rhythm strip:

   a. The rhythm is _____ regular _____ irregular.
   b. The rate is _____ per minute.

2. The ECG pattern is

   a. Atrial fibrillation
   b. Supraventricular tachycardia
   c. Ventricular tachycardia
   d. Sinus tachycardia
   e. Sinus arrhythmia

3. Which of the following statements about this dysrhythmia is true?

   a. It is always a sign of serious heart disease.
   b. It results from an ectopic focus in the ventricle.
   c. It is not associated with decreases in cardiac output.
   d. It indicates disease in the AV junction.
   e. It most commonly occurs in normal individuals who have no clinical evidence of heart disease.

4. One of the *first* measures you might try to treat this problem is

   a. Cardioversion at 50 watt-seconds.
   b. Edrophonium hydrochloride (Tensilon), 10 mg by slow IV push.
   c. Carotid sinus pressure.
   d. Dunk the patient's head in ice water.
   e. Lidocaine, 100 mg IV.

A102

1. The patient's rhythm is perfectly **regular.** The rate is about **230 per minute.**
2. The ECG pattern shows a **supraventricular tachycardia** (answer b). That is a general term, encompassing a number of paroxysmal ·tachycardias (e.g., paroxysmal atrial tachycardia [PAT], paroxysmal nodal tachycardia) that originate from an ectopic focus located in either atrium. In this case, we are probably dealing with PAT, for the history of a sudden onset is quite characteristic of that dysrhythmia, but we won't know for certain until we have tried out a few therapeutic maneuvers and watched the response on the monitor.

    Atrial fibrillation with a rapid ventricular response (answer a) is less likely here because of the precise regularity of the rhythm. Ventricular tachycardia (answer c) also usually shows slight irregularity in rhythm, and the complexes are most often wide and bizarre, like those of the PVCs. Sinus tachycardia (answer d) would rarely be expected to exceed a rate of about 180 per minute. Sinus arrhythmia (answer e) is, by definition, characterized by irregularity of rhythm. Finally, although it was not among the possible answers listed, atrial flutter with a rapid ventricular response is among the diagnoses that must be ruled out here.

3. Paroxysmal atrial tachycardia **most commonly occurs in normal individuals who have no clinical evidence of heart disease** (answer e). It may be precipitated by emotional stress (such as the deadline for the boss's Annual Report!), and usually it does not constitute a serious medical emergency. If, however, it occurs in a patient with coronary artery disease, it can produce angina and infarction; even in normal individuals, the persistence of PAT over several days can lead to heart failure. As noted earlier, the dysrhythmia is due to an ectopic focus in either atrium, not in the ventricles (answer b). Because of the rapid rate, it can be expected to produce significant decreases in cardiac output (answer c), as manifested by a fall in blood pressure.

4. The *first* measure one would try in an attempt to convert this rhythm is **carotid sinus pressure** (answer c). This maneuver is also of diagnostic value, for it can help to distinguish between PAT and other tachycardias, such as paroxysmal atrial flutter or sinus tachycardia. If successful, carotid sinus pressure should produce a sudden and complete conversion from PAT to normal sinus rhythm. In atrial flutter, carotid sinus pressure is more likely to result in a jerky reduction in ventricular rate as the degree of AV block is increased, and flutter waves may then become evident on the ECG; when carotid sinus massage is stopped, one can expect a jerky return to the original ventricular rate. In sinus tachycardia, carotid sinus pressure generally produces a transient, gradual slowing of rate; but, again, the rate rapidly climbs back to its former levels as carotid sinus massage is terminated.

    Carotid sinus massage is performed under constant ECG monitoring, with the patient supine and an IV line securely established. The right carotid sinus is massaged first, for about 10 to 20 seconds. If that fails to convert the rhythm, one may wait a few moments and then try the same maneuver on the left side. NEVER MASSAGE BOTH CAROTID SINUSES SIMULTANEOUSLY!

    Cardioversion (answer a) is not a first-line treatment in the field when the patient is fully conscious and cardiac output is not dangerously compromised. Had this patient been stuporous, however, and showing signs of shock, cardioversion might have been tried (after carotid sinus pressure failed), just in case we were dealing with paroxysmal atrial flutter. Cardioversion would be unlikely to work at all in PAT.

    Edrophonium hydrochloride (Tensilon) is one of the *drugs* for treating PAT (answer b). Like carotid sinus massage, it acts by stimulating the vagus nerve, which in turns slows the heart. If one can accomplish the same thing simply by carotid sinus pressure, one should not use a pharmacologic agent; thus it is always worthwhile to try carotid sinus massage first. If that fails, edrophonium—either by itself or in conjunction with carotid sinus pressure—may be tried.

    Another class of drugs that is sometimes used in an attempt to convert PAT is the vasopressor group, such as metaraminol (Aramine) or phenylephrine (Neo-Synephrine). They presumably work by raising the blood pressure, which in turn stimulates the parasympathetic nervous system and slows the heart. Such drugs are indicated principally in cases where hypotension is a significant part of the clinical picture. Because they may lead to ectopic beats and considerable blood pressure elevation, such drugs are potentially hazardous, especially in the elderly or in the coronary-prone.

    If you answered d to this question, you would not be incorrect. One rather unorthodox method that has been described for converting PAT to sinus rhythm is to immerse the patient's face in ice water. That maneuver is said to elicit the so-called diving reflex, a response that enables animals to slow their heart rate through vagal stimulation when submerged in cold water. The method is quite effective, although it probably is not the ideal first-line treatment in the boss's office, for you might have some trouble explaining what you are doing.

There is no indication for lidocaine (answer e) in this case, for there is no evidence of ventricular irritability.

Patients with recurrent episodes of PAT should be advised to avoid stimulant drugs, such as coffee and tea, as well as to refrain from smoking and avoid situations that produce unwarranted fatigue. They may also be instructed in various maneuvers that they can try themselves in order to convert the dysrhythmia, such as the Valsalva maneuver or facial immersion in ice water, as described above. If you do recommend the latter, just be careful to explain it thoroughly, so that the patient does not misunderstand your intentions when you tell her to ''go soak your head.''

FURTHER READING

Bissett GS et al. The ice bag: A new technique for interruption of supraventricular tachycardia. *J Pediatr* 97:593, 1980.

Brick I. Circulatory response to immersing the face in water. *J Appl Physiol* 21:33, 1966.

Klein HO, Hoffman BF. Cessation of paroxysmal supraventricular tachycardias by parasympathomimetic interventions. *Ann Intern Med* 81:48, 1974.

Levitt MA. Supraventricular tachycardia with aberrant conduction versus ventricular tachycardia: Differentiation and diagnosis. *Am J Emerg Med* 6:273, 1988.

Mehta D et al. Relative efficacy of various physical manoevres in the termination of junctional tachycardia. *Lancet* 1:1181, 1988.

Sperandeo V et al. Supraventricular tachycardia in infants: Use of the ''diving reflex.'' *Am J Cardiol* 51:286, 1983.

Waxman MB et al. Vagal techniques for termination of paroxysmal supraventricular tachycardia. *Am J Cardiol* 46:655, 1980.

Wayne MA. Conversion of paroxysmal atrial tachycardia by facial immersion in ice water. *JACEP* 5:434, 1976.

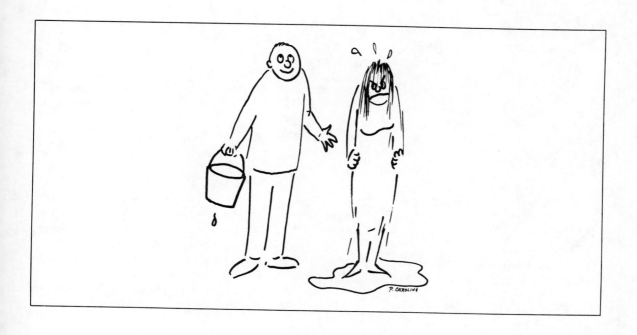

You are called at 4:00 A.M. to see a "man who can't breathe." You arrive at a well-kept ranch house to find a 54-year-old man being restrained by his wife and two daughters. He is in obvious respiratory distress, slightly cyanotic, and coughing up foam. He cannot sit still, and when you try to administer oxygen, he rips off the mask. He is sweating profusely. His pulse is 130 and slightly irregular; respirations are 36 per minute. He will not sit still long enough for you to measure his blood pressure—he keeps getting up and moving around before sinking again into a chair. You manage to get a stethoscope onto his chest for a few seconds, and you hear coarsely bubbling rales in all lung fields.

You contact your base physician by radio and inform him of the situation. Sounding somewhat sleepy, he gives you orders for the following:

a. Oxygen at the highest possible concentration
b. Morphine, 7.5 mg slowly IV
c. Furosemide (Lasix), 80 mg IV
d. Epinephrine, 5 ml of a 1:10,000 solution IV
e. Digoxin, 0.25 mg slowly IV
f. Aminophylline, 250 mg in the IV bag

Which of the above orders should you question?

Match each treatment on the list above (except for the incorrect treatment) with the statement that best describes its therapeutic function:

1. _____ Promotes bronchodilation and also increases the force of cardiac contractions
2. _____ Combats hypoxemia
3. _____ Decreases pulmonary edema by diminishing venous return to the heart; also helps allay anxiety
4. _____ Promotes diuresis of excess fluids
5. _____ Increases the strength of cardiac contractions and thereby improves cardiac output

A103

Our patient, as you have doubtless already figured out, is suffering from severe left heart failure and pulmonary edema. Your base station physician has also figured out the diagnosis, but not being fully awake, he's gotten his orders a bit muddled. The order you should question is **epinephrine** (answer **d**). That is one thing this patient does NOT need at this moment, for his adrenals are probably pouring epinephrine into the bloodstream in response to the enormous stress the patient is experiencing. So inquire politely, "Did you say *epinephrine,* doctor?" and give him a moment to wake up and think about it.

Of course, the base station physician has one enormous advantage: *He* doesn't have to start the IV. And in this patient, getting an IV line in is not going to be any picnic, for the patient is combative and frantic from his hypoxemia. But we will assume that you succeeded brilliantly, and you are now preparing to carry out the physician's (revised) orders. Do you know what the drugs you are giving are for?

1. __f__ Aminophylline   Promotes bronchodilation and also increases the force of cardiac contractions
2. __a__ Oxygen   Combats hypoxemia
3. __b__ Morphine   Decreases pulmonary edema by diminishing venous return to the heart; also allays anxiety
4. __c__ Furosemide   Promotes diuresis of excess fluid
5. __e__ Digoxin   Increases the strength of cardiac contractions and thereby improves cardiac output

The last-mentioned drug, digoxin, should not be used routinely in the field treatment of pulmonary edema. Its onset of action does not occur until 20 minutes after administration, and the maximum therapeutic effect is not seen until 1 to 1½ hours later. Furthermore, if the patient has been taking digitalis at home, your IV dose may push him over the line into digitalis toxicity. Reserve digoxin for circumstances in which transport will be prolonged beyond an hour or so.

FURTHER READING

Abrams J. Vasodilator therapy for chronic congestive heart failure. *JAMA* 254:3070, 1985.

Cohn JN, Fanciosa JA. Vasodilator therapy of cardiac failure. *N Engl J Med* 279:27, 254, 1977.

Dikshit K et al. Renal and extrarenal hemodynamic effects of furosemide in congestive heart failure after acute myocardial infarction. *N Engl J Med* 288:1087, 1973.

Forrester JS, Staniloff HM. Heart failure. *Emerg Med* 16(4):121, 1984.

Francis GS et al. Acute vasoconstrictor response to intravenous furosemide in patients with chronic congestive heart failure. *Ann Intern Med* 103:1, 1985.

Genton R, Jaffe AS. Management of congestive heart failure in patients with acute myocardial infarction. *JAMA* 256:2556, 1986.

Goldberg H, Nakhjavan FK. Pathophysiology, diagnosis, and treatment of heart failure. *Hosp Med* 8(7):8, 1972.

Hoffman JR, Reynolds S. Comparison of nitroglycerin, morphine and furosemide in treatment of presumed pre-hospital pulmonary edema. *Chest* 92:586, 1987.

Levy DB, Pollard T. Failure of the heart. *Emergency* 20(12):22, 1988.

Marantz PR et al. Clinical diagnosis of congestive heart failure in patients with acute dyspnea. *Chest* 97:776, 1990.

Markiewicz W et al. Sublingual isosorbide dinitrate in severe congestive failure. *Cardiology* 67:172, 1981.

McKee PA et al. The natural history of congestive heart failure: The Framingham study. *N Engl J Med* 285:1441, 1971.

Parmley WM. To rescue a failing heart. *Emerg Med* 15(5):179, 1983.

Ramirez A, Abelmann WH. Cardiac decompensation. *N Engl J Med* 290:499, 1974.

Roberts R. Inotropic therapy for cardiac failure associated with acute myocardial infarction. *Chest* 93(1, Suppl):22S, 1988.

Robin ED, Carroll IC, Zelis R. Pulmonary edema. *N Engl J Med* 288:239, 292. 1972.

Tresch DD et al. Out-of-hospital pulmonary edema: Diagnosis and treatment. *Ann Emerg Med* 12:533, 1983.

Wulf-Dirk B, Schupp D. Effect of sublingual nitroglycerin in emergency treatment of severe pulmonary edema. *Am J Cardiol* 41:931, 1978.

A 30-year-old man was a celebrant at a somewhat boisterous party at a friend's second-story apartment. As the evening wore on, and the wine and other spirits flowed, our young man decided to get a breath of fresh air and stepped out onto the fire escape. Unfortunately, he did not see the hibachi, and he tripped, catapulting himself over the balcony and onto the sidewalk below.

When you arrive, you find him lying on the pavement, apparently unconscious, but rousable by shouting his name. His pulse is 90 and regular, blood pressure is 130/90, and respirations are 18. Pupils are equal and reactive. There is a prominent bruise over his left temple and a deformity of the left forearm. Otherwise there is no other evidence of injury, and the patient withdraws all extremities from a painful stimulus.

After immobilizing the patient on a backboard, you are instructed to start an IV.

1. What type of IV is most appropriate in this situation?

   a. D5W at 100 ml per hour
   b. D5W by microdrip infusion set, to keep the vein open
   c. Normal saline solution at 100 ml per hour
   d. Normal saline solution at 200 ml per hour
   e. Colloid, such as plasmanate, at 100 ml per hour

Severe head injury may lead to swelling of the brain (cerebral edema) or bleeding inside the skull, either or both of which can cause an increase in intracranial pressure.

2. What changes in vital signs might suggest that such an increase in intracranial pressure was occurring in this patient?

   a. Rising pulse and rising blood pressure
   b. Rising pulse and falling blood pressure
   c. Slowing of the pulse and rising blood pressure
   d. Slowing of the pulse and falling blood pressure

3. What is the most important single sign to monitor in a head-injured patient while he is under your care?

   a. Whether the pupils are equal
   b. Breathing pattern
   c. Absence of sensation in any extremity
   d. Changes in the state of consciousness
   e. Deep tendon reflexes

A104

1. A patient with a head injury who has no evidence of major hemorrhage elsewhere in the body should receive a minimum of salt and water, lest one precipitate cerebral edema. Thus, an IV line is established solely for the purpose of maintaining a lifeline into the circulation, in the event that resuscitative drugs are needed. For that reason, the most appropriate IV for our patient would be **D5W by microdrip infusion set, to keep the vein open** (answer b). All of the other infusions listed impose too large a fluid or salt and fluid load for a head-injured patient. Should signs of impending shock occur, however, the IV lifeline permits you to switch quickly from D5W to normal saline solution and open the IV wide.

2. An increase in intracranial pressure is often signalled by a **slowing of the pulse and rising blood pressure** (answer c). The increase in intracranial pressure itself usually produces a rise in blood pressure; the bradycardia is usually a secondary phenomenon caused by the vagal stimulation that rapid increases in blood pressure evoke.

    A rising pulse and rising blood pressure (answer a) would be a somewhat unlikely combination, as would a slowing of the pulse and falling blood pressure (answer d). A rising pulse and falling blood pressure (answer b) suggest shock and should prompt a search for sources of hemorrhage elsewhere in the body.

3. All of the signs listed are important, but probably the most important is **d: changes in the patient's state of consciousness.** The neurosurgeon, waiting with his drills and saws in the emergency room, will be extremely eager to know whether the patient's state of consciousness is improving or deteriorating, for that information will help him to decide whether he must operate immediately or whether there is time to observe the patient further. By the time there is unilateral pupillary dilatation (answer a), the patient is already pretty far gone, and changes in the patient's breathing pattern may be a rather late sign as well (answer b).

FURTHER READING

Baxt WG et al. The impact of advanced prehospital emergency care on the mortality of severely brain-injured patients. *J Trauma* 27:365, 1987.

Bouzarth WF. Early management of acute head injury (a surgeon's viewpoint). *EMT J* 2(2):43, 1978.

Caroline NL. *Emergency Care in the Streets* (4th ed.). Boston: Little, Brown, 1991, Ch. 16.

Clifton GL et al. Cardiovascular response to severe head injury. *J Neurosurg* 59:447, 1983.

Cold GE. Does acute hyperventilation provoke cerebral oligaemia in comatose patients after acute head injury? *Acta Neurochir* (Wien) 96:10, 1989.

Davidoff G et al. The spectrum of closed head injuries in facial trauma victims: Incidence and impact. *Ann Emerg Med* 17:6, 1988.

Desai BT et al. Seizures in relation to head injury. *Ann Emerg Med* 12:543, 1983.

Javid M. Head injuries. *N Engl J Med* 291:890, 1974.

Jones CC, McBride MM, Hines LL. New protocols for managing the head injured patient. *Emergency* 12(7):53, 1980.

Jones PW et al. Hyperventilation in the management of cerebral oedema. *Intensive Care Med* 7:205, 1981.

Kenning JA et al. Upright patient positioning in the management of intracranial hypertension. *Surg Neurol* 15:148, 1981.

Lillehei KO, Hoff JT. Advances in the management of closed head injury. *Ann Emerg Med* 14:789, 1985.

Robertson CS et al. Treatment of hypertension associated with head injury. *J Neurosurg* 59:455, 1983.

Rosner MJ et al. Cerebral perfusion pressure, intracranial pressure, and head elevation. *J Neurosurg* 65:636, 1986.

Saul TG, Ducker TB. Management of acute head injuries. *Emergency* 12(2):59, 1980.

Scali VJ et al. Handling head injuries. *Emergency* 21(11):22, 1989.

Seelig JM et al. Traumatic acute subdural hematoma: Major mortality reduction in comatose patients treated within four hours. *N Engl J Med* 304:1151, 1981.

Shields CB. Early management of head injuries. *J Ky Med Assoc* 78:9, 1980.

Smith S. A blow to the head. *Emergency* 22(6):16, 1990.

A 31-year-old purse snatcher raced across a busy street and was struck by a car. The force of the impact lifted him onto the hood of the car, but he then rolled off onto the road and the car ran over him. You find him lying in the street, unconscious, in a pool of blood. He does not appear to be breathing. You open his airway by forward displacement of the mandible, and he begins to breathe spontaneously. You then continue your survey and note that a pulse is present and rapid. There is no obvious injury to the head or neck. Neck veins are collapsed. The chest wall seems somewhat unstable on the right, and there is an open chest wound on the right side. The abdomen has been torn open and loops of bowel protrude. There is instability of the pelvis. Bright red blood is spurting from a large gash in the right upper arm. Both femurs appear to be broken.

Arrange the following steps of management in the appropriate order:

a. Apply military antishock trousers.
b. Cover the eviscerated loops of bowel with bulky dressings soaked in sterile saline.
c. Administer oxygen.
d. Stop the bleeding from the patient's arm with a pressure dressing.
e. Start at least one IV with a large-bore cannula, and run in normal saline wide open.
f. Place the patient on a backboard.
g. Seal off the sucking chest wound.
h. Apply traction splints to both legs.
i. Apply a cervical collar.
j. Start transport.

1. _____
2. _____
3. _____
4. _____
5. _____
6. _____
7. _____
8. _____
9. _____
10. _____

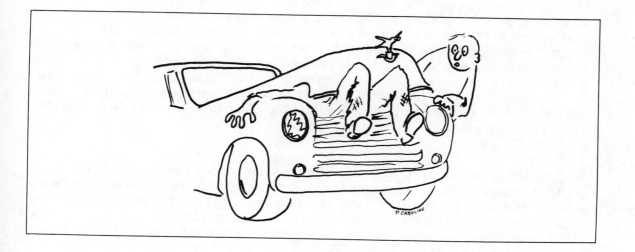

A105

The patient with multiple injuries presents one of the greatest challenges to any health professional, and it requires enormous discipline to approach such a patient in a systematic fashion, for often the most dramatic wounds are not the most important. One must have developed a clearly defined set of priorities in order to provide optimal, orderly care to the multiply injured patient. Those priorities, in general, are as follows:

1. Airway (with cervical spine precautions)
2. Breathing
3. Circulation
4. Spine injuries
5. Open wounds
6. Fractures

With those priorities in mind, let's take a look at how we would manage our banged-up purse snatcher.

1. __g__ Seal off the sucking chest wound.

We have already opened the airway. Our next step is to ensure that the patient is breathing adequately. That will not be possible so long as there is a gaping hole in the patient's chest, so the hole must be sealed off at the earliest possible moment. Remember, though, to check periodically for signs of developing tension pneumothorax.

2. __c__ Administer oxygen.

A major purpose of breathing is to furnish oxygen to the peripheral tissues through the bloodstream. Having sustained an open chest wound, our patient is bound to have a large shunt, and breathing ambient air will not supply him with the oxygen he needs. You have to supply that added oxygen. Breathing is more than simply moving air in and out of the lungs, and oxygenation is a vital part of the breathing process. (Note: If you don't have the oxygen immediately at hand, stop the patient's bleeding before you run back to the vehicle for the oxygen tank. The ABCs should all be accomplished within the first 30 to 60 seconds.)

3. __d__ Stop the bleeding from the patient's arm with a pressure dressing.

Now we move on to the circulation, and arresting major hemorrhage is one of the most crucial aspects of sustaining an adequate circulation. It is counterproductive to spend several minutes at this point trying to start an IV, for while you are fiddling around with the IV equipment, blood is continuing to pour out of the patient's arm onto the ground—and the patient needs that blood more than he needs the equivalent volume of normal saline. So get the bleeding stopped as rapidly as possible.

4. __i__ Apply a cervical collar.

5. __f__ Place the patient on a backboard.

"Wait a minute!" you say. "We haven't finished with the circulation. What about the MAST? What about an IV?" It is a matter of logistics. This patient may have sustained a spine injury; thus we want to minimize the movement to which he is subjected. If we lay the MAST garment flat on the backboard before transferring the patient onto the backboard, we can accomplish two manipulations in a single move. Before we slide our patient onto the backboard, we should maintain his head in axial traction and help stabilize it in position with a cervical collar.

We needn't *immobilize* the patient onto the backboard with straps at this point. The straps will just get in our way as we wrap him in the MAST or attend to his fractures. So full immobilization can wait a moment.

6. __a__ Apply military antishock trousers.

If the MAST is used in your service, now is the time to wrap the patient's legs in the MAST and fasten the patient to the backboard. Needless to say, we don't want to fasten or inflate the abdominal section of the MAST, for it would not be a good idea to put the squeeze on all those loops of bowel that are hanging out. When you get around to inflating the leg sections of the MAST—which will probably be when you are already en route to the hospital—be sure to hold both legs in firm longitudinal traction as you do so.

248

7. ___j___ Start transport.

This is a load-and-go situation, for at least three reasons: The patient is unconscious after an injury; he has an open chest wound; and he probably has a flail chest. So having completed the primary survey and the critical interventions (control of external hemorrhage, sealing off the open chest wound), we have no reason to delay further at the scene. Whatever else we want to do for the casualty, we will have to do en route to the hospital. Remember: EVERY MINUTE OF THE GOLDEN HOUR IS PRECIOUS.

8. ___e___ Start at least one IV with a large-bore cannula, and run in normal saline wide open.

The IV will be much easier to initiate once the MAST has been inflated, for veins that had seemed to disappear will magically pop up in the patient's arm.

9. ___b___ Cover the eviscerated loops of bowel with bulky dressings soaked in sterile saline.

We've taken care of the airway, breathing, and circulation and done as much as we can for the moment for the possible spine injury, so now we turn our attention to open wounds, which must be covered.

10. ___h___ Apply traction splints to both legs.

If there is time, there is no reason why a traction splint cannot be applied over the MAST. If you don't have traction splints, the MAST itself will provide a certain degree of immobilization.

FURTHER READING

Caroline NL. *Emergency Care in the Streets* (4th ed.). Boston: Little, Brown, 1991, Ch. 20.
Caroine NL. *Emergency Medical Treatment: A Text for EMT-As and EMT-Intermediates* (3rd ed.). Boston: Little, Brown, 1991. Ch. 18.

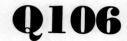

You are called to one of the less savory neighborhoods downtown for a "man down" on the sidewalk. You find a male patient, who appears to be in his 50s, lying unconscious. He is shabbily dressed, unshaven, and exudes a variety of strong aromas, the strongest of which is the aroma of alcohol. There are no obvious signs of injury. Bystanders can tell you only that they think the patient has been lying there "for quite a while."

Which of the following statements about this patient is NOT true?

a. He is in imminent danger of airway obstruction.
b. He should receive 50 ml of 50% glucose.
c. It is safe to assume that he is probably simply drunk, and he needs no specific treatment.
d. He should receive oxygen.
e. He is at high risk to develop aspiration pneumonia.

A106

The correct answer is **c:** It is definitely *not* safe to assume that this patient is simply drunk and therefore requires no specific treatment. MERELY BECAUSE A PATIENT SMELLS OF ALCOHOL, ONE CANNOT AUTOMATICALLY ASSUME THAT ALL HIS SYMPTOMS DERIVE FROM EXCESSIVE ALCOHOL CONSUMPTION. An alcoholic can develop coma from all the same causes of coma in other people—head injury, stroke, hypoglycemia, postictal state of a seizure, and so forth. Indeed, the alcoholic is more prone to many of these conditions than is the average sober citizen. Alcoholics are, for example, very susceptible to head injury, and because they often have defects in their clotting mechanisms as well, even a relatively minor head injury may lead to significant intracranial hemorrhage. Alcoholics tend to be seizure-prone, especially during withdrawal. They are more liable to develop hypoglycemia than the average nondrinker. Excessive intake of alcohol may simply reflect severe depression, and behind that mist of gin vapor may lie a patient who has just swallowed a fistful of sleeping pills. You just can't be sure because the patient can't tell you. Thus it is very risky business indeed to write any comatose patient off as "simply drunk." Too often, "drunks" who have been carted to the local lockup to "sleep it off" have been found dead the next morning—from subdural hematoma, severe hypoglycemia, asphyxia due to airway obstruction, etc.

Every comatose patient is in danger of imminent airway obstruction (answer a), for as the muscles of the jaw go slack, the base of the tongue is more likely to fall back against the posterior pharynx and close off the airway. Furthermore, *every* comatose patient is at significant risk of aspiration (answer e), and if the patient happens to have a stomach full of liquor, or anything else for that matter, the risk of aspiration is even greater. Check for a gag reflex. If it is absent, the patient cannot protect his airway and needs to be intubated. Indeed, it is a pretty safe general rule that any patient who will tolerate endotracheal intubation without bucking or gagging *needs* endotracheal intubation.

Every patient in coma of unknown etiology should receive oxygen (answer d) and 50% glucose (answer b). The brain can do without a lot of things, but it cannot do without oxygen and glucose, even for a few minutes. When a patient is in coma, the brain needs tender loving care. Until you can demonstrate, with appropriate laboratory tests in the hospital, that the arterial PO_2 and the blood sugar are at adequate levels, you have to assume that they are not. Err on the side of caution. You will not do a comatose patient any harm by administering oxygen and glucose; you may do profound harm by withholding that treatment.

FURTHER READING

Alcouloumre E. The intoxicated patient. *Emerg Med Serv* 19(4):65, 1990.
Caroline NL. *Emergency Care in the Streets* (4th ed.). Boston: Little, Brown, 1991, Ch. 27.
Clark DE, McCarthy E, Robinson E. Trauma as a symptom of alcoholism (editorial). *Ann Emerg Med* 14:274, 1984.
Criteria Committee, National Council on Alcoholism. Criteria for the diagnosis of alcoholism. *Ann Intern Med* 77:249, 1972.
Goldfrank LR. A vitamin for an emergency. *Emerg Med* 14(16):113, 1982.
Goldfrank LR. Ask me about alcohol withdrawal. *Emerg Med* 18(6):24, 1986.
Johnson MW. Alcohol-related emergencies. *Emerg Med Serv* 12(3): 51, 1983.
Knott DH, Fink RD, Morgan JC. Beware the patient with alcohol on his breath. *Emerg Med Serv* 6(3):40, 1977.
Lerner WD et al. The alcohol withdrawal syndrome. *N Engl J Med* 313:951, 1985.
Lundberg GD. Ethyl alcohol—ancient plague and modern poison (editorial): *JAMA* 252:1911, 1984.
Maull KI. Alcohol abuse: Its implications in trauma care. *South Med J* 75:794, 1982.
Madden JF. Calming the storms of alcohol withdrawal. *Emerg Med* 22(7):23, 1990.
Niven RG. Alcoholism—a problem in perspective (editorial). *JAMA* 252:1912, 1984.
O'Carroll BM. Alcohol and substance abuse emergencies: Handle with care. *Rescue* 3(5):21, 1990.
Regan TJ. Alcohol and the cardiovascular system. *JAMA* 264:377, 1990.
Scarano SJ. Emergency response: Alcohol-intoxicated patient. *Emerg Med Serv* 8(5):78, 1979.
Sellers EM, Kalant H. Alcohol intoxication and withdrawal. *N Engl J Med* 294:757, 1976.
Siscovick DS et al. Moderate alcohol consumption and primary cardiac arrest. *Am J Epidemiol* 123:499, 1986.
Taigman M. Just another drunk . . . *Emerg Med Serv* 17(8):8, 1988.
Taigman M. The battle scars of booze: Treating the chronic alcoholic. *JEMS* 14(10):45, 1989.
Thrasher MR, Thrasher CL. Prehospital treatment of acute adolescent alcoholism. *Emerg Med Serv* 14(1):32, 1985.
Treatment of alcohol withdrawal. *Med Lett Drug Ther* 28:75, 1986.

A 35-year-old man was the driver of an automobile that struck a lamppost at high speed. He was thrown forward against the steering wheel with sufficient force that his head apparently smashed the windshield. On examination, you find him slumped in the front seat, stuporous and moaning. His skin is cold and clammy. Pulse is 130, weak, and slightly irregular. Blood pressure is 80/60. There are multiple small lacerations on the scalp and forehead. Neck veins are distended to the angle of the jaw. There are bruises on the anterior chest, but there is no instability of the chest wall. Both lung fields are clear, and breath sounds are heard equally bilaterally. Heart sounds are faint. The abdomen is soft and nontender; there are no abdominal bruises. There are minor scratches on the upper extremities, but there is no deformity or limitation of motion in any extremity. This patient is probably suffering from

a. Ruptured spleen
b. Fracture of the femur with massive bleeding into the hip
c. Right-sided tension pneumothorax
d. Cardiac tamponade
e. Right-sided hemothorax

A107

The correct answer is **d: cardiac tamponade.**

In examining this patient, our major diagnostic concern is to find an explanation for his shocklike state. Any of the possibilities listed could lead to hypotension and tachycardia, but several findings on physical examination help us to distinguish among these possibilities.

To begin with, we can probably dismiss femoral fracture (answer b) as an unlikely possibility, for we have found no evidence of deformity or limitation of motion in the extremities. Both tension pneumothorax (answer c) and hemothorax (answer e) are unlikely in view of the normal findings on ausculation of the lungs. Ruptured spleen (answer a) must always be considered in cases of trauma and unexplained hypotension; the fact that there are no bruises over the abdomen does not rule out this possibility, for a good bang to the left lower ribs can also do considerable damage to the spleen. However, the diagnosis of splenic rupture does not help us to explain this patient's distended neck veins, so even if the patient does have a ruptured spleen, we have to look elsewhere to determine what is causing his increased venous pressure.

Among the most common causes of jugular venous distention are (1) right heart failure, (2) increased intrapleural pressure, and (3) cardiac tamponade. We have no reason to suspect that this patient is in right heart failure, and our physical examination has just about ruled out a significant pneumothorax or hemothorax compressing the venae cavae. That leaves us with the third possibility, cardiac tamponade. We have other clues supporting this possibility as well. To begin with, the patient has bruises over his anterior chest, indicating that the mechanism of injury is consistent with myocardial injury. And we were barely able to hear the patient's heart sounds, most likely because they were muffled by an insulating layer of blood.

Having reached the conclusion that the patient has cardiac tamponade, the paramedic should realize that his task is to GET THE PATIENT TO THE HOSPITAL AS RAPIDLY AS POSSIBLE. Unless the blood is evacuated from this patient's pericardial sac SOON, he will die. No two ways about it. And if you have not been trained and authorized to perform pericardiocentesis, you had better get this patient to someone who has. Start oxygen, get him out of the car on a backboard (but do it fast!), and get moving. And be sure to notify the receiving hospital what's in store for them, so they can have a pericardiocentesis tray and ancillary equipment ready for your arrival.

FURTHER READING

Arena AA, Martinez JA, McNulty PA. Problem: Acute cardiac tamponade. *Emerg Med* 16(15):51, 1984.
Callahan M. Acute traumatic cardiac tamponade: Diagnosis and treatment. *JACEP* 7:306, 1978.
Caroline NL. *Emergency Care in the Streets* (4th ed.). Boston: Little, Brown, 1991, Ch. 17.
Conn AKT. Cardiac arrest due to trauma. *Emergency* 11(12):42, 1979.
Forrester JS. Pericardial tamponade. *Emerg Med* 16(4):108, 1984.
Gervin AS, Fischer RP. The importance of prompt transport in salvage of patients with penetrating heart wounds. *J Trauma* 22:443, 1982.
Honigman B et al. Prehospital advance trauma life support for penetrating cardiac wounds. *Ann Emerg Med* 19:145, 1990.
Janeira LF. Cardiac tamponade. *Emergency* 12(2):44, 1980.
McSwain NE. Pericardiocentesis. *Emerg Med* 20(22):102, 1988.
Ramp J, Harkins J, Mason G. Cardiac tamponade secondary to blunt trauma. *J Trauma* 14:767, 1974.

A Boeing 707 has crashed on takeoff at a nearby airport. The first ambulance crew on the scene estimates that there are approximately 60 casualties.

1. Which of the following patients would be bypassed in the FIRST round of triage?

   a. 33-year-old man unconscious and apneic
   b. 50-year-old man in cardiac arrest
   c. 28-year-old woman bleeding massively from an open wound over the left femoral artery
   d. 18-year-old man with an open abdominal wound from which the intestines have eviscerated
   e. 43-year-old man with a sucking chest wound.

2. Approximately 63 ambulances have arrived at the scene from all the neighboring communities. Which of the following patients should be evacuated first?

   a. Patients in cardiac arrest
   b. Patients with open injuries to the chest
   c. Patients with injuries to the face and neck
   d. Patients with blunt abdominal trauma and shock
   e. Those patients who are stabilized first, irrespective of the nature of their injuries

A108

1. All of the injuries listed are considered first priority conditions except for patient **d,** who is suffering from **evisceration.** If he has a good pulse, he should be relegated to third priority; if there are signs of shock or impending shock, he should be seen on the second round of triage. But his injury, unlike the others on the list, does not constitute an IMMEDIATE (i.e., within seconds) threat to life. Therefore his treatment can be briefly postponed.

2. We have managed to assemble 63 ambulances for an estimated 60 casualties. Under circumstances where there are a sufficient number of evacuation vehicles, the principle of evacuation is that **THOSE PATIENTS WHO ARE STABILIZED FIRST ARE EVACUATED FIRST** (answer **e**). Had there been a shortage of ambulances, we would have had to assign our priorities somewhat differently. The "walking wounded" would have been moved to the end of the line, while patients a, b, and c (cardiac arrest, open chest injuries, injuries to the face and neck) would be moved to first evacuation priority. Patient d, with blunt abdominal trauma and impending shock, would be a very close second, depending upon the degree to which his shock had been temporarily stabilized in the field.

Table 3. Priorities of Treatment in Triage

Priority Group	Problem	Treatment			
		1st Round Triage	2nd Round Triage	3rd Round Triage	4th Round Triage
First	Airway obstruction	Airway opened manually	Endotracheal intubation; cricothyrotomy		
	Sucking chest wound	Sealed manually	Sealed with occlusive dressing; O_2	Chest tube with Heimlich valve	
	Apnea	Mouth-to-mouth ventilation	Bag-valve-mask with O_2	Continue artificial ventilation	
	Cardiac arrest*	External cardiac compressions (ECC)	Continue ECC; start IV; O_2	Drugs; defibrillation	
	Exsanguinating hemorrhage	Manual control of bleeding; MAST	IV infusions; O_2		
	Tension pneumothorax		O_2; needle decompression	Chest tube with Heimlich valve	
	Pericardial tamponade		O_2; ECC	Evacuate blood from pericardium	
	Impending shock		O_2; MAST	IV infusions	
	Massive hemothorax		O_2	Chest tube	
Second	Head injury			Secure airway; O_2	Stabilize cervical spine
	Evisceration			IV; cover viscera	
	Open fractures			Dress wounds	Splint
	Spinal injuries			Immobilize	
Third	Lesser fractures, wounds				Splint; dress wounds

*Only if there are a sufficient number of rescuers to spare two people for CPR; if shorthanded, bypass patients in cardiac arrest.

FURTHER READING

Butman AM. The challenge of casualties en masse. *Emerg Med* 15(7):110, 1983.
Haynes BE et al. A prehospital approach to multiple-victim incidents. *Ann Emerg Med* 15:458, 1986.
Kelly JT. Model for pre-hospital disaster response. *J World Ass Emerg Disaster Med* 1:80, 1986.
Koehler JJ et al. Prehospital index: A scoring system for field triage of trauma victims. *Ann Emerg Med* 15:178, 1986.
Mathews TP. Triage 81. *J World Assn Emerg Disaster Med* 1:153, 1985.
Rund DA, Rausch TS. *Triage.* St. Louis: Mosby, 1981.
Schwartz TJ. Model for pre-hospital disaster response. *J World Assn Emerg Disaster Med* 1:78, 1986.

You are called to a see a 6-year-old child because he has a very high fever. His mother tells you that he became ill about 4 hours ago and has been complaining of a severe sore throat. He won't take anything to eat or drink because he says it hurts to swallow.

You find the child sitting upright in bed, crying and drooling noticeably. He appears very frightened. His axillary temperature is 104°F (40°C). His respirations are 30 and shallow, and there is flaring of his nostrils on inhalation. His chest is clear.

Which of the following is NOT part of the management of this child?

a. Administer humidified oxygen.
b. Start IV line with D5/½ normal saline.
c. Carefully examine the throat to determine whether the epiglottis is swollen.
d. Transport the child to the hospital in a sitting position without delay.

A109

This child presents a classic picture of acute obstructive supraglottic laryngitis (*epiglottitis*), and he is in imminent danger of complete airway obstruction. Do *not* mess around with his throat (answer **c**)! NEVER, NEVER, NEVER PLACE A TONGUE BLADE, THERMOMETER, OR ANY OTHER INSTRUMENT INTO THE MOUTH OF A PATIENT SUSPECTED TO HAVE EPIGLOTTITIS UNLESS YOU ARE TRAINED, EQUIPPED, AUTHORIZED, AND PREPARED TO DO AN IMMEDIATE TRACHEOSTOMY! Even slight manipulations of this child's throat may cause precipitous further swelling and complete closure of his upper airway.

Humidified oxygen (answer a) is indicated, for the child is showing signs of respiratory distress (tachypnea, flaring of the nostrils). An IV line is desirable (answer b), both as a lifeline in the event of cardiac arrest and as a route for fluids, but don't bother with it if you are close to the hospital or if getting the IV in will significantly delay transport. The child needs to reach a medical facility as soon as possible. He should be transported sitting up (answer d); he probably won't let you transport him in any other position.

FURTHER READING

Bass JW et al. Sudden death due to acute epiglottitis. *Pediatr Infect Dis* 4:447, 1985.

Chaisson RE et al. Clinical aspects of adult epiglottitis. *West J Med* 144:700, 1986.

Costigan DC, Newth DJL. Respiratory status of children with epiglottitis with and without an artificial airway. *Am J Dis Child* 137:139, 1983.

Diaz JH, Lockhart CH. Early diagnosis and airway management of acute epiglottitis in children. *South Med J* 75:399, 1982.

Dierking BH. Respiratory distress! *Emergency* 21(1):27, 1989.

Losek JD et al. Epiglottitis: Comparison of signs and symptoms in children less than 2 years old and older. *Ann Emerg Med* 19:55, 1990.

Mauro RD et al. Differentiation of epiglottitis from laryngotracheitis in the child with stridor. *Am J Dis Child* 142:679, 1988.

Schuh S, Huang A, Fallis JC. Atypical epiglottitis. *Ann Emerg Med* 17:168, 1988.

Sendi K, Crysdale WS. Acute epiglottitis: Decade of change—a 10-year experience with 242 children. *J Otolaryngol* 16:196, 1987.

Tintinalli J. Respiratory stridor in the young child. *JACEP* 5:195, 1976.

Zillger JJ et al. Assessment of intubation in croup and epiglottitis. *Ann Otol Rhinol Laryngol* 91:403, 1982.

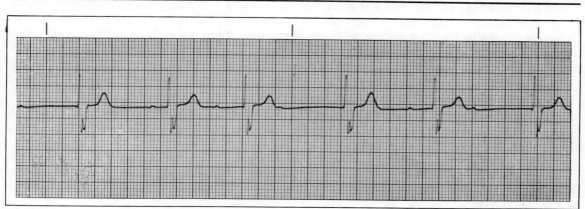

Figure 15

Your patient is a 52-year-old executive who has been feeling ill since shortly after lunchtime, when he developed "indigestion." He complains of a feeling of fullness and tightness in the epigastrium and says he feels nauseated. He states that he has been under treatment for high blood pressure, and he takes Diuril and Aldomet regularly. He denies any allergies. On physical examination, he is pale, apprehensive, and diaphoretic. His pulse is strong, blood pressure is 140/90, and respirations are 16. There is no jugular venous distention. The chest is clear, and heart sounds are well heard. There is no peripheral edema. A portion of his ECG is shown in Figure 15.

1. Examine the rhythm strip:

    a. The rhythm is _____ regular _____ irregular.
    b. The rate is _____ per minute.

2. The rhythm is

    a. Junctional rhythm
    b. First-degree AV block
    c. Wenckebach second-degree AV block
    d. Second-degree AV block (Mobitz type II)
    e. Complete heart block (third-degree AV block)

3. The pattern on the ECG reflects events in the heart and, in this case, suggests

    a. There is disease or injury in the area of the AV junction.
    b. There is an inferior wall myocardial infarction.
    c. The patient has had a previous myocardial infarction.
    d. There is accelerated conduction through the AV node.
    e. There is an aberrant pathway of conduction through the AV junction.

4. The treatment of this patient in the field is

    a. Transthoracic cardiac pacemaker.
    b. Oxygen, IV lifeline, and transport.
    c. Oxygen, IV, atropine, and transport.
    d. Oxygen, IV, isoproterenol, and transport.
    e. No treatment is required.

A110

1. The patient's rhythm is **irregular.** The rate is approximately **60 per minute.**
2. The rhythm is **Wenckebach** (answer **c**), with its classic pattern of progressive prolongation of the P–R interval until there is a P wave not followed by a QRS complex, together with progressive shortening of the R–R intervals. It is not a junctional rhythm (answer a), for P waves are clearly evident. In first-degree AV block (answer b), there is simply a fixed prolongation of the P–R interval beyond 0.2 seconds; there are no dropped beats. Mobitz type II second-degree block (answer d) usually shows a fixed degree of block—i.e., 2:1, 3:1—and thus the R–R intervals tend to remain fairly constant. Complete heart block (answer e) is characterized by a lack of any relationship between the P waves and QRS complexes.
3. Any degree of heart block suggests that there is **disease or injury in the area of the AV junction** (answer **a**); thus the electric impulses arriving from the atria are delayed or entirely prevented from reaching the ventricles.

   There is good reason to believe, from this patient's predominantly gastrointestinal symptoms, that he has had an inferior wall myocardial infarction (answer b), but confirmation of that hunch requires a full 12-lead ECG, as would any conclusions regarding previous myocardial infarctions (answer c).

   Conduction through the AV junction is certainly NOT accelerated in this patient (answer d); quite the contrary, it is considerably delayed and every few beats blocked altogether. An aberrant pathway of conduction through the AV junction (answer e), as in the Wolff-Parkinson-White (WPW) syndrome, would be expected to produce an abnormality in the shape of the P–R interval, such as the characteristic delta wave of WPW.
4. The treatment of this patient in the field is simply to **administer oxygen, establish an IV lifeline** (just in case), **and transport** him to the hospital (answer **b**). He does not have symptomatic bradycardia; he in conscious, alert, and not hypotensive. Thus there is no indication for measures to speed up his heart rate, such as a transthoracic pacemaker (answer a), atropine (answer c), or isoproterenol (answer d). However, some treatment *is* required (answer e)—treatment with the most important drug you carry for use in acute myocardial infarction: oxygen.

FURTHER READING

Bilitch M. *A Manual of Cardiac Arrhythmias.* Boston: Little, Brown, 1971.

Diamond NJ. Recognition of type 1 second degree atrial ventricular block during incomplete atrial ventricular dissociation in acute inferior myocardial infarction. *JACEP* 6:308, 1977.

Dubin D. *Rapid Interpretation of EKGs* (3rd ed.). Tampa: Cover, 1974.

Langendorf R, Cohen H, Gozo EG. Observations on second degree atrioventricular block, including new criteria for the differential diagnosis between type I and type II block. *Am J Cardiol* 29:111, 1972.

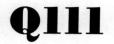

It's one of those days when nothing seems to go right. The oxygen tank ran out in the middle of a resuscitation, and when you went to get another one, you tripped over the defibrillator. The ambulance had a flat tire on the way back from the hospital. A patient vomited into your new demand valve. And now, 10 minutes before the end of your shift, you get a call for a "possible OB."

The woman is a "multip" in her ninth month of pregnancy, and her contractions are less than 2 minutes apart. So much for getting off duty on time. You and your partner quickly set her up for delivery at home, and in minutes, the baby is on the way.

1. You note that the umbilical cord is wrapped around the baby's neck. You should

   a. Push the baby gently back into the birth canal, so that the cord can untangle itself.
   b. Immediately clamp the cord and cut it.
   c. Gently try to unwrap the cord from the baby's neck; if that fails, clamp the cord and cut it.
   d. Leave the cord alone; it will not interfere with the birth of the baby.

2. Having successfully dealt with the problem of the umbilical cord, you find yourself holding a squalling baby girl. You suction out the infant's airway, wrap her in a sterile blanket, and patiently wait for the delivery of the placenta. Fifteen minutes pass, and the placenta is nowhere to be seen. You should

   a. Prepare the mother for transport to the hospital.
   b. Exert firm, steady traction on the umbilical cord to pull the placenta out.
   c. Probe manually into the vagina and attempt to remove the placenta.
   d. Pack the vagina firmly with bulky, sterile pads and move on to the hospital.

A111

1. The correct answer is **c: Gently try to unwrap the cord from the baby's neck; if that fails, clamp the cord and cut it.** In most cases, the maneuver will be successful, and one needn't immediately cut the cord in what may be a less than optimal spot (answer b). Certainly one should not try to push the baby back into the birth canal if she is trying to make her way out (answer a); just slow her down a bit while you untangle the cord from her neck. If you leave it there (answer d), it can strangle her or tear as she whizzes out into the world.

2. If the placenta fails to deliver within about 15 minutes after delivery of the baby, one should **prepare the mother for transport to the hospital** (answer a). DO NOT pull on the umbilical cord in an attempt to deliver the placenta (answer b) nor should you go fishing around blindly in the vagina for the placenta (answer c) or insert packs therein (answer d). Just place some sanitary pads between the mother's legs, put her supine on a stretcher, and start moving on to the hospital. But be prepared in case the placenta delivers while en route.

FURTHER READING

Anderson B, Shapiro B. *Emergency Childbirth Handbook.* Albany, NY: Delmar, 1979.
Emergence emergencies. *Emerg Med* 4(9):89, 1972.
Harris BA. Dealing with a difficult delivery. *Emerg Med* 16(11):22, 1984.
Kilgore JR. Management of an obstetric patient by the EMT. *EMT J* 4(2):50, 1980.
Nixon RG. Third trimester obstetric complications. Part III: Problems during fetal delivery. *Emerg Med Serv* 10(5):80, 1981.
Williams C. Emergency childbirth. *Emerg Med Serv* 14(3):100, 1985.
Wojslawowicz JM. Emergency childbirth for emergency medical technicians. *EMT J* 1(4):66, 1977.

You are called for a "man down" in a busy downtown area. Upon arrival at the scene, you find a man who appears to be in his middle 50s lying on the sidewalk in front of a department store. Bystanders state that several minutes before your arrival the patient had a "fit." Now he is groggy and confused, but he responds to voice.

1. Which of the following may have been the cause of this patient's seizure? (There may be more than one correct answer.)

   a. Stroke
   b. Head trauma
   c. Hypoxia
   d. Hypoglycemia
   e. Failure to take prescribed antiseizure medications.

2. The patient appears to be waking up gradually, and after a few minutes he is able to give you his name and address and to answer questions coherently. Which of the following would NOT be appropriate in the management of the patient at this time?

   a. Administer oxygen.
   b. Start an IV line to keep the vein open.
   c. Monitor the patient's cardiac rhythm.
   d. Administer diazepam (Valium), 5 to 10 mg IV.
   e. Transport the patient to the hospital in the supine position.

A112

1. The correct answer is **a, b, c, d, and e:** All of the situations listed may be the cause of seizures, and until one has more information, one has to take all of these possibilities into consideration. Stroke (answer a) and head trauma (answer b) can lead to seizures either immediately after the insult or even years later as a result of residual scar tissue in the damaged area of the brain. Hypoxia (answer c) is an important cause of seizures, and a convulsion from that source may occur after a relatively transient episode of cerebral ischemia, such as might occur during a few moments of cardiac dysrhythmia. A whole variety of neurologic symptoms may be seen in hypoglycemia (answer d); in addition to seizures, one may see confusion, bizarre behavior, and even coma. Finally, the failure of a known epileptic to take his prescribed medications (answer e) is among the most common causes of seizure.

2. The administration of diazepam (Valium) would NOT be appropriate in the management of this patient at this time (answer **d**). So far, he has had only a single seizure, from which he appears to be recovering adequately, and there is no need to give central nervous system depressant drugs—with all their possible hazards—in the management of an isolated seizure. It *is* a good idea to get an IV lifeline established (answer b), just in case the patient does have another seizure while under your care; for in that situation, you probably will be instructed to administer diazepam, and the tonic-clonic phase of a seizure is not the optimal time to try to start an IV.

   Since we still don't know what caused this patient's seizure, we want to cover all bets. The possibility of hypoxia makes it desirable to administer oxygen (answer a), while the possibility that the patient's seizure was secondary to a cardiac dysrhythmia that compromised blood flow to the brain is a good enough indication for cardiac monitoring (answer c). The patient should be transported in a position that will optimize cerebral perfusion, i.e., supine (answer e). Don't let him get up and walk away, even if he says he is feeling just dandy now. A patient who has had a seizure should be fully evaluated at the hospital.

FURTHER READING

Bader T. Telling pseudoseizures from true. *Emerg Med* 17(13):41, 1985.
Barber JM. EMT checkpoint: Seizures. *EMT J* 2(1):75, 1978. 18:965, 1984.
Bernat JL. Getting a handle on an adult's first seizure. *Emerg Med* 21(1):20, 1989.
Caroline NL. *Emergency Care in the Streets* (4th ed.). Boston: Little, Brown, 1991, Ch. 24.
Curry HB. Fits and faints: Causes and cures. *Emerg Med* 14(3):70, 1982.
Finelli PF, Cardi JK. Seizures as a cause of fracture. *Neurology* 39:858, 1989.
Gress D. Stopping seizures. *Emerg Med* 22(1):22, 1990.
Parrish GA, Skiendzielewski JJ. Bilateral posterior fracture-dislocations of the shoulder after convulsive status epilepticus. *Ann Emerg Med* 14:264, 1985.
Riley TL. Epilepsy—or merely hyperventilation? *Emerg Med* 14(14):162, 1982.
Waldhour RH. Management of the epileptic patient. *EMT J* 2(1):71, 1971.

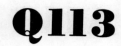

It is the second day of the summer's first real heat wave, and you are called in the mid-afternoon to a construction site, where one of the workers lies writhing on the ground, crying in pain. He states that the pain began about 2 hours ago as a dull ache in his right side and has become progressively worse. It is cramping in nature and radiates into his right groin. He denies any significant medical problems in the past. On physical examination, he is in marked distress and thrashing about on the ground. His skin is warm and moist. Pulse is 110, blood pressure is 150/90, and respirations are 20. There is moderate tenderness to palpation over the right flank, just below the rib margin. Otherwise there are no abnormal physical findings.

Which of the following is NOT part of the treatment of this patient?

a. Start an IV with normal saline, and run it in wide open.
b. Apply but do not inflate military antishock trousers.
c. Give morphine, 0.1 mg per kilogram slowly IV.
d. Transport the patient to the hospital in a position of comfort.

A113

Our construction worker is manifesting a typical picture of renal colic, and his pain is most likely due to the obstruction of his right ureter by a stone. During the first few hot days of summer, one is likely to see a whole rash of such cases, for most people have not yet increased their fluid intake to meet the changing climatic demands, and renal colic tends to develop in susceptible individuals under conditions of moderate dehydration.

This patient is not in any imminent danger of shock, and thus the application of military antishock trousers is entirely unnecessary in this case (answer **b**). He does, however, need a lot of fluids (answer a), both to correct his dehydration (and thereby minimize the possibility of further stone formation) and to help him pass the stone lodged in his ureter. He also needs strong analgesia (answer c), for the pain of renal colic can be the most excruciating pain that a person can suffer. Our patient's pain is fairly typical: originating in the flank and radiating into the groin, with associated right costovertebral angle tenderness. Sometimes the pain of renal colic will radiate into the leg as well. It is characteristic for the patient to thrash around as he attempts to find a position in which the pain is minimal. He should be permitted to assume whatever position is most comfortable for him during transport (answer d).

FURTHER READING

Edna TH et al. Acute ureteral colic and fluid intake. *Scand J Urol Nephrol* 17:175, 1983.
Flannigan GM et al. Indomethacin—an alternative to pethidine in ureteric colic. *Br J Urol* 55:6, 1983.
Klein LA et al. The emergency management of patients with ureteral calculi and fever. *J Urol* 129:938, 1983.
Sjodin JG. Clinical experience of indomethacin in pain from ureteral stone. *Scand J Urol Nephrol* 75:35, 1983.
Williams HE. Nephrolithiasis. *N Engl J Med* 290:33, 1974.

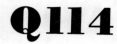

While playing Frisbee on the beach one fine summer day, you notice a small commotion taking place about 100 yards down the shore. Running to investigate, you find a 20-year-old man who has just been pulled from the water lying unconscious on the sand. He does not appear to be breathing, and his color is slate gray. You should

a. Quickly turn him to his side to drain the water out of his lungs.
b. Turn him over prone and use the back pressure/arm lift (Holger Nielsen) technique of artificial ventilation.
c. Keep him supine and use the chest pressure/arm lift (Silvester) method of resuscitation.
d. Tilt his head back, and if that maneuver fails to produce spontaneous breathing, start mouth-to-mouth ventilation.
e. Straddle the patient and perform a Heimlich maneuver to get the water out of his lungs.

After you have been working on the patient for just a few moments, he begins to revive, and within 2 or 3 minutes he is fully conscious and alert and states he feels perfectly fine. You should

a. Have him run up and down the beach for a few minutes to get his circulation going again.
b. Give him some water or juice to drink, since he is bound to be dehydrated.
c. Tell him that it's all right to stay at the beach, so long as he doesn't exert himself.
d. Instruct him to go home and rest there for a day or two.
e. See to it that he is taken to the hospital, preferably by ambulance, for evaluation.

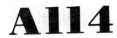

A114
If the patient is apneic, one should immediately **open his airway by backward tilt of the head,** and if he does not resume spontaneous breathing, **start mouth-to-mouth ventilation** (answer d). Maneuvers designed to force water out of the lungs, such as rolling the patient to the side (answer a) or performing a Heimlich maneuver (answer e) are simply a waste of time. To begin with, if the patient has been submerged for only a short time (and we can assume that this is the case, for there is no indication that he has suffered cardiac arrest yet, only respiratory arrest), there is unlikely to be any water in his lungs at all. In the first moments of near drowning, reflex laryngospasm usually occurs and effectively seals off the lower airway from aspiration of water. There *is,* however, likely to be water in the patient's stomach—a lot of water—and the Heimlich maneuver carries a significant risk of displacing that water into the posterior oropharynx, from where it can be easily aspirated. Secondly, even if there were water in the patient's lungs, neither rolling him to the side nor a Heimlich maneuver nor, for that matter, hanging him upside down by his toes is likely to remove that water. All those maneuvers will simply waste precious minutes, during which the patient could be receiving artificial ventilation and a new lease on life.

The Holger Nielsen and Silvester methods of artificial ventilation (answers b and c) went out with the rumble seat. Studies carried out in the 1950s demonstrated that those techniques could not move adequate volumes of air in and out of the lungs, while excellent tidal volumes could be achieved through the use of mouth-to-mouth ventilation. Furthermore, the Holger Nielsen and Silvester techniques provide no means of maintaining the airway in an open position during ventilation, while mouth-to-mouth ventilation enables the rescuer to keep the victim's head in a backward tilt position and thereby prevent recurrent airway obstruction.

Every near-drowning victim should be **evaluated in the hospital,** even when the victim seems to have recovered completely at the scene (answer **e**). Delayed pulmonary edema is not uncommon in near drowning, and for that reason alone near-drowning victims deserve careful monitoring for at least 24 hours in the hospital. The victim should NOT be left at the scene (answer c) or instructed to go home and rest (answer d); he needs to be in a medical setting where treatment will be immediately available if late complications develop. Running around the beach (answer a) will NOT "get his circulation going again." To begin with, there is no evidence that there was anything wrong with this patient's circulation in the first place. And running will simply exhaust him and add to whatever element of metabolic acidosis remains from the near-drowning episode. He should remain sitting quietly until the ambulance arrives.

It is NOT a good idea to give such a patient anything by mouth (answer b), for the danger of vomiting remains, even after resuscitation. Fluids, if needed at all, should be provided by the intravenous route as soon as the ambulance arrives with the necessary equipment. The ambulance crew should consult their base station physician for orders in this regard.

FURTHER READING
Cairns FJ. Deaths from drowning. *NZ Med J* 97:65, 1984.
Dietz PE, Baker SP. Drowning: Epidemiology and prevention. *Am J Pub Health* 64:303, 1974.
Harries MG. Clinical course of 61 serious immersion incidents. *Disaster Med* 1:263, 1983.
Harries MG. Drowning in man. *Crit Care Med* 9:407, 1981.
Hooper HA. Near drowning. *Emergency* 12(5):75, 1980.
Jacobson WK et al. Correlation of spontaneous respiration and neurologic damage in near-drowning. *Crit Care Med* 11:487, 1983.
Modell JH. Near-drowning. *Int Anesthesiol Clin* 15:107, 1977.
Modell JH. Is the Heimlich maneuver appropriate as first treatment in drowning? *Emerg Med Serv* 10(6):63, 1981.
Ornato JP. The resuscitation of near-drowning victims. *JAMA* 256:75, 1986.
Redding JS. Historic vignettes concerning resuscitation from drowning. In Safar P and Elam JO (Eds.), *Advances in Cardiopulmonary Resuscitation.* New York: Springer-Verlag, 1977, pp. 276–280.
Safar P. The failure of manual artificial respiration. *J Appl Physiol* 14:84, 1959.
Safar P, Escarrage L, Elam J. A comparison of the mouth-to-mouth and mouth-to-airway methods of artificial respiration with the chest pressure-arm lift methods. *N Engl J Med* 258:671, 1958.
Sarnaik AP et al. Near-drowning: Fresh, salt, and cold water immersion. *Clin Sports Med* 5:33, 1986.
Redding JS. Drowning and near-drowning. *Postgrad Med* 74:85, 1983.
Redmond AD et al. Resuscitation from drowning. *Arch Emerg Med* 1:113, 1984.

The call comes in as a "man who has gone crazy," and the dispatcher directs you to a telephone booth near the outskirts of town. There you find a very excited young woman, with her three small children huddled around her. She gestures toward a house down the street and states that her husband is inside with a gun and is threatening to kill anyone who comes near him. He came home from work today "completely crazy." She has never seen him like this before.

You should

a. Enter the house alone and try to reason with the husband.
b. Enter the house with the wife and try to reason with the husband.
c. Keep the wife and children in a safe place and call the police.
d. Inform the wife that this is not a medical problem and that there is nothing you can do to help.

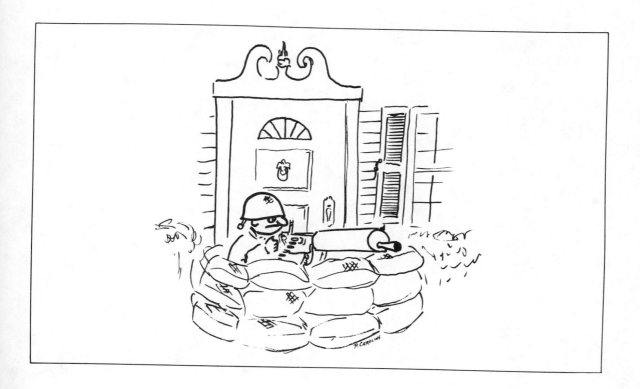

A115

The violent, homicidal patient is a potential danger to all those around him, including the paramedic team. It is a matter for the police, not a paramedic, to deal with such an individual (answer c). Trying to reason with a violent, crazed individual—especially when he has a gun and you don't—is sheer folly (answer a), nor should you expose the man's wife to that danger (answer b). Your job is to see to it that the wife and children are safe and to provide them with whatever comfort you can, until others are available to assume that role. Your base hospital may be able to help you put the family in touch with a community social service agency that can be of assistance. Simply to announce that this is not a medical problem and drive away (answer d) is to display a callous and irresponsible attitude that is entirely inappropriate in a health professional. When someone calls for an ambulance, he or she is expressing a need for help. If you cannot supply this help, it is part of your job to assist the caller in finding the the person or agency who can.

FURTHER READING

Bassuk EL, Fox SS, Prendergast KJ. *Behavioral Emergencies: A Field Guide for EMTs and Paramedics.* Boston: Little, Brown, 1983.

Dick T. Rules of restraint. *JEMS* 5(7):22, 1980.

Dick T. Gloves without fingers: Using stockinette as a restraint. *JEMS* 14(12):25, 1989.

Dubin WR. Evaluating and managing the violent patient. *Ann Emerg Med* 10:481, 1981.

Dubin WR et al. Rapid tranquilization of the violent patient. *Am J Emerg Med* 7:313, 1989.

Gorski T. Managing the violent patient. *Emerg Med Serv* 10(5):6, 1981.

Infantino JA. Controlling violent patients. *Emerg Med Serv* 13(5):23, 1984.

Leisner K. Managing the pre-violent patient. *Emerg Med Serv* 18(7):18, 1989.

Lipscomb WR. Acute paranoia. *Emerg Med* 6(2):268, 1974.

Makadon HJ, Gerson S, Ryback R. Managing the care of the difficult patient in the emergency unit. *JAMA* 252:2585, 1984.

Nordberg N. Hate in the streets. *Emerg Med Serv* 18(8):24, 1989.

Rund DA. Emergency management of the difficult patient. *Emerg Med Serv* 13(3):17, 1984.

Taylor C. Domestic violence: The medical response. *Emerg Med Serv* 3(5):35, 1984.

The violent patient. *Emerg Med* 15(9):26, 1983.

STEP ON A CRACK AND BREAK YOUR BACK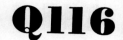

Which of the following patients should be assumed to have suffered an injury to the spine and should therefore be immobilized on a long backboard? (There may be more than one correct answer.)

a. A 35-year-old man who was the driver of a car that struck a wall at 55 mph and who suffered a head injury. The patient is unconscious.
b. A 20-year-old man who dove into a shallow pool and struck his head on the bottom. He is conscious and can move all extremities.
c. A 50-year-old house painter who fell from a scaffolding on the second floor. He is conscious and can move all extremities.
d. A 42-year-old pedestrian who was struck by a bus. He is conscious and complaining of numbness and tingling in both his legs.

A116

The correct answers are **a, b, c,** and **d:** *All* of the patients should be assumed to have suffered an injury to the spine and should therefore be immobilized on a long backboard.

When evaluating the possibility of spinal injury, one must rely heavily on an assessment of the *mechanisms of the injury;* by the time symptoms develop, the chances of recovering motor and sensory function have considerably decreased. Thus any patient who has suffered an injury that *could* have produced trauma to the spine should be assumed to have a spine injury until proved otherwise. The time to immobilize such a patient is *before* you have moved him and he begins complaining that he can no longer move his legs.

Patient a sustained a head injury severe enough to produce unconsciousness in a situation of marked deceleration forces. He is thus an excellent candidate for cervical spine damage. He needs a cervical collar, and he should be packaged and removed from the vehicle with short and long backboards.

Patient b suffered a classic diving injury of the sort that too often leads to quadriplegia. Don't be lulled into a false sense of security by the fact that he can move all his extremities. Injudicious movement of this patient could change that situation in minutes. Get enough help so that he can be logrolled onto his side, with his spine kept in alignment, while a long backboard is slid beneath him, and immobilize him well.

A patient who falls from a height (patient c) may give his spine a tremendous jolt. Once again, it is of no practical significance in the field that our house painter can move all his extremities. Because of the manner in which he sustained his injury, we must assume that he suffered damage to his spine until this possibility can be ruled out by x-ray and other studies in the hospital.

The prospects for our pedestrian who was struck by a bus (patient d) are less optimistic, for he has already developed symptoms of spinal cord compression. Nonetheless, everything possible must be done to avoid aggravating his injury further, and he too should be securely immobilized on a backboard before any attempt is made to move him.

FURTHER READING

Anast GT. Fractures and injuries of the cervical spine. *EMT J* 2(3):36, 1978.

Anderson DK et al. Spinal cord injury and protection. *Ann Emerg Med* 14:816, 1985.

Barber JM. EMT checkpoint: Spinal cord injury and neurogenic shock. *EMT J* 2(3):69, 1978.

Bayless P, Ray VG. Incidence of cervical spine injuries in association with blunt head trauma. *Am J Emerg Med* 7:139, 1989.

Bourn S. Tell the spinal fanatics to "back off." *JEMS* 15(5):73, 1990.

Byun HS et al. Severe cervical injury due to break dancing: A case report. *Orthopedics* 9:550, 1986.

Caroline NL. *Emergency Care in the Streets* (4th ed.). Boston: Little, Brown, 1991, Ch. 16.

Caroline NL. *Emergency Medical Treatment: A Text for EMT-As and EMT-Intermediates* (3rd ed.). Boston: Little, Brown, 1991, Ch. 14.

Davidson JSD, Birdsell DC. Cervical spine injury in patients with facial skeletal trauma. *J Trauma* 29:1276, 1989.

Dula DJ. Trauma to the cervical spine. *JACEP* 8:504, 1979.

Gopalakrishnan KC, El Masri WS. Fractures of the sternum associated with spinal injury. *J Bone Joint Surg* [*Br*] 68B:178, 1986.

Guthkelch AN et al. Patterns of cervical spine injury and their associated lesions. *West J Med* 147:428, 1987.

Hadley MN et al. Pediatric spinal trauma: Review of 122 cases of spinal cord and vertebral column injuries. *J Neurosurg* 68:18, 1988.

In diving injuries . . . *Emerg Med* 14(13):139, 1982.

Jackson DW et al. Cervical spine injuries. *Clin Sports Med* 5:373, 1986.

McCabe JB, Angelos MG. Injury to the head and face in patients with cervical spine injury. *Am J Emerg Med* 2:333, 1984.

O'Malley KF, Ross SE. The incidence of injury to the cervical spine in patients with craniocerebral injury. *J Trauma* 28:1476, 1988.

Reiss SJ et al. Cervical spine fractures with major associated trauma. *Neurosurgery* 18:327, 1986.

Ruge JR et al. Pediatric spinal injury: The very young. *J Neurosurg* 68:25, 1988.

A call at 3:00 A.M. to the Happy Hollow Senior Citizens' Home, for a "possible stroke." The night manager, a very nervous little man, hurries you upstairs to room 212, where Mr. and Mrs. Ryan reside. The manager tells you that they are both in their late 70s and "have never given us any trouble before." When you enter the room, you find Mr. Ryan, who is apparently the patient, shuffling about in a somewhat dazed state. Mrs. Ryan tells you that he had seemed fine when they went to bed, but that he wakened about half an hour ago very confused. He takes "blood pressure pills" but otherwise has had no major medical problems.

On examination, you find Mr. Ryan wholly confused and disoriented. He also seems quite restless. His skin is pale, cool, and somewhat clammy. Pulse is 44 and occasionally irregular, blood pressure is 180/110, and respirations are 30. There is no evidence of head trauma. There has been cataract surgery on the right, but the left pupil is reactive. There is no jugular venous distention. Auscultation of the chest reveals rales at both bases and about halfway up the chest. Heart sounds are well heard. The abdomen is soft. There is no peripheral edema, and the patient moves all extremities equally.

Which of the following is NOT part of the management of this patient?

a. Administer oxygen in high concentration.
b. Start an IV with D5W to keep the vein open.
c. Administer morphine, 5 mg very slowly IV (1 mg at a time).
d. Monitor cardiac rhythm.
e. Transport the patient supine to the hospital.

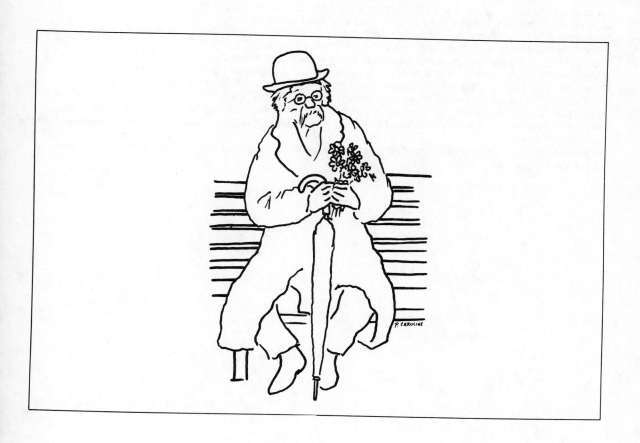

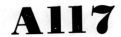**A117**

Really, you aren't going to compel this gentleman to lie flat all the way to the hospital, are you (answer **e**)? The poor man is suffering from pulmonary edema secondary to left heart failure; he needs to be sitting upright, preferably with his legs dangling, not lying supine so that his whole vascular volume can collect in his lungs.

How do we know he's in left heart failure? Forget about what the manager told you ("possible stroke"), and LOOK AT THE PATIENT! He has a hypertensive history, which already predisposes him to left-sided heart failure. He is tachypneic, and his lungs are full of rales. How much more evidence do you want?

Don't be fooled by the patient's confusion. He has every right to be confused: His brain isn't getting enough oxygen, and thus you'd better give him some (answer a). You will need the IV line (answer b) to administer medications, such as the morphine (answer c) indicated for his pulmonary edema—not to mention the atropine you may have to administer immediately afterward if his pulse drops any further. The patient's bradycardia and irregularities in pulse are by themselves sufficient indication to monitor his cardiac rhythm (answer d), even if he weren't in heart failure. Don't be surprised if you find signs of acute myocardial infarction; AMI frequently presents in the elderly simply as confusion or heart failure, without any chest pain.

The moral of this story is twofold:

1. MANY SERIOUS ILLNESSES IN THE ELDERLY PRESENT SIMPLY AS CONFUSION.
2. WHEN ALL ELSE FAILS, EXAMINE THE PATIENT.

FURTHER READING

Aronow WS. Prevalence of presenting symptoms of recognized acute myocardial infarction and of unrecognized healed myocardial infarction in elderly patients. *Am J Cardiol* 60:1182, 1987.

Bayer AJ et al. Changing presentation of myocardial infarction with increasing old age. *J Am Geriatr Soc* 34:263, 1986.

Bosker G, Sequeira M. The 60-second geriatric assessment. *Emerg Med Serv* 17(7):17, 1988.

Eckstein D. Common symptoms and complaints of the elderly. *J Am Geriatr Soc* 21:440, 1973.

Eliastam M. Elderly patients in the emergency department. *Ann Emerg Med* 18:1222, 1989.

Garvin JM. Caring for the geriatric patient. *Emerg Med Serv* 9(2):75, 1980.

Gerson LW, Skvarch L. Emergency medical service utilization by the elderly. *Ann Emerg Med* 11:610, 1982.

Judd RL. Caring for the elderly. *Emergency* 21(6):38, 1989.

Kapoor W et al. Syncope in the elderly. *Am J Med* 80:419, 1986.

Kincaid DT, Botti RE. Myocardial infarction in the elderly. *Chest* 64:170, 1973.

Lipowski ZJ. Delirium in the elderly patient. *N Engl J Med* 320:578, 1989.

McMahan FJ et al. What special problems do geriatric patients present? *Emerg Med Serv* 14(2):19, 1985.

Moscovitz HL. Old hearts: The same but different. *Emerg Med* 8:53, 1976.

Muller RT et al. Painless myocardial infarction in the elderly. *Am Heart J* 119:202, 1990.

Rockwood K. Acute confusion in elderly medical patients. *J Am Geriatr Soc* 37:150, 1989.

Rowe JW, Besdine RW. *Health and Disease in Old Age.* Boston: Little, Brown, 1982.

Schanzer HR. The emergencies of old age. *Emerg Med* 17(21):59, 1985.

Taylor BW. Altered factors in the assessment of the geriatric patient. *Emerg Med Serv* 14(2):26, 1985.

Wilson LB, Simson SP, Baxter CR (eds.). *Handbook of Geriatric Emergency Care.* Baltimore: University Park Press, 1984.

Wroblewski M et al. Symptoms of myocardial infarction in old age: Clinical case retrospective and prospective studies. *Age Aging* 15:99, 1986.

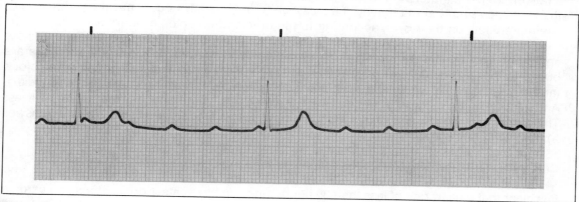

Figure 16

You are called to a downtown bank, where the chief loan officer has collapsed at his desk. You find him slumped in his chair, surrounded by several highly nervous co-workers. The patient is breathing stertorously and has a very slow pulse. His skin is pale and clammy. Pupils are equal and reactive, and the chest is clear. The monitor shows the rhythm in Figure 16.

1. Examine the rhythm strip:

   a. The rhythm is _____ regular _____ irregular.
   b. The rate is _____ per minute.

2. This ECG pattern is

   a. Sinus arrest
   b. Wenckebach
   c. (Mobitz II) second-degree AV block
   d. Complete heart block
   e. Slow atrial flutter

3. The probable reason for this patient's unconsciousness is

   a. Cerebrovascular accident (stroke)
   b. Inadequate cardiac output
   c. Acute myocardial infarction
   d. Hypoglycemia
   e. High peripheral resistance

4. Which of the following is NOT part of the management of this patient?

   a. Immediately get the patient out of the chair and place him supine on the floor.
   b. Administer oxygen.
   c. Start an IV with 250 ml of D5W, and add 1 mg of isoproterenol to the bag; run at approximately 0.5 to 1.0 ml per minute.
   d. Administer atropine, 1 mg IV.
   e. Administer lidocaine, 100 mg IV to abolish the PVCs.
   f. Notify the hospital to have a pacemaker ready in the emergency room.

A118

1. The patient's rhythm is **regular.** The rate is **less than 30 per minute.**
2. The ECG pattern is **complete heart block** (answer **d**). The atria are contracting merrily away at a rate of 125 per minute, but the electric impulses are not getting through the AV junction, so the ventricles simply aren't getting the message from the sinus node. Thus the ventricles are beating entirely on their own, according to the orders of an ectopic ventricular focus.

   If there were sinus arrest (answer a), we would expect to see a few dropped P waves here and there, but the P wave rate is perfectly regular, and the only P waves we don't see are buried in the QRS complexes. In Wenckebach (answer b) or full-blown second-degree block (answer c), there is a predictable relationship between the P waves and the QRS complexes. And in atrial flutter (answer e), we don't see P waves at all, but rather sawtooth flutter waves.
3. The probable reason for the patient's unconsciousness is **inadequate cardiac output** (answer **b**). Recalling our equation:

   CARDIAC OUTPUT = STROKE VOLUME × HEART RATE

   it is clear that a heart rate of less than 30 per minute can have catastrophic effects on cardiac output. This patient is unconscious because there isn't enough blood going to his head, and there is no need to search for further explanations, such as stroke (answer a) or hypoglycemia (answer d).
4. All of the measures mentioned are part of the patient's management *except* lidocaine for PVCs (answer **e**): THOSE AIN'T PVCs!! Granted, they are ectopic, but those ventricular beats are the only source of cardiac output this patient has—so don't try to abolish those beats with lidocaine unless you're in the mood for a very long exercise in external cardiac compression! As is, you may have to initiate chest compressions on this patient should the measures you take to increase his heart rate fail.

   Get the patient flat as rapidly as possible to promote blood flow to his brain (answer a), and administer oxygen (answer b) so that what blood does reach the brain will provide the maximum oxygen supply. Isoproterenol (answer c) and atropine (answer d) are administered in an attempt to speed up the heart rate, until a pacemaker can be inserted in the hospital (answer f).

FURTHER READING

American Heart Association. Standards and guidelines for cardiopulmonary resuscitation (CPR) and emergency cardiac care (ECC). *JAMA* 255:2905, 1986.

Atkins JM et al. Ventricular conduction blocks and sudden death in acute myocardial infarction: Potential indications for pacing. *N Engl J Med* 288:281, 1973.

Bandy R, Orban DJ, Geiderman JM. Application of the Cardiotrak™ pacemaker monitor to prehospital care. *Ann Emerg Med* 10:579, 1981.

Caroline NL. *Emergency Care in the Streets* (4th ed.). Boston: Little, Brown, 1991, Ch. 23.

Falk RH et al. External noninvasive cardiac pacing in out-of-hospital cardiac arrest. *Crit Care Med* 11:779, 1983.

Jaggarao NSV et al. Use of an automated external defibrillator-pacemaker by ambulance staff. *Lancet* 2:73, 1982.

Kastor JA. Atrioventricular block. *N Engl J Med* 292:462 and 292:572, 1975.

Marriott HJL. What's the meaning of arrhythmias after MI? *Emerg Med* 14(14):120, 1982.

Roberts JR, Greenberg Jl. Emergency transthoracic pacemaker. *Ann Emerg Med* 10:600, 1981.

A 62-year-old woman was a front-seat passenger in an automobile that was struck from behind by a truck moving at high speed. The woman was not wearing a seat belt and was thrown through the front windshield, sustaining multiple lacerations.

You find her wandering in a dazed state a few yards from the automobile. She is covered with blood, and there are obvious lacerations over her face and arms. There is also a prominent bruise on the right forehead. She is spitting out blood, and some teeth appear to be missing. There is a large laceration over the region of the left jugular vein. Physical examination is otherwise negative.

1. The penetrating injury to the patient's neck must be sealed immediately because an open neck injury carries the danger of a life-threatening complication. This potential complication is

   a. Paraplegia
   b. Air embolism
   c. Thyroid damage
   d. Subcutaneous emphysema
   e. Aspiration of a foreign body

2. Which of the following statements regarding the type of injury this patient sustained are true and which are false?
   a. Massive trauma to the face is likely to be associated with injury to the cervical spine and thus requires that the patient be immobilized accordingly.

      TRUE   FALSE

   b. One should not waste time at the scene searching for lost teeth or broken dentures, since these are unlikely to be of any use to the patient.

      TRUE   FALSE

   c. Clear fluid draining from the patient's nose after a head injury suggests that the patient has sustained a skull fracture.

      TRUE   FALSE

A119

1. Open injuries to the neck may permit air to be sucked into the great veins and thereby result in fatal **air embolism** (answer **b**). While thyroid damage (answer c) and subcutaneous emphysema (answer d) may also occur, they are not life-threatening complications. The likelihood of injury to the cervical spine is neither increased nor decreased by the fact that the neck injury is open, and, besides, cervical spine damage would be more apt to produce quadriplegia than paraplegia (answer a). Aspiration of a foreign body through the wound (answer e) will not take place so long as the trachea is intact, and we have no evidence that there has been tracheal penetration in this patient.

2. TRUE-FALSE questions:
   a. Massive trauma to the face is likely to be associated with injury to the cervical spine and thus requires that the patient be immobilized accordingly.

   TRUE. Forces sufficient to cause significant facial injury must be assumed sufficient to have caused cervical spine injury as well. In the case of our patient, that means applying a cervical collar (after sealing off her neck wound!) and immobilizing her on a long backboard. The fact that she is up wandering around does not rule out the possibility of cervical spine damage, and one should not wait for signs of spine injury to occur before making a decision to immobilize such a patient.

   b. One should not waste time at the scene searching for lost teeth or broken dentures, since these are unlikely to be of any use to the patient.

   FALSE! It isn't at all a waste of time to try to find lost teeth or dentures. Dislodged teeth, if carefully preserved and transported in a carton of milk or in sterile dressings soaked with sterile saline, can often be reimplanted by dental surgeons. Dentures can be enormously helpful in ensuring proper alignment when a fractured mandible must be wired in position.

   c. Clear fluid draining from the patient's nose after a head injury suggests that the patient has sustained a skull fracture.

   TRUE. The drainage of clear fluid from a patient's nose in the context of head injury suggests possible fracture of the cribiform plate of the skull, a very thin, bony structure separating the nasal cavity from the brain behind it.

FURTHER READING

Barrs DM, Kern EB. Acute nasal trauma: Emergency room care of 250 patients. *J Fam Pract* 10:225, 1980.
Carducci B, Lowe RA, Dalsey W. Penetrating neck trauma: Consensus and controversies. *Ann Emerg Med* 15:208, 1986.
Chamberlain JH, Goerig AC. Rationale for the treatment and management of avulsed teeth. *J Am Dent Assoc* 101:471, 1980.
Champion HC. The penetrated neck. *Emerg Med* 15(14):259, 1983.
Frame SB. Stab wound to the larynx. *Emerg Med* 20(9):62, 1988.
Hendler BH. The sites and signs of maxillofacial trauma. *Emerg Med* 16(6):23, 1984.
Kalish M. Airway management in maxillofacial trauma. *Emerg Med Serv* 18(6):42, 1989.
Krasner PR. Management of avulsed teeth. *Emerg Med Serv* 18(6):31, 1989.
Landeen JM. Emergency management of the maxillofacial-injured patient. *Emergency* 10(6):42, 1978.
Lapeyrolerie FM. Emergency dental considerations. *Emergency* 10(12):50, 1978.
Lind GL, Spiegel EH, Munson ES. Treatment of traumatic tooth avulsion. *Anesth Analg* 61:469, 1982.
Manson PN, Kelly KJ. Evaluation and management of the patient with facial trauma. *Emerg Med Serv* 18(6):22, 1989.
Medford HM, Curtis JW. Acute care of severe tooth fractures. *Ann Emerg Med* 12:364, 1983.
Sarri P. Emergency care of dento-facial injuries. *J Prehosp Med* 2(2):35, 1988.
Wender RW, Swerdloff M, Alexander SA. Prehospital treatment of dental injuries. *Emerg Med Serv* 8(5):10, 1979.

COMING APART AT THE SEAMS

You are called late at night to the home of a 58-year-old executive, who is complaining of a very severe, "tearing" pain in his back and abdomen. He states that he has been having back pain for several months but that none of the doctors he consulted were able to find the cause. On physical examination, he appears pale and anxious. Pulse is 110 and regular, blood pressure is 110/90, and respirations are 18. There is no jugular venous distention. The chest is clear and heart sounds are well heard. The abdomen is soft, and there is a moderately tender, pulsating mass palpable. There is no peripheral edema.

    Which of the following is NOT part of the management of this patient?

a. Start an IV line with normal saline, and run it initially to keep the vein open.
b. Apply but do not inflate military antishock trousers (MAST).
c. Administer nitrous oxide/oxygen.
d. Administer norepinephrine (Levophed) by titrated IV infusion.
e. Notify the hospital to have a surgical team standing by.

A120

Our executive is showing signs of an expanding abdominal aortic aneurysm and may be in acute danger of rupture. An aneurysm is an abnormal widening of the arterial wall, often into a large bulge or sac. This attenuated area of aortic wall may rupture under the enormous stresses of systolic thrust, and the results may be rapidly catastrophic, with exsanguination into the abdomen. Our patient's pain suggests that his aneurysm is already leaking.

Norepinephrine (Levophed) or any other measures to raise the blood pressure are contraindicated in this patient (answer **d**), for they will only increase the tension on the weakened area of the aorta. An IV line should be started, so that it will be available for massive fluid infusion in the event of aneurysmal rupture and sudden hypotension (answer a). Similarly, the MAST should be applied but not inflated, as a precautionary measure (answer b), so that it can be deployed rapidly should a sudden drop in blood pressure occur. Nitrous oxide is a good analgesic in this case (answer c), for it will not have deleterious effects on the patient's blood pressure or mask the patient's symptoms and signs, which the surgeons must evaluate carefully when the patient arrives in the emergency department. Finally, in a case of this sort, one must assume that rupture of the aneurysm may occur at any moment, and thus a surgical team should be standing by at the hospital, in the event that the patient must be taken immediately to the operating room (answer e).

FURTHER READING
The four faces of aneurysm. *Emerg Med* 8(5):140, 1976.
Tintinalli JE. Ruptured aortic aneurysm. *JACEP* 4:440, 1975.

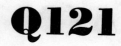

Your patient is a 37-year-old woman who complains of the sudden onset of severe dyspnea. She denies any pain, nausea, dizziness, or paresthesias. Her medical history is unremarkable. Her regular medications include vitamin pills and birth control pills. She smokes 1½ packs of cigarettes a day. She has no known allergies. On physical examination, she appears to be in acute respiratory distress. Her pulse is 140 and regular, blood pressure is 100/70, and respirations are 32 and labored. There is no jugular venous distention, lungs are clear, and breath sounds are equal bilaterally. The abdomen is soft, and there is no pedal edema. The ECG shows only sinus tachycardia.

The most likely cause of this patient's dyspnea is

a. Hyperventilation syndrome
b. Acute pulmonary embolism
c. Left heart failure with pulmonary edema
d. Spontaneous pneumothorax
e. Acute asthmatic attack

A121

The correct answer is **b: acute pulmonary embolism.** There are many factors that predispose a person to develop pulmonary embolism—among them, prolonged bed rest, deep venous insufficiency of the legs, major fractures to the long bones, and, at least according to some studies, birth control pills. Women over 35 who take birth control pills and who also smoke are particularly at risk for embolic phenomena. The most notable feature of our patient's story is the absence of any significant medical history or even significant findings, save for tachycardia, on physical examination. That is often the case in pulmonary embolism, which may present simply as unexplained dyspnea, tachycardia, hypotension, or a combination thereof.

This patient is NOT presenting a typical picture of hyperventilation syndrome (answer a): She has none of the paresthesias (tingling sensations) usually associated with the condition, and her relative hypotension would be difficult to explain on the basis of hyperventilation alone. Nor is there any evidence for left heart failure with pulmonary edema (answer c). The woman has no cardiac history, and her lungs are entirely free of the rales one would expect in pulmonary edema. Spontaneous pneumothorax (answer d) could present as sudden dyspnea, and there could be associated tachycardia and hypotension as well, but the presence of equal breath sounds on both sides of the chest argues strongly against this diagnosis. Finally, an acute asthmatic attack (answer e) would be very unusual in a 37-year-old woman who gives no history of asthma or allergic conditions. Furthermore, her lungs are clear, and an asthmatic attack severe enough to produce marked dyspnea would be expected to be associated with significant wheezing.

FURTHER READING

Bell WR, Simon TL, DeMets DL. The clinical features of submassive and massive pulmonary emboli. *Am J Med* 62:355, 1977.

Cooke DH. Focusing in on pulmonary embolism. *Emerg Med* 17(9):86, 1985.

Goodall RJR et al. Clinical correlations in the diagnosis of pulmonary embolism. *Ann Surg* 191:219, 1980.

Huet Y et al. Hypoxemia in acute pulmonary embolism. *Chest* 88:829, 1985.

McGlynn TJ, Hamilton RW, Moore R. Pulmonary embolism: 1979. *JACEP* 8:532, 1979.

Park H et al. Pulmonary embolism. *Emerg Med Serv* 4(5):33, 1975.

Sabiston DC. Pathophysiology, diagnosis and management of pulmonary embolism. *Am J Surg* 138:384, 1979.

Sutton GC, Honey M, Gibson RV. Clinical diagnosis of acute massive pulmonary embolism. *Lancet* 1:271, 1979.

Thrombi and emboli: Finding them, fighting them. *Emerg Med* 8(11):142, 1976.

Williams MH. Pulmonary embolism. *Emerg Med* 16(4):135, 1984.

A 33-year-old man was struck down and run over by a car that went through a red light at an intersection. You find him lying on the street, surrounded by a mob of curious bystanders. He is conscious, moaning in pain, and complaining of severe thirst. His skin is pale, cold, and moist. Pulse is 130, blood pressure is 90/60, and respirations are 30 and shallow. There is no evidence of injury to the head or neck. There is no jugular venous distention. There are no bruises on the chest, and the chest wall is stable. Breath sounds are clear and equal bilaterally. Heart sounds are well heard. There is a tire-tread mark across the patient's abdomen, and the abdomen is rigid to palpation. There is some deformity in the left midthigh. Otherwise the extremities show no obvious injury.

1. Which of the following is NOT part of the management of this patient?

   a. Administer oxygen.
   b. Allow the patient to drink as much water as he craves until you can get an IV started.
   c. Keep the patient flat.
   d. Apply military antishock trousers.
   e. Start at least one IV line using a large-bore cannula, and administer normal saline solution with the IV(s) wide open.

2. Which of the following statements about blunt trauma to the abdomen are true and which are false?

   a. Blunt abdominal trauma may cause devastating injury to internal organs with few external signs.

      TRUE   FALSE

   b. Blunt trauma to the right upper quadrant is very likely to produce injury to the spleen.

      TRUE   FALSE

   c. Frontal impact injuries to the abdomen may cause rupture of a full bladder.

      TRUE   FALSE

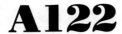**A122**

1. Answer **b** is NOT part of the management of this patient. No patient who has sustained trauma to the abdomen or who is in shock for any other reason should be permitted to take anything by mouth. Indeed, no critically ill or injured patient should be allowed food or fluids by mouth, for this will only increase the risk of vomiting and aspiration, either during transport or during induction of anesthesia in the operating room. All of the other measures listed (answers a, c, d, and e) are part of the standard management of hemorrhagic shock.

   KEEP CRITICALLY ILL AND INJURED PATIENTS NPO.

2. TRUE-FALSE questions:
   a. Blunt abdominal trauma may cause devastating injury to internal organs with few external signs.

      TRUE, VERY TRUE. Beneath an innocent-looking bruise (or perhaps no bruise at all) may lie a wasteland of blood and mangled tissue. So don't be lulled into complacency by an abdominal wall that looks uninjured. The patient's general appearance and vital signs may give you much more information as to the extent of damage hidden from view within the peritoneal cavity.

   b. Blunt trauma to the right upper quadrant is very likely to produce injury to the spleen.

      FALSE. It can happen, but it is not "very likely." If you answered "true" to this question, go back and review your anatomy charts: The spleen lies in the *left* upper quadrant and thus is more apt to be disrupted by left-sided injuries or by injuries to the left lower ribs.

   c. Frontal impact injuries to the abdomen may cause rupture of a full bladder.

      TRUE. And that's another good reason why it's not a good idea to drink before you drive. The classic injury producing bladder rupture occurs when a drunken driver with a full bladder gets hurled forward against the steering wheel, but any significant blunt trauma to the lower abdomen in the context of a full bladder can cause this injury.

FURTHER READING

Asbun HJ et al. Intra-abdominal seatbelt injury. *J Trauma* 30:189, 1990.
Bietz DS. Abdominal injuries. *Emergency* 10(12):30, 1978.
Caroline NL. *Emergency Care in the Streets* (4th ed.). Boston: Little, Brown, 1991, Ch. 18.
Cwinn AA et al. Prehospital advanced trauma life support for critical blunt trauma victims. *Ann Emerg Med* 16:399, 1987.
Denis R et al. Changing trends with abdominal injury in seatbelt wearers. *J Trauma* 23:1007, 1983.
Edwards FJ. Liver trauma. *Emerg Med Serv* 19(3):28, 1990.
Fiedler MD et al. A correlation of response time and results of abdominal gunshot wounds. *Arch Surg* 12:902, 1986.
Freeark RJ. Penetrating wounds of the abdomen. *N Engl J Med* 291:186, 1974.
Frentz GD, Lang EK. Problem: Bladder injury. *Emerg Med* 15(12):111, 1983.
Mackersie RC et al. Intra-abdominal injury following blunt trauma: Identifying the high-risk patient using objective risk factors. *Arch Surg* 124:809, 1989.
McSwain N. Visual examination for blunt abdominal trauma. *JACEP* 6:56, 1977.
Murr PC et al. Abdominal trauma associated with pelvic fracture. *J Trauma* 20:919, 1980.
Pennell TC. Hepatic trauma: An overview. *Emerg Med Serv* 6(5):68, 1977.
Pons PT et al. Prehospital advanced trauma life support for critical penetrating wounds to the thorax and abdomen. *J Trauma* 25:828, 1985.
Thompson D, Adams SL, Barrett J. Relative bradycardia in patients with isolated penetrating abdominal trauma and isolated extremity trauma. *Ann Emerg Med* 19:268, 1990.
Vayer JS et al. Absence of a tachycardic response to shock in penetrating intraperitoneal injury. *Ann Emerg Med* 17:227, 1988.
Ward KR, Sullivan RJ, Zelenak RR. Isolated blunt splenic trauma. *Emerg Med* 21(1):73, 1989.
Whitehurst AW, Resnick M. The kidney and trauma: Diagnosis and treatment. *Emerg Med Serv* 5(6):30, 1976.

A 24-year-old woman ingested 50 pills from a bottle of over-the-counter sleep medication about 15 minutes before you arrived. You find her alert and weeping. Pulse is 100, blood pressure is 120/80, and respirations are 16 per minute. Pupils are slightly dilated but reactive. The remainder of the physical examination is unremarkable.

Which of the following statements regarding this case is TRUE?

a. Ingested poisons or drugs usually pass quickly through the stomach into the small intestine, where most of the absorption of the agent takes place.
b. Gastric lavage through a nasogastric tube will be a more effective means of emptying the patient's stomach than will be the induction of vomiting.
c. The FIRST step in treating this patient is to administer an antidote.
d. If you give syrup of ipecac, you should not administer activated charcoal.
e. If you administer syrup of ipecac, the correct dose for this patient is 5 ml PO.

A123

Answer **a** is true. **Ingested drugs or poisons usually pass quickly through the stomach into the small intestine, where most of the absorption of the agent takes place.**

Why then, you ask, do we bother trying to empty the stomach? The reason is that, in any given case, it is very difficult to know how quickly the drug or poison has passed into the intestinal tract and how much still remains in the stomach. Many factors may delay gastric emptying: pain, anxiety, disease, even the ingested agent itself. If there is any doubt whether a residual of the agent remains in the stomach, it is worthwhile to try to remove it.

Answer **b** is NOT true. Vomiting is a much more effective means of emptying the stomach than is gastric lavage and is thus to be preferred unless there are specific contraindications.

Alas, specific antidotes (answer **c**) are rare indeed, and even when they do exist, first priority always goes to maintaining vital functions (A, B, C . . .) and trying to remove whatever residual of the drug may remain in the stomach.

Activated charcoal should NOT be withheld when giving syrup of ipecac (answer **d**). To the contrary, charcoal should be given as soon as possible to the poisoned patient, whether or not syrup of ipecac is also to be administered. In fact, some authorities now recommend skipping the syrup of ipecac altogether and giving activated charcoal only.

The adult dosage of syrup of ipecac is 30 ml PO. If you give our patient 5 ml, you may wait a long time before she shows an inclination to vomit (answer **e**).

FURTHER READING

Albertson T et al. Superiority of activated charcoal alone compared with ipecac and activated charcoal in the treatment of acute toxic ingestions. *Ann Emerg Med* 18:101, 1989.

Auerback PS et al. Efficacy of gastric emptying: Gastric lavage versus emesis induced with ipecac. *Ann Emerg Med* 15:692, 1986.

Caroline NL. *Emergency Care in the Streets* (4th ed.). Boston: Little, Brown, 1991, Ch. 27.

Eason J et al. Efficacy and safety of gastrointestinal decontamination in the treatment of oral poisoning. *Pediatr Clin North Am* 26:827, 1979.

Flomenbaum NE, Hoffman R. GI evacuation: Is it still worthwhile? *Emerg Med* 22(2):80, 1990.

Freedman GE, Pasternak S, Krenzelok EP. A clinical trial using syrup of ipecac and activated charcoal concurrently. *Ann Emerg Med* 16:164, 1987.

Grande GA et al. The effect of fluid volume on syrup of ipecac emesis time. *Clin Toxicol* 25:473, 1987.

Greensher J et al. Ascendency of the black bottle (activated charcoal). *Pediatrics* 80:949, 1987.

Ipecac syrup and activated charcoal for treatment of poisoning in children. *Med Lett* 21:70, 1979.

Katona BG et al. The new black magic: Activated charcoal and new therapeutic uses. *J Emerg Med* 5:99, 1987.

Krenzelok EP et al. Preserving the emetic effect of syrup of ipecac with concurrent activated charcoal administration: A preliminary study. *Clin Toxicol* 24:159, 1986.

Krenzelok EP et al. Effectiveness of commercially available aqueous activated charcoal products. *Ann Emerg Med* 16:1340, 1987.

Kulig K et al. Management of acutely poisoned patients without gastric emptying. *Ann Emerg Med* 14:562, 1985.

Levy DB. Activated charcoal update. *Emergency* 20(6):16, 1988.

Levy DB. Syrup of ipecac review. *Emergency* 21(12):20, 1989.

McNamara RM et al. Efficacy of charcoal carthartic versus ipecac in reducing serum acetaminophen in a simulated overdose. *Ann Emerg Med* 18:934, 1989.

Mofenson HC. Benefits/risks of syrup of ipecac. *Pediatrics* 77:551, 1986.

Park GD et al. Expanded role of charcoal therapy in the poisoned and overdosed patient. *Arch Intern Med* 146:969, 1986.

Tandberg D, Diven BG, McLeod JW. Ipecac-induced emesis versus gastric lavage: A controlled study in normal adults. *Am J Emerg Med* 4:205, 1986.

Tenenbein M. Inefficiency of gastric emptying procedures. *J Emerg Med* 3:133, 1985.

Tenenbein M, Cohen S, Sitar DS. Efficacy of ipecac-induced emesis, orogastric lavage, and activated charcoal for acute drug overdose. *Ann Emerg Med* 16:838, 1987.

It's one of those miserable days of late summer—temperature in the 90s and ambient humidity about 95 percent—when you get a call for a "man down" outside the main downtown hotel. You arrive to find several construction workers, who are building an addition to the hotel, crowded around one of their colleagues. They inform you that he is a "new man on the job" and that he "just collapsed" about 15 minutes earlier.

The patient appears to be in his middle 30s. He is lying on the ground and seems delirious. His skin is very hot, pink, and dry. Pulse is 140 and strong, blood pressure is 150/90, and respirations are 28 and deep. There is no evidence of trauma, and the remainder of the physical examination is unremarkable.

Among the following possible treatments, select those that you think are appropriate for this patient.

a. Immediately strip off most of his clothing, and begin cooling him by any means available.
b. Administer oxygen.
c. Start an IV with D5W as a lifeline.
d. Start at least two IVs with normal saline, and run them wide open.
e. Administer norepinephrine (Levophed) to raise the patient's blood pressure.
f. Administer 50% glucose, 20 ml IV.
g. Administer atropine, 0.01 mg per kilogram IV.
h. Administer mannitol, 12.5 gm IV.
i. Administer chlorpromazine (Thorazine), 25 mg IM.

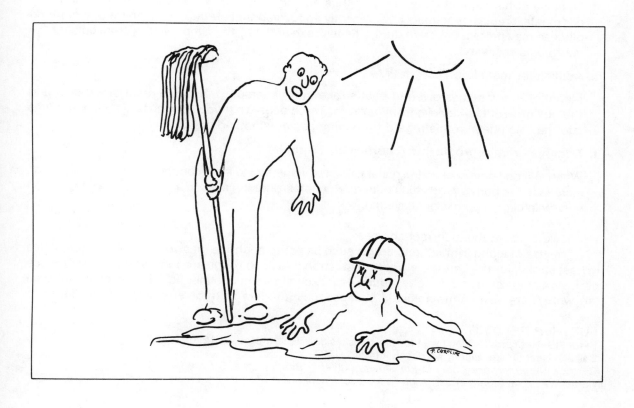

A124

Our construction worker presents a classic case of exertional heat stroke. He has been doing strenuous work under conditions of high temperature and humidity, and perhaps with poor acclimatization (he's the "new man on the job")—conditions under which it is very difficult to dissipate heat effectively from the body. Ordinarily, heat is lost from the body by radiation, but as the ambient temperature increases, the body becomes progressively more dependent upon sweating as a mechanism for ridding itself of excess heat. When there is high humidity as well, however, evaporation of sweat from the body surface ceases to be an effective means of heat dissipation, and the stage is set for heat stroke, a dire medical emergency.

Among the list of treatment options presented, the appropriate measures for this patient are

a. Immediately strip off most of his clothing, and begin cooling him by any means available.

Do not delay one instant! Use whatever you can find at the scene to begin cooling the patient down—e.g., a hose, buckets of water. As soon as the patient is in the ambulance, use convection and evaporation for cooling (i.e., spray and fan). Continue until his rectal temperature has fallen to 38.3°C. Massage the patient's flanks to eliminate stasis in the peripheral circulation and prevent peripheral vasoconstriction.

b. Administer oxygen.

Patients with heat stroke are apt to develop pulmonary abnormalities, and while shunt has not been a prominent problem in this condition, the very high metabolic rate probably warrants oxygen supplementation. Start oxygen therapy as soon as is convenient, but don't let it delay or interfere with cooling the patient, which is the single most important aspect of his immediate management.

c. Start an IV with D5W as a lifeline.

At the moment, our patient appears to be adequately perfused. A significant number of patients with heat stroke are NOT dehydrated, and overaggressive fluid administration in heat stroke may lead to pulmonary edema. The keep-open line gives us the option of piggybacking in saline and infusing it rapidly should the need arise; it also provides us with a lifeline for the administration of drugs.

f. Administer 50% glucose, 20 ml IV.

Not a bad idea at all. To begin with, the patient's energy requirements are vastly increased because of his high temperature, and thus additional fuel may be helpful. Furthermore, experimental studies in animals have recently suggested that elevated concentrations of blood glucose may protect the brain during heat stroke and may thus improve the prospects for full neurologic recovery.

h. Administer mannitol, 12.5 gm IV.

Mannitol is sometimes given in heat stroke in an attempt to promote renal blood flow and thereby protect the kidneys from damage. The glucose that you administered a few minutes ago may also help in this regard by serving as an osmotic diuretic.

i. Administer chlorpromazine (Thorazine), 25 mg IM.

When you do begin cooling the patient, it will be important to try to control shivering, for shivering increases the body's production of heat. Phenothiazine drugs, such as chlorpromazine, can be very helpful in suppressing shivering.

A word about the incorrect choices:

The use of alpha sympathetic drugs, such as norepinephrine (answer e), is NOT a good idea in heat stroke, for the peripheral vasoconstriction that such drugs produce would simply reduce perfusion of the skin and thereby reduce heat exchange. Anticholinergic drugs, such as atropine (answer g), are also contraindicated because they interfere with the sweating mechanism.

FURTHER READING

Birrer RB. Heat stroke: Don't wait for the classic signs. *Emerg Med* 20(12):9, 1988.
Brill JC. Heat stroke. *Emerg Med Serv* 6(4):44, 1977.
Caroline NL. *Emergency Care in the Streets* (4th ed.). Boston: Little, Brown, 1991, Ch. 31.
Carter WA. Heat emergencies: A guide to assessment and management. *Emerg Med Serv* 9(4):29, 1980.

Clowes GHA, O'Donnell TF. Heat stroke. *N Engl J Med* 291:564, 1974.

Cummins P. Felled by the heat. *Emerg Med* 15(12):94, 1983.

Forester D. Fatal drug-induced heat stroke. *JACEP* 7:243, 1978.

Graham BS et al. Nonexertional heatstroke: Physiologic management and cooling in 14 patients. *Arch Intern Med* 146:87, 1986.

Hanson PG. Exertional heat stroke in novice runners. *JAMA* 242:154, 1979.

Hart GR et al. Epidemic classical heat stroke: Clinical characteristics and course of 28 patients. *Medicine* 61:189, 1982.

Jones TS. Morbidity and mortality associated with the July 1980 heat wave in St. Louis and Kansas City, Mo. *JAMA* 247:3327, 1982.

Kerstein MD. Heat illness in hot/humid environment. *Milit Med* 151:308, 1986.

Kilbourne EM et al. Risk factors for heatstroke. *JAMA* 247:3362, 1982.

Knochel JP. Environmental heat illness: An eclectic review. *Arch Intern Med* 133:841, 1974.

Knochel JP. Dog days and siriasis—how to kill a football player. *JAMA* 233:513, 1975.

Kunkel DB. The ills of heat. Part I: Environmental causes. *Emerg Med* 18(14):173, 1986.

Larkin JT. Treatment of heat-related illness. *JAMA* 245:570, 1981.

Parks FB, Calabro JJ. Hyperthermia: Performing when the heat is on. *JEMS* 15(8):24, 1990.

Sawka MN et al. Influence of hydration level and body fluids on exercise performance in the heat. *JAMA* 252:1165, 1984.

Slovis CM, Anderson GF, Casolaro A. Survival in a heat stroke victim with a core temperature in excess of 46.5°C. *Ann Emerg Med* 11:269, 1982.

Sprung CL. Heat stroke: Modern approach to an ancient disease. *Chest* 77:461, 1980.

Stine RJ. Heat illness. *JACEP* 8:154, 1979.

Surpure JS. Heat-related illness and the automobile. *Ann Emerg Med* 11:263, 1982.

Tintinalli JE. Heat stroke. *JACEP* 5:525, 1976.

Wettach JE, Smith DS, Stalling CE. EMS protocol for management of heat emergencies during a heat wave in an urban population. *EMT J* 5(5):328, 1981.

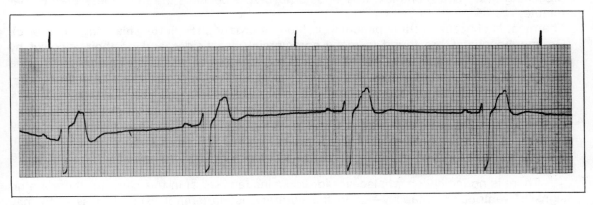

Figure 17

You are called to the Green Gardens Nursery to attend to a worker who has suddenly taken ill. The manager tells you that his employee seemed fine when he arrived for work this morning, but he became very ill after disinfecting greenhouse no. 3. You find the worker in the manager's office, being restrained in a chair by two other gardeners. He is confused, agitated, and drooling profusely. His skin is pale and diaphoretic. Pulse is strong. Blood pressure is 146/80; respirations are 28. Pupils are somewhat constricted. Neck veins are flat. There are scattered wheezes in the chest. Bowel sounds are hyperactive, and there are occasional twitches of the extremities. The patient's rhythm strip is shown in Figure 17.

1. Examine the patient's rhythm strip:

    a. The rhythm is _____ regular   _____ irregular.
    b. The rate is _____ per minute.

2. The ECG pattern is

    a. Normal sinus rhythm
    b. Sinus bradycardia
    c. Junctional rhythm
    d. Wenckebach second-degree AV block
    e. Complete heart block

3. The most likely cause of this patient's problem is

    a. Acute myocardial infarction
    b. Cerebrovascular accident (stroke)
    c. Organophosphate poisoning
    d. Psychiatric disturbance
    e. Carotid sinus syndrome

4. Besides oxygen, what other drug should you administer to this patient?

    a. Lidocaine, 100 mg IV bolus
    b. Isoproterenol (Isuprel), 5 μg per minute IV
    c. Atropine, 2 mg IM plus 1 mg IV
    d. Morphine, 5 to 10 mg slowly IV
    e. Diazepam (Valium), 5 mg slowly IV

A125

1. The patient's rhythm is **regular.** The rate is approximately **40 per minute.**
2. The ECG pattern is **sinus bradycardia** (answer b). It is sinus because there is a normal P wave preceding every QRS complex; it is sinus *bradycardia* because the rate is less than 60 per minute.
3. The most likely cause of this patient's problem is **organophosphate poisoning** (answer c). Organophosphates are found in many commercial insecticides and do their mischief by potentiating the action of acetylcholine at the neuromuscular junction—thereby putting the victim in a state of unremitting parasympathetic stimulation. All of the signs we detected—drooling, confusion, sweating, bradycardia, pupillary constriction, bowel hyperactivity—are indications of parasympathetic nervous system stimulation.
4. The drug of choice for organophosphate poisoning is **atropine** (answer c), starting with 2 mg IM and 1 mg IV. The dose should be repeated until signs of atropinization (dry mouth, increased pulse) are apparent, and sometimes very large doses—in the range of 40 mg—will be required over a 24-hour period.

   There is no indication whatsoever for lidocaine (answer a) in this case, for there are no signs of ventricular irritability—quite the contrary. Isoproterenol (Isuprel, answer b) may speed up the patient's heart rate somewhat, but his bradycardia is not his problem; it is only a sign of his problem, and isoproterenol will do nothing to reverse the other systemic manifestations of parasympathetic system overactivity. Morphine is the last thing this patient needs (answer d), for morphine has its own parasympathetic stimulating effects. The patient's wheezes may indeed be due to a degree of pulmonary edema, or at least to hypersecretion in the respiratory tract, but morphine is not the answer. Once the patient is fully atropinized, his hypersecretion should cease; meanwhile, treat his shunt with oxygen.

   If diazepam (Valium) is indicated at all (answer e), it is for all the nervous people around the patient. The patient himself does not need it. He is agitated and twitching on account of the poison in his system, and once you reverse the effects of that poison, he will calm down.

   Don't forget that organophosphate poisons are absorbed through the skin, and this patient will need to be washed down thoroughly, from head to toe, with soap and water. If you are only a short distance from the hospital, his bath can be deferred until you get there. Otherwise you're going to have to strip him and hose him down before you leave the scene.

FURTHER READING

Done AK. Nerve gases in the war against pests. *Emerg Med* 5(5):250, 1973.
Done AK. Autonomic toxicology primer. *Emerg Med* 15(13):134, 1983.
Done AK. Autonomics unravelled: I. Cholinergics. *Emerg Med* 15(14):287, 1983.
Heath DF. *Organophosphate Poisons.* Oxford: Pergamon, 1961.
Midtling JE et al. Clinical management of field worker organophosphate poisoning. *West J Med* 142:514, 1985.
The toxic effects of agriculture. *Emerg Med* 16(11):119, 1984.
Wyckoff DW et al. Diagnostic and therapeutic problems of parthion poisonings. *Ann Intern Med* 68:875, 1968.

The call comes in as a "woman bleeding" in a suburban neighborhood about 15 minutes away. Arriving at the scene, you are ushered into the bedroom by a distraught husband and find an obviously pregnant woman lying in bed. She states that she is in her ninth month and that during the past hour she has been passing considerable quantities of bright red blood through her vagina. She denies any pain. She says that this is her first pregnancy, and she is afraid she will lose the baby.

On physical examination, you find her pale and anxious. Her skin is cool and moist. Pulse is 130, blood pressure is 80 systolic, and respirations are 28. Neck veins are collapsed. The chest is clear. Heart sounds are well heard. The abdomen is soft and nontender. Fetal heart sounds are audible.

1. Which of the following would NOT be part of the management of this patient?

   a. Administer oxygen.
   b. Apply military antishock trousers (leg sections only).
   c. Start at least one IV with a large-bore cannula, and run in normal saline wide open.
   d. Do a vaginal examination to determine whether the baby is crowning and thus whether there is time to get to the hospital.
   e. Notify the hospital of your situation and your estimated time of arrival.

2. This patient's condition is called

   a. Abruptio placenta
   b. Placenta previa
   c. Prolapsed umbilical cord
   d. Breech delivery

A126

1. One should NEVER, NEVER, NEVER do a vaginal examination on a woman with third trimester bleeding; thus answer **d** is NOT part of the management of this patient. Vaginal examination may dislodge the placenta and lead to uncontrollable exsanguinating hemorrhage. Our patient is already in shock, and it will be difficult enough to get her to the hospital alive without adding to the problem. She needs oxygen (answer a) because of her poor tissue perfusion, and she needs volume, which can be provided by intravenous infusions (answer c). The hospital must be notified that you are coming so that they can set up an operating room and summon the necessary staff to be ready when you arrive (answer e).

2. Our patient is in all probability suffering from **placenta previa** (answer b), i.e., a situation in which the placenta, rather than the baby's head, is the presenting part. While it may be very difficult to distinguish clinically between placenta previa and abruptio placenta (premature separation of a normally implanted placenta from the uterine wall, answer a), there are certain features of this patient's case that suggest the former. First of all, her bleeding is painless; in abruptio placenta, there is more likely to be pain of varying severity. Secondly, our patient stated that she passed bright red blood, which is more characteristic of placenta previa; in abruptio placenta, passage of dark blood is more common. On physical examination, our patient's abdomen (and uterus) was soft, and fetal heart sounds were audible; in abruptio placenta, the uterus is more likely to be firm or rigid, and fetal heart sounds may not be heard. None of those distinctions are absolute, but taken together they make us lean more toward a diagnosis of placenta previa. It should be noted, however, that both conditions—placenta previa and abruptio placenta—may be rapidly fatal, and thus it is of academic interest in the field to distinguish between them. ANY CASE OF THIRD TRIMESTER BLEEDING MUST BE CONSIDERED A DIRE MEDICAL EMERGENCY, AND THE PATIENT SHOULD BE TRANSPORTED AS SOON AS POSSIBLE TO A MEDICAL FACILITY.

   Neither prolapsed umbilical cord (answer c) nor breech delivery (answer d) usually presents as third trimester bleeding. Prolapsed umbilical cord is the situation in which the umbilical cord is the presenting part; in breech delivery, some part of the baby other than the head is the presenting part. Those situations present their own hazards, but exsanguination is not usually one of them.

FURTHER READING

Anderson B, Shapiro B. *Emergency Childbirth Handbook.* Albany, NY: Delmar, 1979.

Boulton FE et al. Obstetric haemorrhage: Causes and management. *Clin Haem* 14:683, 1985.

Celebrezze EM. Third trimester predelivery hemorrhage. *Emergency* 13(10):48, 1981.

Emergence emergencies. *Emerg Med* 4(9):89, 1972.

Kaunitz AM et al. Causes of maternal mortality in the United States. *Obstet Gynecol* 65:605, 1985.

Kilgore JR. Management of an obstetric patient by the EMT. *EMT J* 4(2):50, 1980.

Nixon RG. Third trimester obstetric complications. Part I: Antepartum hemorrhage and fetal distress. *Emerg Med Serv* 10(3):53, 1981.

Williams C. Emergency childbirth. *Emerg Med Serv* 14(3):100, 1985.

Wojslawowicz JM. Emergency childbirth for emergency medical technicians. *EMT J* 1(4):66, 1977.

You are called to the scene of an accident in which a car plowed into the side of a semitrailer. The driver of the truck appears unhurt, but you find the driver of the car slumped forward over the steering wheel, unconscious, and breathing stertorously. His pulse is strong.

Arrange the following steps of management in the correct order:

a. Remove the patient from the car on the long backboard.
b. Administer oxygen.
c. One rescuer holds the patient's head and neck steady in neutral position.
d. Slide the short backboard behind the patient and strap him to it.
e. Establish an open airway, with minimal extension of the patient's neck.
f. Maneuver the patient so that he is lying on the long backboard.
g. Apply a cervical collar.

1. _____
2. _____
3. _____
4. _____
5. _____
6. _____
7. _____

A127

Removing a patient from a wrecked vehicle in an orderly fashion is vitally important. But did you remember to attend to his airway and oxygenation first?

1. __e__ Establish an open airway, with minimal extension of the patient's neck.
2. __b__ Administer oxygen.
3. __c__ One rescuer holds the patient's head and neck steady in neutral position.
4. __g__ Apply a cervical collar.
5. __d__ Slide the short backboard behind the patient and strap him to it.
6. __f__ Maneuver the patient so that he is lying on the long backboard.
7. __a__ Remove the patient from the car on the long backboard.

FURTHER READING

Anast GT. Fractures and injuries of the cervical spine. *EMT J* 2(3):36, 1978.
Anderson DK et al. Spinal cord injury and protection. *Ann Emerg Med* 14:816, 1985.
Aprahamian CA et al. Experimental cervical spine injury model: Evaluation of airway management and splinting techniques. *Ann Emerg Med* 13:584, 1984.
Bourn S. Tell the spinal fanatics to "back off." *JEMS* 15(5):73, 1990.
Caroline NL. *Emergency Care in the Streets* (4th ed.). Boston: Little, Brown, 1991, Ch. 16.
Caroline NL. *Emergency Medical Treatment: A Text for EMT-As and EMT-Intermediates* (3rd ed.). Boston: Little, Brown, 1991, Ch. 14.
Cline JR et al. A comparison of methods of cervical immobilization used in patient extrication and transport. *Trauma* 25:649, 1985.
Dick T. Spider's embrace: The Idaho answer to backboard straps. *JEMS* 14(8):26, 1989.
Dula DJ. Trauma to the cervical spine. *JACEP* 8:504, 1979.
Graziano AF et al. A radiographic comparison of prehospital cervical immobilization methods. *Ann Emerg Med* 16:1127, 1987.
Grundy D et al. ABC of spinal cord injury: Early management and complications. *Br Med J* I.292:44, 1986. II.292:123, 1986.
Herzenberg JE et al. Emergency transport and positioning of young children who have an injury of the cervical spine. *J Bone Joint Surg [Am]* 71A:15, 1989.
Holley J, Jorden R. Airway management in patients with unstable cervical spine fractures. *Ann Emerg Med* 18:1237, 1989.
Howell JM et al. A practical radiographic comparison of short board technique and Kendrick extrication device. *Ann Emerg Med* 18:943, 1989.
Huerta C, Griffith R, Joyce SM. Cervical spine stabilization in pediatric patients: Evaluation of current techniques. *Ann Emerg Med* 16:1121, 1987.
Jackson DW et al. Cervical spine injuries. *Clin Sports Med* 5:373, 1986.
Little NE. In case of a broken neck. *Emerg Med* 21(9):22, 1989.
Marsden AK. Emergency cervical splints—their value and limitation. *Disaster Med* 1(2):197, 1983.
McCabe JB, Nolan DJ. Comparison of the effectiveness of different cervical immobilization collars. *Ann Emerg Med* 15:50, 1986.
McGuire RA et al. Spinal instability and the log-rolling maneuver. *J Trauma* 27:525, 1987.
Podolsky S et al. Efficacy of cervical spine immobilization methods. *J Trauma* 23:461, 1983.
Rimel R et al. Prehospital treatment of the patient with spinal cord injuries. *EMT J* 3(4):49, 1979.
Smith M, Bourn S, Larmon B. Ties that bind: Immobilizing the injured spine. *JEMS* 14(4):28, 1989.
Swain A et al. ABC of spinal cord injury: At the accident. *Br Med J* 291:1558, 1985.
Wolf AL. Initial management of brain- and spinal-cord injured patients. *Emerg Med Serv* 18(6):35, 1989.

1. You are sitting in a steak house enjoying a quiet meal on your night off when you notice a man a few tables away performing a bizarre pantomime. His mouth is wide open and he seems to be trying to talk, but he is completely silent. His complexion is becoming an alarming shade of blue, and he appears to be struggling. Then he collapses to the floor. The most likely cause of his behavior is

   a. He has had a heart attack.
   b. He has suffered a spontaneous pneumothorax.
   c. He found a cockroach in his coleslaw.
   d. He is having an epileptic seizure.
   e. He choked on a piece of meat.

2. The following week, again on your night off, you are dining at an elegant seafood restaurant. Your companion has just finished her shrimp cocktail when she begins complaining of itching. You notice that her eyes look rather puffy, and her voice is becoming quite hoarse. She is most likely suffering from

   a. A heart attack
   b. A severe allergic reaction (anaphylaxis)
   c. Tonsillitis
   d. Choking on a piece of shrimp
   e. Flea bites

   In this case, the single most important medication that should be administered immediately is

   a. Epinephrine
   b. Diphenhydramine (Benadryl)
   c. Morphine
   d. Atropine

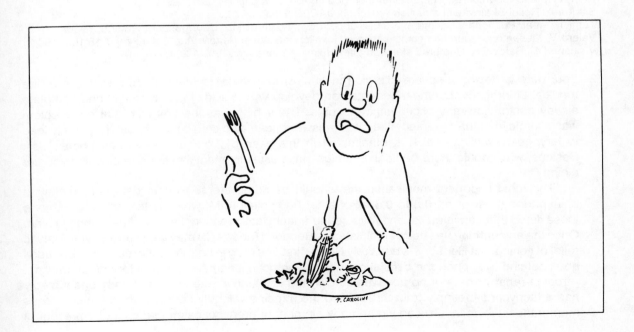

P. CAROLINE

A128

1. The tip-off in this question is that the patient is COMPLETELY SILENT, which is a very good indication that something is preventing the passage of air through his vocal cords. Certainly, most patients suffering a heart attack (answer a) or a spontaneous pneumothorax (answer b) and in such apparent distress would cry out. And just as certainly, someone who finds a cockroach in his coleslaw (answer c) would have something to say on the subject. Even the epileptic patient (answer d) is likely to give a gasp or cry as a premonitory sign of a seizure (besides, the patient has simply collapsed; there is no mention of tonic-clonic movements). Thus the correct answer is **e**: This patient has **choked on a piece of meat,** which is now obstructing his upper airway to the degree that he cannot utter a sound.

   It should not have taken you more than a few seconds to reach that conclusion, for you don't have very much time if you want to save this man's life. Complete airway obstruction can be expected to lead to cardiac arrest within a very few minutes, and irreversible brain damage will follow shortly thereafter if ventilation and circulation are not promptly restored. Since it's your night off, and you didn't happen to bring your laryngoscope and Magill forceps with you to dinner, you have only your two hands to work with. If the obstructing bolus of food cannot be readily reached and removed with your fingers, and if a few sharp blows to the patient's back don't do the trick, immediately straddle the patient and perform a swift, upward compression of the upper abdomen (Heimlich maneuver).
   Moral: DON'T TALK WITH YOUR MOUTH FULL.

FURTHER READING

Addy DP. The choking child: Back bangers against front pushers. *Br Med J* 286:536, 1983.
American Heart Association. Standards and guidelines for cardiopulmonary resuscitation (CPR) and emergency cardiac care (ECC). *JAMA* 255:2905, 1986.
Day RL. Differing opinions on the emergency treatment of choking. *Pediatrics* 71:976, 1983.
Day RL et al. Choking: The Heimlich abdominal thrust vs back blows: An approach to measurement of inertial and aerodynamic forces. *Pediatrics* 70:113, 1982.
Eller WC, Haugen RK. Food asphyxiation—restaurant rescue. *N Engl J Med* 289:81, 1973.
Gann DS. Emergency management of the obstructed airway. *JAMA* 243:1141, 1980.
Guildner CW, Williams D, Subitch T. Airway obstruction by foreign material: The Heimlich maneuver. *JACEP* 5:675, 1976.
Haugen RK. The cafe coronary: Sudden deaths in restaurants. *JAMA* 186:142, 1963.
Hoffman JR. Treatment of foreign body obstruction of the upper airway. *West J Med* 136:11, 1982.
Meredith MJ. Rupture of the esophagus caused by the Heimlich maneuver (letter). *Ann Emerg Med* 15:106, 1986.
Mittleman RE, Wetli CV. The fatal cafe coronary. *JAMA* 247:1285, 1982.
Orlowski JP. Vomiting as a complication of the Heimlich maneuver. *JAMA* 258:512, 1987.
Redding JS. The choking controversy: Critique of evidence on the Heimlich maneuver. *Crit Care Med* 7:475, 1979.
Robison P et al. Heimlich maneuver in children. *Tex Med* 81(6):60, 1985.
Ruben H, MacNaughton FI. The treatment of food choking. *Practitioner* 221:725, 1978.
Sladen A. Relief of airway obstruction (editorial). *JACEP* 5:710, 1976.
Tami TA et al. Pulmonary edema and acute upper airway obstruction. *Laryngoscope* 96:506, 1986.
Valero V. Mesenteric laceration complicating a Heimlich maneuver (letter). *Ann Emerg Med* 15:105, 1986.
Visintine RE, Baick CH. Ruptured stomach after Heimlich maneuver. *JAMA* 234:415, 1975.

2. Your date is having a severe allergic reaction, or **anaphylaxis** (answer **b**), and this is a dire medical emergency. Laryngeal edema can develop very quickly in such cases, and complete airway obstruction may occur within minutes. The itching was the first clue that her problem was allergic in nature; granted, flea bites (answer e) can also cause itching, but they rarely lead to laryngeal swelling, which is manifested in this case by your date's sudden hoarseness. Besides, why should there be fleas in a high-class establishment like the one at which you are dining?

   The most important medication that should be administered to your date immediately is epinephrine (answer a), 0.3 to 0.5 ml of a 1:1,000 solution IM, which is the only drug among those listed that can interrupt and reverse the anaphylactic responses your date is manifesting. Once the epinephrine has been administered, Benadryl (answer b) may be given for symptomatic relief of itching, but Benadryl is definitely NOT a first-line drug in anaphylactic reactions; Benadryl does nothing to support the circulation, reverse bronchospasm, or interrupt laryngeal swelling. Atropine (answer d) is of no use whatsoever in this situation; the patient already undoubtedly has a tachycardia, simply from stress, and the atropine will only serve to dry out her mucous membranes, which in turn can worsen any element of bronchospasm that might be present. If you chose to administer morphine (answer c), your date may die more peacefully, but she *will* probably die, for you have done nothing to reverse the allergic process; to the contrary, you have simply helped accelerate the development of hypotension and shock.

Remember: ANAPHYLAXIS REQUIRES EPINEPHRINE. Accept no substitutes.

FURTHER READING

Allergic to what he eats. *Emerg Med* 19(2):20, 1987.

Austen KF. Systemic anaphylaxis in the human being. *N Engl J Med* 291:661, 1974.

Barach EM et al. Epinephrine for treatment of anaphylactic shock. *JAMA* 251:2118, 1984.

Busse WW. Anaphylaxis: Diagnosis and management. *Emerg Med Serv* 5(2):44, 1976.

Caroline NL. *Emergency Care in the Streets* (4th ed.). Boston: Little, Brown, 1991, Ch. 26.

Casale TB, Keahey TM, Kaliner M. Exercise-induced anaphylactic syndromes. *JAMA* 255:2049, 1986.

Fischer M et al. Volume replacement in acute anaphylactoid reactions. *Intensive Care* 7:375, 1979.

Frazier CA. Food allergy emergencies. *Emerg Med Serv* 12(2):71, 1983.

Fries JH. Peanuts: Allergic and other untoward reactions. *Ann Allergy* 48:220, 1982.

Hooper HA. Allergic reactions. *Emergency* 11(4):32, 1979.

Kaliner MA. Calling a halt to anaphylaxis. *Emerg Med* 21(6): 51, 1989.

Kelly JF, Patterson R. Anaphylaxis: Cause, mechanisms, and treatment. *JAMA* 227:1431, 1974.

Levy DB. Anaphylaxis. *Emergency* 21(4):42, 1989.

Lucke WC, Thomas H. Anaphylaxis: Pathophysiology, clinical presentations and treatment. *J Emerg Med* 1:83, 1983.

Morrow DH, Luther RR. Anaphylaxis: Etiology and guidelines for management. *Anesth Analg* 55:493, 1976.

Perkin RM, Anas NG. Mechanisms and management of anaphylactic shock not responding to traditional therapy. *Ann Allergy* 54:202, 1985.

Raebel M. Potentiated anaphylaxis during chronic beta-blocker therapy. *Drug Intell Clin Pharm* 22:720, 1988.

Roth R. Allergic response. *Emergency* 22(6):28, 1990.

Scheffer AL. Anaphylaxis. *J Allergy Clin Immunol* 75:227, 1985.

Schwartz HJ, Sher Th. Anaphylaxis to penicillin in a frozen dinner. *Ann Allergy* 52:342, 1984.

Vaneslow NA. Minutes to counter anaphylaxis. *Emerg Med* 20(15):121, 1988.

Yuninger JW et al. Fatal food-induced anaphylaxis. *JAMA* 260:1450, 1988.

James H. Taylor

A lazy morning of late August. The call comes in as a "very sick man" on a small farm just outside the city. You arrive at an old, broken-down farmhouse on a small, scrubby plot of land, and a woman, apparently the patient's wife, waves you in the door. On a shabby cot inside, a man is lying in obvious distress. With difficulty, he tells you that about an hour ago, while in the outhouse, he felt a sudden pain around his scrotum and shortly thereafter he started getting severe pains in his abdomen. He has a headache, and he has vomited twice.

On physical examination, you find the patient to be restless, diaphoretic, and in apparent respiratory distress. Pulse is 120 and regular, blood pressure is 110/70, and respirations are 20. The pupils are equal and reactive. There is no neck vein distention. The chest is clear, and heart sounds are well heard. The abdomen is rigid and boardlike, but it does not seem to be tender to palpation.

Which of the following drugs may provide the patient with some temporary relief of his abdominal pain?

a. Atropine, 0.1 mg IV
b. Potassium chloride, 100 mEq IV
c. Sodium chloride, 100 ml IV of normal saline
d. Calcium gluconate, 10 ml of a 10% solution IV
e. Sodium bicarbonate, 50 ml IV

A129

With whom did the farmer have a clandestine meeting in the outhouse? If you guessed it was a black widow spider, you are probably correct. Black widow spiders like to hang around in sheds, woodpiles, basements, and outhouses and are most usually found in these locales from April to October. Most of the time, a person who has been bitten by a black widow spider cannot give you a definite history of having been bitten; he will simply report having felt a sudden sting or prick, followed by numbness or paresthesias in the area. The numbness may gradually spread, and it is often followed by excruciating abdominal pain, sweating, headache, and respiratory distress. On physical examination, it may be nearly impossible to find the bite itself, although an examiner with very sharp eyes may detect tiny red fang marks at the site.

Victims of black widow spider bites require supportive care, with primary attention to the airway and adequate intravenous fluids. Significant relief of pain may sometimes be afforded by the administration of **calcium gluconate IV** (answer **d**). Atropine at the dose listed is unlikely to have any effect at all (answer a). A dose of 100 mEq of potassium chloride will provide quite permanent relief of pain (answer b), for it will almost certainly cause immediate and refractory cardiac arrest. Sodium chloride (answer c) may have some placebo effect, but otherwise it is of no particular usefulness, except as a source of intravenous volume. There is no reason to give sodium bicarbonate (answer e) because acidosis is not in general part of the clinical picture in black widow spider bites.

FURTHER READING

Of bites and stings. *Emerg Med* 15(11):121, 1983.

Frazier CA. Emergency treatment of insect stings and bites. *Emerg Med Serv* 6(4):8, 1977.

Key GF. A comparison of calcium gluconate and methocarbamol (Robaxin) in the treatment of latrodectism (black widow spider envenomation). *Am J Trop Med Hyg* 30:273, 1981.

Kobernick M. Black widow spider bite. *Am Fam Phys* 29:241, 1984.

Rauber A. Black widow spider bites. *J Toxicol Clin Toxicol* 21:473, 1984.

Wasserman G. Wound care of spider and snake envenomations. *Ann Emerg Med* 17:1331, 1988.

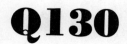

You are assisting in the delivery of a baby, and the procedure has gone smoothly. A lusty baby boy was delivered without difficulty. While the placenta is delivering, however, the mother begins complaining of shortness of breath. Your partner, who is positioned at the mother's vertex to protect her airway in the event of vomiting, reports that her carotid pulse is about 130 and she looks very pale. Her respiratory rate is 30. You notice that the blood coming from the vagina has become much darker than it was.

   You should

a. Administer oxygen at a high concentration to the mother, and transport her to the hospital as soon as possible.
b. Intubate the mother's trachea.
c. Insert a chest tube.
d. Assist respirations with a bag-valve-mask.
e. Have the mother breathe into a paper bag.

A130 Mother seems to have suffered a pulmonary embolism, which is suggested by the sudden onset of dyspnea, tachypnea, and tachycardia. When pulmonary embolism occurs in the context of childbirth, it may be due to a blood clot or to amniotic fluid that has leaked into the mother's circulation. The net effect of either is the same: shunt and hypoxemia. Thus this patient needs **oxygen** in a high concentration (answer **a**). There is little more you can do for her in the field.

There is no indication to intubate this woman's trachea at the moment; she is awake and fully able to protect her own airway (answer b). Nor does she need ventilatory assistance (answer d); she is already breathing more than adequately on her own. There is no reason to suspect that this woman has suffered a pneumothorax, so there is no indication to insert a chest tube (answer c). And, while her respiratory rate is rapid, she is not suffering from hyperventilation in the strict sense of that term. She is breathing rapidly because she is hypoxemic and trying to get more oxygen; having her rebreathe into a paper bag will not improve her situation (answer e).

FURTHER READING

Bell WR, Simon TL, DeMets DL. The clinical features of submassive and massive pulmonary emboli. *Am J Med* 62:355, 1977.

Cooke DH. Focusing in on pulmonary embolism. *Emerg Med* 17(9):86, 1985.

Dismuke SE, Wagner EH. Pulmonary embolism as a cause of death. *JAMA* 255:2039, 1986.

Goodall RJR et al. Clinical correlations in the diagnosis of pulmonary embolism. *Ann Surg* 191:219, 1980.

Hoellerich VL et al. Diagnosing pulmonary embolism using clinical findings. *Arch Intern Med* 146:1699, 1986.

Huet Y et al. Hypoxemia in acute pulmonary embolism. *Chest* 88:829, 1985.

Langdon RW, Swicegood WR, Schwartz DA. Thrombolytic therapy of massive pulmonary embolism during prolonged cardiac arrest using recombinant tissue-type plasminogen activator. *Ann Emerg Med* 18:678, 1989.

McGlynn TJ, Hamilton RW, Moore R. Pulmonary embolism: 1979. *JACEP* 8:532, 1979.

Palmer LB, Schiff MJ. Pulmonary embolism and venous thrombosis. *Emerg Med* 20(15):37, 1988.

Park H et al. Pulmonary embolism. *Emerg Med Serv* 4(5):33, 1975.

Sabiston DC. Pathophysiology, diagnosis and management of pulmonary embolism. *Am J Surg* 138:384, 1979.

Stein PD et al. History and physical examination in acute pulmonary embolism in patients without preexisting cardiac or pulmonary disease. *Am J Cardiol* 47:218, 1981.

Sutton GC, Honey M, Gibson RV. Clinical diagnosis of acute massive pulmonary embolism. *Lancet* 1:271, 1979.

Valenzuela TD. Pulmonary embolism. *Ann Emerg Med* 17:209, 1988.

Williams MH. Pulmonary embolism. *Emerg Med* 16(4):135, 1984.

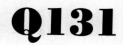

A 30-year-old man was the driver of a car that struck a truck head-on. The car shows extensive damage to the front end, a bent steering column, and a smashed front windshield. The patient has some small lacerations on his face, but he is conscious and alert. His pulse is 120, blood pressure is 90/60, and respirations are 26 and shallow. There is evidence of multiple rib fractures on the left and a fractured left patella. Sensation is intact in all extremities.

Which of the following statements about this patient are true and which are false?

a. He probably has a significant shunt and should receive oxygen.

    TRUE   FALSE

b. There is no need for spinal immobilization, since the patient shows no signs of spine injury.

    TRUE   FALSE

c. There is a high probability of left hip fracture.

    TRUE   FALSE

d. If the patient's pulse is regular and he has no history of cardiac problems, there is no need to monitor his cardiac rhythm.

    TRUE   FALSE

e. In view of the injuries already detected, there is good reason to suspect injury to the spleen.

    TRUE   FALSE

A131

a. He probably has a significant shunt and should receive oxygen.

TRUE. This patient has acute respiratory insufficiency; that is clear simply from observing the rate and depth of his respirations. And he has good reason to have acute respiratory insufficiency: He's got multiple rib fractures on the left side, and it is very difficult to break several ribs without doing some damage to the lung beneath them. Thus the chances are very good that beneath those fractured ribs are areas of lung where alveoli are filled with blood or collapsed altogether, and more and more alveoli will collapse as the patient continues his shallow breathing. It takes periodic deep breaths to inflate the lungs fully, and this patient is not going to take deep breaths because of the pain that a deep inhalation would cause him. The net effect is that there are areas of lung that are not being ventilated, even though blood is continuing to circulate through those areas—and that spells shunt. This patient, then, definitely should receive oxygen.

b. There is no need for spinal immobilization, since the patient shows no signs of spine injury.

FALSE! If you wait until the patient does show signs of spine injury, you've lost the ball game. One must always consider the *mechanisms of injury,* and any patient who has been in an accident that *could* have produced a spinal injury should be presumed to have a spinal injury until proved otherwise. Our patient is certainly in that category, having been involved in an automobile accident with massive acceleration-deceleration forces. He deserves a backboard. If it turns out later that his spine is in marvelous shape—fine, you haven't lost anything. But it is better to immobilize 1,000 patients who don't have spinal injury than to miss one who does.

c. There is a high probability of left hip fracture.

TRUE. Again, look at the mechanisms of injury. The patient has a fracture of the left patella. That tells you that a force was probably applied along the longitudinal axis of the left femur (since the patient was sitting at the time), and one must consider the possibility that the impact that fractured the patella also dislocated or fractured the hip as the force of impact was propagated down the femur. Injuries of this sort often come in pairs, or even groups; when you see one (the patellar fracture, for example), you should look for the other (the hip fracture, in this example). We shall return to this point in answer e.

d. If the patient's pulse is regular and he has no history of cardiac problems, there is no need to monitor his cardiac rhythm.

FALSE! Once again, look at the mechanisms of injury. This patient was hurled forward with sufficient force to bend the steering column, smash the windshield with his head, and break several ribs. That is good enough reason to presume that his myocardium also took a pounding. Trauma to the myocardium is often missed because people don't look for it; there may be few signs or symptoms of cardiac injury on initial examination. Nonetheless, myocardial contusion can produce all the same complications as myocardial infarction, including a variety of cardiac dysrhythmias. The type of dysrhythmia seen is somewhat dependent upon the site of the injury; right-sided chest trauma more often results in atrial dysrhythmias and heart block, while left-sided and frontal chest trauma are more apt to produce ventricular fibrillation. But you'll never know about it if you're not monitoring the patient. Remember: ANY PATIENT WHO HAS SUSTAINED MAJOR CHEST WALL TRAUMA HAS A MYOCARDIAL CONTUSION UNTIL PROVED OTHERWISE. Treat him as you would a patient with acute myocardial infarction, with constant electrocardiographic monitoring.

e. In view of the injuries already detected, there is good reason to suspect injury to the spleen.

TRUE. Again, think in terms of injuries that go together: In this case, the pathologic pair consists of multiple rib fractures on the left side and ruptured spleen. Recall that the spleen sits tucked up in a corner of the left upper quadrant of the abdomen, just beneath the lower left ribs. A force sufficient to fracture those ribs is also more than sufficient to rupture the spleen. Furthermore, our patient has signs of significant hypovolemia: tachycardia and hypotension. He is losing blood somewhere, and one good bet is that he is bleeding into his abdomen. If this is so, the spleen has to be high on the list of potential sources.

FURTHER READING

Baxt WG et al. The failure of prehospital trauma prediction rules to classify trauma patients accurately. *Ann Emerg Med* 18:1, 1989.

Cales RH. Injury severity determination: Requirements, approaches, and applications. *Ann Emerg Med* 15:1427, 1986.

Champion HR et al. Assessment of injury severity: The triage index. *Crit Care Med* 8:201, 1980.

Champion HR et al. Trauma score. *Crit Care Med* 9:672, 1981.

Champion HR. Field triage of trauma patients (editorial). *Ann Emerg Med* 11:160, 1982.

Champion HR et al. The effect of medical direction on trauma triage. *J Trauma* 28:235, 1988.

Champion HR et al. A revision of the trauma score. *J Trauma* 29:623, 1989.

Ferko JG. The triage factor. *Emergency* 20(8):44, 1988.

Gormican SP. CRAMS scale: Field triage of trauma victims. *Ann Emerg Med* 11:132, 1982.

Kane G et al. Empirical development and evaluation of prehospital trauma triage instruments. *J Trauma* 25:482, 1985.

Knopp R et al. Mechanism of injury and anatomic injury as criteria for prehospital trauma triage. *Ann Emerg Med* 17:895, 1988.

Knudson P, Frecceri CA, DeLateur SA. Improving the field triage of major trauma victims. *J Trauma* 28:602, 1988.

Koehler JJ et al. Prehospital index: A scoring system for field triage of trauma victims. *Ann Emerg Med* 15:178, 1986.

Koenig WJ. Management of severe multiple trauma. *Emergency* 11(2):27, 1979.

Larkin J, Moylan J. Priorities in the management of trauma victims. *Crit Care Med* 3:192, 1975.

Moreau M et al. Application of the trauma score in the prehospital setting. *Ann Emerg Med* 14:1049, 1985.

Morris JA et al. The trauma score as a triage tool in the prehospital setting. *JAMA* 256:1319, 1986.

Nixon RG. Assessment of the trauma patient. *Emerg Med Serv* 8(2):50, 1979.

Ornato J et al. Ineffectiveness of the trauma score and the CRAMS scale for accurately triaging patients to trauma centers. *Ann Emerg Med* 14:1061, 1985.

Rogers LF. Common oversights in the evaluation of the patient with multiple injuries. *Skel Radiol* 12:103, 1984.

Spoor JE. Trauma responses: Beyond the ABCs. *Emergency* 12(2):33, 1980.

Spoor JE. Multiple trauma (from the scene to the surgeon). *Emerg Med Serv* 10(3):38, 1981.

Timberlake GA. Trauma in the golden hour. *Emerg Med* 19(20):79, 1987.

Trunkey DD. Is ALS necessary for pre-hospital trauma care? *J Trauma* 24:86, 1984.

Trunkey DD. Trauma: The first hour. *Emerg Med* 16(5):93, 1984.

A 24-year-old man was involved in an altercation in which knives were deployed freely. You find him lying stuporous in an alley behind a bar. There is an impressive pool of blood around him. His skin is gray, cold, and clammy. Vital signs are pulse of 128, blood pressure 88 systolic, respirations 28 and shallow. There is no evidence of injury to the head or neck; jugular veins are collapsed. There are a few superficial lacerations on the anterior chest, but no evidence of deep chest wounds. Breath sounds are well heard bilaterally. Examination of the abdomen reveals a 12-inch-long, diagonal laceration on the anterior abdominal wall, through which several loops of bowel have emerged. There is also a deep slash on the anterior left thigh, and bright red blood is spurting from it.

1. Which of the following is NOT part of the appropriate management of this patient?

   a. Administer oxygen.
   b. Apply military antishock trousers (MAST).
   c. Start at least one IV with a large-bore cannula and normal saline solution, and run it wide open.
   d. Start a dopamine infusion at a rate of 16 μg/kg/min.
   e. Keep the patient at physiologic temperature.

2. How would you manage this patient's abdominal wound?

   a. Rinse the eviscerated loops of bowel thoroughly with sterile saline, replace them carefully into the abdominal cavity, and cover the wound with a dry, sterile dressing.
   b. Do not waste time rinsing the eviscerated loops of bowel, but simply replace them as rapidly as possible into the abdominal cavity and cover the wound with a dry, sterile dressing.
   c. Do not attempt to replace the eviscerated loops of bowel; leave them outside the abdominal cavity and cover with a dry, sterile dressing.
   d. Do not attempt to replace the eviscerated loops of bowel; leave them outside the abdominal cavity and cover with bulky, sterile dressings that have been soaked in sterile saline.

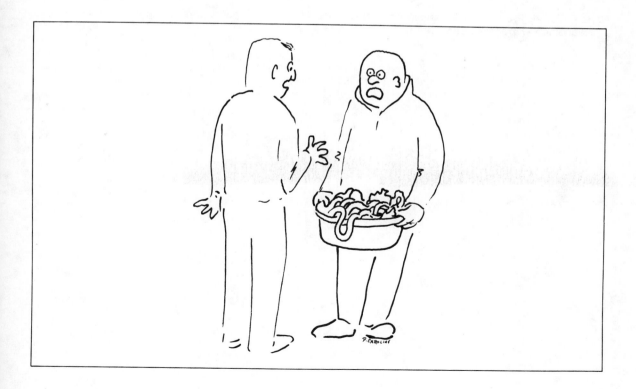

A132

1. A dopamine infusion (answer **d**) is NOT part of the appropriate management of this patient. He is hypotensive because of massive blood loss, not because of any defect in his mechanisms of vasoconstriction. Indeed, at this moment he is probably in a state of diffuse, near maximal vasoconstriction (witness his gray, cold skin). Thus the alpha effects of dopamine are not called for here. Nor do we need its beta effects, for there is no reason to believe that there is any intrinsic problem with a 24-year-old man's heart. His problem is severe hypovolemia secondary to blood loss, and what he needs is volume replacement.

   Oxygen (answer a), intravenous volume replacement (answer c), and maintenance of the patient at physiologic temperature (answer e, which generally means simply covering him with a blanket) are all part of the standard treatment for a patient in shock. What about the military antishock trousers, though (answer b)? Is it wise, you ask, to apply circumferential pressure to the abdomen when the patient's intestines are hanging out? No, it isn't wise. You are absolutely correct. And for that reason, we won't fasten or inflate the abdominal segment, but only the two leg segments. The MAST may still help by applying pressure over the site of arterial bleeding in the left thigh (which, of course, we have already covered with a bulky, sterile dressing). The MAST in this instance will make a fine pressure dressing and help promote hemostasis.

2. The most appropriate management of this patient's abdominal wound is answer **d**: **Do not attempt to replace the eviscerated loops of bowel; leave them outside the abdominal cavity and cover with bulky, sterile dressings that have been soaked in sterile saline.** Certainly no attempt should be made to replace the eviscerated organs in the abdominal cavity (answers a and b), for that carries the risk of further damage to the intestines and practically guarantees the introduction of bacteria into the peritoneal cavity, no matter how conscientiously you rinse off the loops of bowel. Dry dressings over the eviscerated bowel loops (answer c) will only aggravate the injury to these organs, which should be kept moist.

FURTHER READING

Asbun HJ et al. Intra-abdominal seatbelt injury. *J Trauma* 30:189, 1990.

Bietz DS. Abdominal injuries. *Emergency* 10(12):30, 1978.

Caroline NL. *Emergency Care in the Streets* (4th ed.). Boston: Little, Brown, 1991, Ch. 18.

Edwards FJ. Liver trauma. *Emerg Med Serv* 19(3):28, 1990.

Freeark RJ. Penetrating wounds of the abdomen. *N Engl J Med* 291:186, 1974.

Majernick TG et al. Intestinal evisceration resulting from a motor vehicle accident. *Ann Emerg Med* 13:633, 1984.

Moore JB, Moore EE, Thompson JS. Abdominal injuries associated with penetrating trauma in the lower chest. *Am J Surg* 140:724, 1980.

Pons PT et al. Prehospital advanced trauma life support for critical penetrating wounds to the thorax and abdomen. *J Trauma* 25:828, 1985.

It's one of those weeks. Prices are rising, the local football team just lost the division championship, and it's been raining for days. Small wonder then that in the course of the week, you are called to attend to patients who have overdosed with the following agents:

a. Meperidine (Demerol)
b. Amitriptyline (Elavil)
c. Amphetamines (e.g., Dexedrine)
d. Phenobarbital (Nembutal)
e. Digitalis
f. Aspirin

Among your cases were the patients described below. Match each case with the drug from the above list that could account for the clinical picture (i.e., match the patient with the drug on which he overdosed):

1. _____ A 45-year-old man is found semistuporous in his apartment, where he lives alone. A friend tells you that the patient has been under psychiatric care for depression. The patient is restless and seems to be hallucinating. There is prominent twitching of his muscles, and deep tendon reflexes are hyperactive. His skin is very dry and cold. Pulse is 120 and slightly irregular, blood pressure is 130/80, and respirations are 16. Pupils are dilated. The remainder of the physical examination is unremarkable.

2. _____ A 28-year-old woman, who recently lost her job, is found unconscious at home by friends. On examination, you find her responsive only to painful stimuli, to which she reacts with a few slurred mumbles before she lapses back into sleep. Her pulse is 100 and regular, blood pressure is 90/70, and respirations are 8 per minute and shallow. Her skin is warm and dry. Pupils are widely dilated and poorly reactive. Reflexes cannot be elicited.

3. _____ A 25-year-old man is found unconscious in his apartment. He does not respond to painful stimuli. The skin is slightly bluish. Pulse is 40 and regular, blood pressure is 80 systolic, and respirations are 6 per minute. Pupils are pinpoint. There is vomitus around the patient's mouth. The muscles seem flaccid.

4. _____ A 16-year-old boy is found unconscious by his parents. He appears to be delirious when you arrive, and his skin is quite hot and wet. Pulse is 140 and regular, blood pressure is 100/60, and respirations are 30 and deep.

Listed below are treatment routines for different types of overdose. Indicate beside each the number of the case described above for which the treatment would be appropriate.

a. _____ Open the airway. Administer oxygen and assist ventilations. Start an IV line with normal saline, and run it in rapidly. Intubate the trachea. Administer 50% glucose, 50 ml IV. Administer sodium bicarbonate, 1 to 2 ampules IV. Insert a nasogastric tube, lavage the stomach, and instill activated charcoal.

b. _____ Start an IV with normal saline. Administer sodium bicarbonate, 2 to 4 mEq per kilogram IV. Sponge the patient with lukewarm water.

c. _____ Administer oxygen. Start an IV line with normal saline and 40 mEq of potassium. Give physostigmine, 2 mg IV over 2 to 3 minutes.

d. _____ Open the airway. Administer oxygen and assist ventilations. Start an IV line with normal saline. Administer naloxone (Narcan), 0.8 mg diluted in 9 ml saline slowly IV.

311

A133

The general principles of management are basically the same for all cases of overdose—maintain an airway, ensure effective breathing and oxygenation, support the circulation—but there are often additional measures of specific value in specific overdoses. In order to apply these specific measures, one must be able to recognize the signs of overdose with various agents. Sometimes the presence of an empty medicine bottle at the scene will provide an important clue, but don't trust the label on the bottle if the clinical picture doesn't fit.

What did they ingest?

1. **__b__** Our 45-year-old man who is twitching and hyperreflexic took the **amitriptyline** (Elavil), a tricyclic antidepressant drug that, together with antihistamines, belladonna alkaloids (like atropine), and certain plants (jimsonweed), is classed as an anticholinergic. That is to say, it opposes the actions of the parasympathetic, or cholinergic, nervous system. Thus our patient's pulse is rapid (due to blocking effects on the vagus nerve), his skin is dry (due to inhibition of sweating), and his pupils are dilated. There is a specific antidote for anticholinergic poisoning, which we will find in the second part of this question.

2. **__d__** Our 28-year-old lady who tried to end it all after she lost her job has gotten into the **phenobarbital** bottle. Her clinical picture is somewhat nonspecific and could be the picture of almost any overdose with a depressant/hypnotic drug, although the dilated pupils and hypotension are suggestive of barbiturate overdose. Anyway, none of the other drugs on our list would account for all of her clinical signs.

3. **__a__** Our 25-year-old man has tried to do himself in with **meperidine** (Demerol), and he is showing classic signs of narcotic overdose: bradycardia, hypotension, respiratory depression, and pinpoint pupils. Don't be fooled by the fact that there are no needle tracks on his arms; not all narcotics are taken intravenously.

4. **__f__** Our 16-year-old overdosed on **aspirin** and also presents a fairly classic picture: delirium, fever, tachycardia, and hyperventilation (due to metabolic acidosis—salicylates are acids, after all).

And what do we do for them?

a. **__2__** Our young lady with barbiturate overdose gets mainly supportive care. We have to protect her airway because she is comatose and can't do it herself. We will give her oxygen and assist her ventilations, since she doesn't appear to be breathing very adequately on her own. We shall empty her stomach, just in case there are still a few pills remaining there. We give 50% glucose because this is part of the care of any patient in coma where the etiology is not 100 percent certain. And we shall give sodium bicarbonate, which promotes the excretion of phenobarbital though the kidneys.

b. **__4__** For the aspirin overdose, the care is also supportive—with attention to maintaining the airway and circulation. He probably does not need oxygen, for there is nothing wrong with his respiratory function at this point. This patient gets sodium bicarbonate because of his severe metabolic acidosis. And we sponge him down on account of his fever in order to lessen the possibility of febrile convulsions.

c. **__1__** For our amitriptyline overdose, there is a specific antidote in addition to general supportive measures, and that is physostigmine. Physostigmine is a parasympathetic stimulating drug; thus it opposes the effects of parasympathetic blockers (i.e., of anticholinergics). The patient is still awake enough that we can probably forego intubation for the moment, and besides, his restlessness and hallucinations might make intubation a rather harrowing exercise. If you wanted to give this patient 50% glucose, no one would fault you, for hypoglycemia can produce many bizarre neurologic syndromes, and simply because the patient has a known psychiatric history we cannot automatically rule out the possibility that he also has a diabetic history.

d. **__3__** Naloxone (Narcan) is a specific antidote for narcotic overdose and can, by itself, reverse all of the adverse effects of narcotics taken in excess. Thus it is the drug of choice for our young man who took meperedine.

Why didn't we intubate him? After all, he was deeply comatose and unable to protect his airway properly. Indeed, he has already vomited and probably aspirated.

All very true. The problem is that, if we are correct in our diagnosis of meperidine overdose, we can expect our patient to wake up very quickly after we administer the naloxone. And just as quickly, he will reach up and yank out the endotracheal tube that we took so much trouble to insert. And he'll have every right to pull it out, for when he is wide awake, he no longer has any need of it. So we'll hold off on intubation and see what naloxone accomplishes. If that, or 50% glucose, fails to wake him promptly, then we ought to intubate him without further delay.

FURTHER READING

General
Bourne PG. *Acute Drug Abuse Emergencies.* New York: Academic, 1976.
Comstock EG et al. Assessment of the efficacy of activated charcoal following gastric lavage in acute drug emergencies. *J Toxicol* 19:149, 1982.
Done AK. The toxic emergency: Signs, symptoms, and sources. *Emerg Med* 14(1):42, 1982.
Levy G. Gastrointestinal clearance of drugs with activated charcoal. *N Engl J Med* 307:676, 1982.
Ragno RE et al. Effect of ethanol ingestion on outcome of drug overdose. *Crit Care Med* 10:180, 1982.
Turner BM. Drug use: Myths, reality, and problems for EMS. *Emerg Med Serv* 12(3):49, 1983.
Wright N. An assessment of the unreliability of the history given by self-poisoned patients. *Clin Toxicol* 16:381, 1980.

Anticholinergic Overdose
Bessen HA et al. Effect of respiratory alkalosis in tricyclic antidepressant overdose. *West J Med* 139:373, 1983.
Callaham M. Tricyclic antidepressant overdose. *JACEP* 8:413, 1979.
Callaham M. Admission criteria for tricyclic antidepressant ingestion. *West J Med* 137:425, 1982.
Greenland P et al. Cardiac monitoring in tricyclic antidepressant overdose. *Heart Lung* 105:856, 1981.
Manoguerra AS, Ruiz E. Physostigmine treatment of anticholinergic poisoning. *JACEP* 5:125, 1976.
Molloy DW et al. Use of sodium bicarbonate to treat tricyclic antidepressant-induced arrhythmias in a patient with alkalosis. *Canad Med Assoc J* 130:1457, 1984.
Noble J, Matthew H. Acute poisoning by tricyclic antidepressants: Clinical features and management of 100 patients. *Clin Toxicol* 2:403, 1969.
Orr DA et al. Tricyclic antidepressant poisoning and prolonged external cardiac massage during asystole. *Br Med J* 283:1107, 1981.
Pentel P et al. Incidence of late arrhythmias following tricyclic antidepressant overdose. *Clin Toxicol* 18:543, 1981.

Barbiturate Overdose
Berg MJ et al. Acceleration of the body clearance of phenobarbital by oral activated charcoal. *N Engl J Med* 307:642, 1982.
Costello JB et al. Treatment of massive phenobarbital overdose with dopamine diuresis. *Arch Intern Med* 141:938, 1981.
Done AK. The toxic emergency: To sleep, perchance to die. *Emerg Med* 7(9):277, 1975.
Matthew H. Barbiturates. *Clin Toxicol* 8:495, 1975.
McCarron MM et al. Short-acting barbiturate overdosage: Correlation of intoxication score with serum barbiturate concentration. *JAMA* 248:55, 1982.
Pond SM et al. Randomized study of the treatment of phenobarbital overdose with repeated doses of activated charcoal. *JAMA* 251:3104, 1984.
Robinson RR et al. Treatment of acute barbiturate intoxication. *Mod Treat* 8:561, 1971.

Narcotic Overdose
Bradberry JC et al. Continuous infusion of naloxone in the treatment of narcotic overdose. *Drug Intell Clin Pharm* 15:945, 181.
Cuss FM et al. Cardiac arrest after reversal of effects of opiates with naloxone. *Br Med J* 288:363, 1984.
Handal KA, Schauben JL, Salamone FR. Naloxone. *Ann Emerg Med* 12:438, 1983.
Kersh ES. Narcotic overdosage. *Hosp Med* 10(3):8, 1974.
Kersh ES, Schwartz LK. Narcotic poisoning: An epidemic disease. *Am Fam Physician* 8:90, 1973.
Moore RA et al. Naloxone: Underdosage after narcotic poisoning. *Am J Dis Child* 134:156, 1980.
Tandberg D, Abercrombie D. Treatment of heroin overdose with endotracheal naloxone. *Ann Emerg Med* 11:443, 1982.

Salicylate Overdose
Andrews HB. Salicylate poisoning. *Am Fam Physician* 8:102, 1973.
Burton BT et al. Comparison of activated charcoal and gastric lavage in the prevention of aspirin absorption. *J Emerg Med* 1:411, 1984.
Curtis RA et al. Efficacy of ipecac and activated charcoal/cathartic prevention of salicylate absorption in simulated overdose. *Arch Intern Med* 144:48, 1984.
Done AK. Aspirin revisited. *Emerg Med* 9(9):51, 1977.
Gaudreault P et al. The relative severity of acute versus chronic salicylate poisoning in children: A clinical comparison. *Pediatrics* 70:566, 1982.

Heffner JE et al. Salicylate-induced pulmonary edema: Clinical features and prognosis. *Ann Intern Med* 95:405, 1981.

Hill JB. Current concepts: Salicylate intoxication. *N Engl J Med* 288:1110, 1973.

Prescott LF et al. Diuresis or urinary alkalinisation for salicylate poisoning? *Br Med J* 285:1383, 1982.

Walters JS et al. Salicylate-induced pulmonary edema. *Radiology* 146:289, 1983.

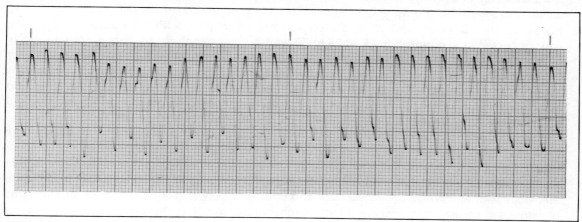

Figure 18

The call comes in simply as a "man down," and you are directed to a drinking establishment in one of the less savory neighborhoods of the city. You park the ambulance beneath a glittering neon light proclaiming the virtues of several unclad ladies, and you enter a smoky "cocktail lounge" illuminated with flashing lights in dozens of colors and shaking under the din of disco music. The manager quickly diverts your attention from the young ladies on stage and leads you to a corner of the lounge, where a middle-aged man lies unconscious on the floor. His complexion appears alternately quite green, then orange, then purple, thanks to the lighting. He is not breathing, and no pulse is palpable. While your partner begins CPR, you apply the quick-look paddles of your defibrillator to the patient's chest and note the rhythm shown on the ECG tracing in Figure 18.

1. The ECG pattern is

   a. Ventricular fibrillation
   b. Supraventricular tachycardia
   c. Ventricular tachycardia
   d. Sinus tachycardia
   e. Asystole

2. At this stage, what is your next step in the management of this patient?

   a. Start an IV with D5W, and administer lidocaine, 100 mg by bolus.
   b. Start an IV with D5W, and administer epinephrine, 5 to 10 ml of a 1:10,000 solution, and bicarbonate, 50 to 100 ml IV.
   c. Start an IV with D5W, and administer calcium chloride, 5 ml of a 10% solution IV.
   d. Administer a lusty thump to the patient's chest.
   e. Countershock at 25 to 50 watt-seconds.

3. Having accomplished the above, which of the steps listed in question 2 would you do next?

A134

1. The ECG pattern is **ventricular tachycardia** (answer **c**), and even if it were supraventricular tachycardia (answer **b**), in these circumstances you would treat it as ventricular tachycardia. Our patient is, if not clinically dead, much closer to clinical death than most of us would like to come, and saving his life will require more than a few squeezes on the carotid sinus.

2. Having started CPR and determined the nature of the rhythm with the quick-look paddles, your next step is to **countershock at 25 to 50 watt-seconds** (answer **e**). This is one of the few instances in which immediate countershock is indicated in *unwitnessed* "cardiac arrest," for although the patient's pulse is not palpable, he does in fact have a cardiac rhythm, and this suggests that he has not been apneic long enough to produce profound hypoxemia and acidosis. Thus the chances of successfully converting his rhythm are still good, and there is no point in losing several minutes trying to get the IV in (answers a, b, and c).

   Chest thump has been reported to convert ventricular tachycardia (answer d); it is thought to create a few watt-seconds of electricity that act on the myocardium as shock from a defibrillator would. But if you have a defibrillator and its paddles are already on the chest, there is little point in beating up the patient to convert his rhythm when you can do the same job more efficiently with electronic equipment. Chest thump should probably be reserved for situations of witnessed cardiac arrest where a monitor/defibrillator is not immediately available.

3. Once you deliver the countershock, your next step is to **start an IV with D5W and administer lidocaine** (answer **a**). If countershock was successful, lidocaine will help stabilize the rhythm; if unsuccessful, lidocaine may increase the chances that the next shock is more effective. If you do not obtain an effective rhythm with 1 or 2 countershocks (first at about 50 watt-seconds, second at 400) your partner will have to continue CPR while you get the IV in.

FURTHER READING

American Heart Association. Standards and guidelines for cardiopulmonary resuscitation (CPR) and emergency cardiac care (ECC). *JAMA* 255:2906, 1986.

Baerman JM et al. Differentiation of ventricular tachycardia from supraventricular tachycardia with aberration: Value of the clinical history. *Ann Emerg Med* 16:40, 1987.

Bilitch M. *A Manual of Cardiac Arrhythmias.* Boston: Little, Brown, 1971.

Bluxhas J et al. Ventricular tachycardia in myocardial infarction: Relation to heart rate and premature ventricular contractions. *Eur Heart J* 6:745, 1985.

Campbell RWF. Treatment and prophylaxis of ventricular arrhythmias in acute myocardial infarction. *Am J Cardiol* 52:55C, 1983.

Caroline NL. *Emergency Care in the Streets* (4th ed.). Boston: Little, Brown, 1991, Ch. 23.

DeSouza N et al. Evaluation of warning arrhythmias before paroxysmal ventricular tachycardia during acute myocardial infarction in man. *Circulation* 60:814, 1979.

Dubin D. *Rapid Interpretation of EKGs* (3rd ed.). Tampa: Cover, 1974.

Frank MJ. Restoring ventricular rhythm. *Emerg Med* 15(2):51, 1983.

Levitt MA. Supraventricular tachycardia with aberrant conduction versus ventricular tachycardia: Differentiation and diagnosis. *Am J Emerg Med* 6:273, 1988.

Morady F. et al. Clinical symptoms in patients with sustained ventricular tachycardia. *West J Med* 142:341, 1985.

Northover BJ. Ventricular tachycardia during the first 72 hours after acute myocardial infarction. *Cardiology* 69:149, 1982.

Schaeffer WA, Cobb LA. Recurrent ventricular fibrillation and modes of death in out-of-hospital ventricular fibrillation. *N Engl J Med* 293:259, 1975.

Tye K et al. R on T or R on P phenomenon? Relation to the genesis of ventricular tachycardia. *Am J Cardiol* 44:632, 1979.

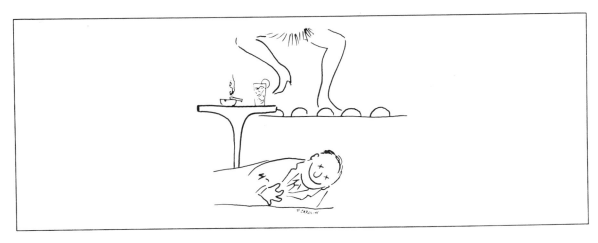

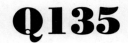

In an explosion in a munitions factory, a 24-year-old worker was struck in the right chest by flying debris and developed a sucking chest wound. The paramedic team caring for the patient applied an occlusive dressing to close the wound, started an infusion, and began administering oxygen. After about 10 minutes, the patient's blood pressure began to fall, his pulse rate increased, and he began showing signs of restlessness and extreme respiratory distress.

1. What has probably happened?

   a. The patient suffered a pulmonary embolism.
   b. The patient developed a tension pneumothorax on the right.
   c. The patient developed pulmonary edema from fluid overload.
   d. The patient developed oxygen toxicity.
   e. The patient is simply suffering from extreme pain.

2. How would you treat this complication?

   a. Administer oxygen under positive pressure.
   b. Give Lasix and discontinue the infusion to combat fluid overload.
   c. Momentarily release the occlusive dressing covering the open chest wound.
   d. Discontinue oxygen administration.
   e. Give a nitrous oxide/oxygen combination to relieve the patient's pain.

A135

1. The correct answer is **b**: The patient has developed a **tension pneumothorax on the right.** How did this happen? Clearly the debris that made a hole in the patient's chest also injured the lung beneath and apparently created a wound in the lung that acted as a one-way valve. When the patient inhaled, air escaped from the lung, through the one-way valve, into the pleural space; when he exhaled, the air could not flow back into the lung, and since you had closed off the chest with an occlusive dressing, it could not escape through the chest wall either. With each inhalation, a little more air collected in the right pleural space, causing progressive buildup of pressure within the pleural space and progressive compression of lung tissue. Small wonder the patient is in respiratory distress.

   Why did he become hypotensive? Because the increased pressure in the pleural cavity also tends to collapse the vena cava and thus to inhibit venous return to the heart; as this happens, cardiac output falls and hypotension may occur. If you had looked closely, you would have noticed that the patient's neck veins had become distended—another reflection of the increased pressure on the vena cava.

2. The treatment for this situation is to **momentarily release the occlusive dressing covering the open chest wound** (answer c) in order to allow the air under pressure to escape from the pleural cavity. This patient will require a chest tube as soon as possible, but until he gets one, keep one side of the occlusive dressing untaped so that air under pressure can be vented out of the chest through the open side of the dressing.

Let us look for a moment at the incorrect answers. While hypotension, tachycardia, and respiratory distress are all consistent with a diagnosis of pulmonary embolism (answer 1a), we have no reason to suspect that this has occurred. As far as we know, the patient had no underlying conditions that would have predisposed him to the development of pulmonary embolism (e.g., prolonged immobilization or thrombophlebitis in his legs), and there is nothing about his injury that would suggest a pulmonary embolism either, for he had no massive fractures (which can produce fat embolism). Pulmonary edema from fluid overload (answer 1c) would be highly unlikely in this situation for a number of reasons. First of all, it would be very difficult in the space of 10 minutes, with a single IV line, to give a sufficient volume of fluid to send anyone into pulmonary edema; indeed, in this time period, you have probably scarcely replaced the patient's blood loss. Furthermore, a young patient can tolerate considerable fluid volumes without experiencing heart failure.

There is virtually no possibility that this patient has developed oxygen toxicity, i.e., pathologic changes in the lung caused by the administration of high concentrations of oxygen (answer 1d). Oxygen toxicity is seen only in cases where a patient has been maintained for many hours, or even days, on high inhaled-oxygen concentrations. There is no danger in administering high oxygen concentrations to an adult for short periods (i.e., up to 12–18 hours).

The patient undoubtedly *is* suffering from a great deal of pain (answer 1e), but that does not sufficiently explain the degree of his respiratory distress or hypotension, and a cause must be sought elsewhere. Restlessness too is always an indication to check for hypoxemia.

As to the incorrect answers regarding treatment, the administration of oxygen under positive pressure (answer 2a) should rarely be undertaken in a patient with a significant chest injury unless he has a chest tube in place; oxygen under positive pressure can precipitate a pneumothorax in a damaged lung or worsen an existing pneumothorax. As mentioned above, this patient does not have a problem of fluid overload—quite the contrary—and thus it would be entirely inappropriate to give him Lasix and discontinue his infusion (answer 2b). It is also entirely inappropriate to discontinue oxygen administration (answer 2d); this patient probably has a high degree of shunt and needs oxygen in high concentrations. Finally, although nitrous oxide/oxygen combinations are very effective in the treatment of pain, they are contraindicated in any situation where pneumothorax is suspected (answer 2e) because nitrous oxide tends to collect in dead air spaces and thus will worsen a pneumothorax.

FURTHER READING

Cannon WB, Mark JBD, Jamplis RW. Pneumothorax: A therapeutic update. *Am J Surg* 142:26, 1981.
Darin JC. The diagnosis and treatment of chest injuries. *EMT J* 2(2):52, 1978.
Gauthier RK. Thoracic trauma. *Emerg Med Serv* 13(3):28, 1984.
Thoracic trauma. *Emerg Med* 12(19):69, 1980.

You are called to see a 58-year-old man who, according to his wife, "just stopped speaking." You find him conscious and alert, but evidently anxious, and intermittently crying. He does not answer questions, but he is able to follow commands. His right arm is flaccid, and he staggers when he tries to walk.

1. Which of the following statements about this patient is TRUE?

   a. There is no need to monitor his cardiac rhythm, since his problem is neurologic, not cardiac.
   b. He should receive oxygen and be transported supine to the hospital.
   c. The fact that he is anxious and weeping suggests that he is suffering from a psychiatric problem.
   d. The fact that the patient staggers indicates that he has probably been imbibing alcohol.

2. Indicate which of the following statements about cerebrovascular accident (CVA), or stroke, are true and which are false.

   a. Stroke may occur in young people, especially young women taking birth control pills.

   TRUE   FALSE

   b. Stroke always presents as paralysis on one side of the body and disturbances of speech.

   TRUE   FALSE

   c. Some patients will experience a series of transient "little strokes" in the weeks or months preceding their CVA.

   TRUE   FALSE

A136

1. The correct answer is **b**: This patient should **receive oxygen and be transported supine to the hospital.** Furthermore, contrary to what is stated in answer a, there is a very good reason to monitor this patient's cardiac rhythm: An ECG may reveal a cardiac dysrhythmia or an otherwise silent myocardial infarction that caused this patient's stroke by producing a decrease in cardiac output.

   The fact that our patient is anxious and weeping does NOT suggest that he is suffering from a psychiatric problem (answer c). Under the circumstances, this is a normal and entirely appropriate response. Imagine how you would feel if you suddenly found yourself paralyzed on one side of your body and couldn't even communicate your distress in words. There can be few experiences more terrifying and more depressing, and this patient has every reason in the world to cry.

   The most likely reason that our patient is staggering is because of weakness or paralysis in his right leg, NOT because he is intoxicated (answer d).

2. Now to our quiz about stroke in general:
   a. Stroke may occur in young people, especially young women taking birth control pills.

      TRUE. While most cases of stroke occur in the over-50 generation, as a result of underlying cardiovascular or cerebrovascular disease, strokes can and do sometimes occur in younger people, and women taking birth control medications are considered to be at greater risk than are other persons of the same age.

   b. Stroke always presents as paralysis on one side of the body and disturbances of speech.

      FALSE. This is the classic stroke presentation, but it is by no means the only one. Stroke may present as hemiplegia alone, without speech disturbance, or as speech disturbance alone, without hemiplegia. Or it may present as the sudden development of confusion or coma. There may be only a sensory loss on one side or just weakness of one leg. Depending on the size and location of the ischemic area in the brain, there may be significant departures from the classic clinical picture. Whenever there is a fairly sudden development of a neurologic deficit, stroke must be considered among the possible causes.

   c. Some patients will experience a series of transient "little strokes" in the weeks or months preceding their CVA.

      TRUE. Such "little strokes" are referred to as transient ischemic attacks (TIAs). They occur most commonly in the early morning when the patient is awakening and usually pass within a few minutes, although they may last several hours. Thus the patient may complain, for example, that during the past few weeks he has several times had difficulty speaking or moving his arm when he wakened from sleep, but that after lying in bed for a while, he found that the problem went away. Any patient telling such a story must be considered at high risk of developing a stroke in the near future and should be evaluated fully in the hospital.

FURTHER READING

Alberts MJ, Bertels C, Dawson D. An analysis of time of presentation after stroke. *JAMA* 263:65, 1990.

Barber JM. EMT checkpoint: Management of the patient with suspected stroke. *EMT J* 4(3):69, 1980.

Caroline NL. *Emergency Care in the Streets* (4th ed.). Boston: Little, Brown, 1991, Ch. 24.

Edmeads J. Strategies in stroke. *Emerg Med* 15(4):163, 1983.

Jacobs FL. Stroke: Emergency assessment and management. *Emerg Med Serv* 14(2):41, 1985.

Komrad MS et al. Myocardial infarction and stroke. *Neurology* 34:1403, 1984.

Klag MJ et al. Decline in US stroke mortality: Demographic trends and antihypertensive treatment. *Stroke* 20:14, 1989.

Lavin P. Management of hypertension in patients with acute stroke. *Arch Intern Med* 146:66, 1986.

Marler JR et al. Morning increase in onset of ischemic stroke. *Stroke* 20:473, 1989.

Mikolich JR et al. Cardiac arrhythmias in patients with acute cerebrovascular accidents. *JAMA* 246:1314, 1981.

Myers MG et al. Cardiac sequelae of acute stroke. *Stroke* 13:838, 1982.

Parsons-Smith BG. First aid for acute cerebral stroke. *Practitioner* 223:553, 1979.

Ross GS, Klassen R. The stroke syndrome. Part 1: Pathogenesis. *Hosp Med* 9:3, 1973.

Ross GS, Klassen R. The stroke syndrome. Part 2: Clinical and diagnostic aspects. *Hosp Med* 9:55, 1973.

Samuels MA. All about stroke. *Emerg Med* 18(6):94, 1986.

Walshaw MJ, Pearson MG. Hypoxia in patients with acute hemiplegia. *Br Med J* 288:15, 1984.

At 2:15 in the morning, you are summoned to a shabby tenement for a "possible OB." The woman has had eight successful pregnancies previously and now is having contractions 2 minutes apart. With the graduates of her eight previous pregnancies standing around you watching intently, you immediately prepare the patient for delivery. And none too soon, for within moments you are holding a baby boy in your hands, amidst wild cheers from the audience.

1. Sixty seconds after the birth of the infant, you evaluate him to determine the Apgar score. You find the following:

   Color: body pink, extremities blue
   Pulse: 80
   Reflex irritability: cries when stimulated
   Muscle tone: actively moving
   Respiratory effort: good, strong cry

   What is baby's Apgar score?

2. The placenta is delivered shortly thereafter, but there is still a moderate amount oɪ bleeding. Several measures may be used to promote uterine contraction and thereby control bleeding. Which of the following is NOT among the measures you can use to promote uterine contraction?

   a. Start an IV and add 10 units of oxytocin (Pitocin) to the intravenous bag.
   b. Begin a dopamine infusion at 3 μg/kg/min.
   c. Gently massage the abdomen over the uterus.
   d. Put the baby to the mother's breast.

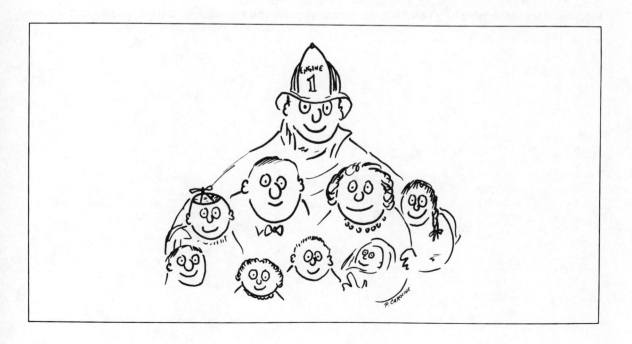

A137

Table 4. Apgar Scoring System

Clinical Sign	Points Given According to Status		
	0 Points	1 Point	2 Points
A Appearance (color)	Pale, blue	Body pink, extremities blue	Completely pink
P Pulse (heart rate)	Absent	Below 100	Over 100
G Grimace (reflex irritability)	No response	Grimaces	Cries
A Activity (muscle tone)	Limp	Some flexion of extremities	Active motion
R Respiratory effort	Absent	Slow, irregular	Good, strong cry

1. The scoring system devised by Virginia Apgar is designed to evaluate a baby's vital functions shortly after birth. One minute after the complete birth of the infant, certain signs are assessed and given a score of 0, 1, or 2, according to the criteria in Table 4.

   Now let's total up the score on our baby:

Color: body pink, extremities blue	= 1
Pulse: 80	= 1
Reflex irritability: cries when stimulated	= 2
Muscle tone: actively moving	= 2
Respiratory effort: good, strong cry	= 2

   APGAR SCORE   8

2. There is no place for dopamine (answer **b**) in the management of this woman. At the dose listed, dopamine is a beta sympathetic drug and would simply cause peripheral arterial vasodilation. All of the other measures listed do promote uterine contraction, which, by squeezing down on the blood vessels that had connected the uterus to the placenta, shuts off flow through those vessels and thereby diminishes bleeding.

FURTHER READING

Anderson B, Shapiro B. *Emergency Childbirth Handbook.* Albany, NY: Delmar, 1979.
Boulton FE et al. Obstetric haemorrhage: Causes and management. *Clin Haem* 14:683, 1985.
Harris BA. Dealing with a difficult delivery. *Emerg Med* 16(11):22, 1984.
Kilgore JR. Management of an obstetric patient by the EMT. *EMT J* 4(2):50, 1980.
Nixon RG. Third trimester obstetric complications. Part II: Eclampsia and postpartum hemorrhage. *Emerg Med Serv* 10(4):52, 1981.
Williams C. Emergency childbirth. *Emerg Med Serv* 14(3):100, 1985.
Wojslawowicz JM. Emergency childbirth for emergency medical technicians. *EMT J* 1(4):66, 1977.

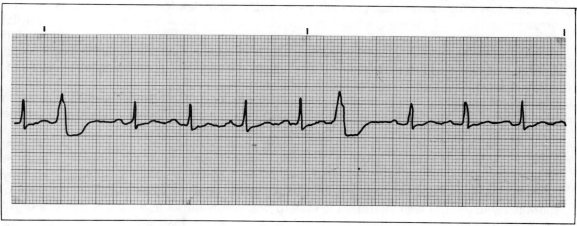

Figure 19

You are summoned to a political rally where a 40-year-old candidate for city council became ill while delivering a speech. You find the patient in the backstage area of a large auditorium, sitting in a chair, with his tie pulled loose and his shirt collar open. He states that while he was making his most crucial point about the dangers of inflation, he began to feel a "squeezing" in his chest and became somewhat sick to his stomach. He denies any significant past medical history. He denies any allergies, and he takes no medications regularly. On physical examination, he is pale, diaphoretic, and anxious. His pulse is strong, blood pressure is 150/80, and respirations are 18. There is no jugular venous distention. The chest is clear. Heart sounds are well heard. There is no peripheral edema. A portion of the patient's ECG is shown in Figure 19.

1. Examine the patient's rhythm strip:

   a. The rhythm is _____ regular _____ irregular.
   b. The rate is _____ per minute.

2. The *underlying* rhythm is

   a. Normal sinus rhythm
   b. Junctional rhythm
   c. Sinus arrhythmia
   d. Atrial fibrillation
   e. Second-degree AV block

3. Which of the following is NOT part of the management of this patient?

   a. Administer oxygen.
   b. Start an IV with D5W.
   c. Administer lidocaine, 100 mg by IV bolus followed by infusion at 2 to 3 mg per minute.
   d. Administer morphine, 5 to 10 mg by slow IV titration.
   e. Transport the patient in a supine position to the hospital.

4. Certain types of PVCs are always regarded as dangerous, even if they occur in individuals not having a myocardial infarction. Other kinds of PVCs may be benign in healthy individuals. Which of the following types of PVCs do NOT require immediate treatment with lidocaine if detected in an otherwise healthy individual?

   a. A PVC falling on the T wave
   b. One PVC seen during 15 minutes of monitoring
   c. Three PVCs in a row
   d. Multifocal PVCs
   e. More than 15 PVCs per minute

A138

1. The patient's rhythm is slightly **irregular.** The rate in this strip, taking into account the ectopic beats, is **90 per minute;** the underlying rate is 75 per minute.

2. The underlying rhythm is **normal sinus** (answer **a**), for there is a P wave preceding every QRS complex (save for the two ectopic beats) and a QRS complex following every P wave. The presence of normal P waves rules out the possibility of junctional rhythm (answer b) or atrial fibrillation (answer d). The basic regularity of the rhythm is, by definition, inconsistent with sinus arrhythmia (answer c). In second-degree block (answer e), one would expect to find some P waves that are not conducted, i.e., P waves without QRS complexes following them, and that is not the case in the rhythm strip shown.

3. The patient should be transported in a semisitting position to the hospital, for in that position cardiac work is minimized and breathing is most comfortable. Thus, transport in a supine position is NOT part of the management of this patient (answer **e**).

   If you were very wide awake, you might also have answered d to this question, i.e., that administration of morphine is NOT part of the management of our candidate. His story of gastrointestinal symptoms is suggestive of an *inferior* wall myocardial infarction, and many cardiologists prefer *not* to give morphine under those circumstances because morphine is more likely in inferior wall infarction to lead to bradyarrhythmias and various degrees of AV block. Nitrous oxide/oxygen is probably a safer analgesic in this case.

4. **One PVC seen during 15 minutes of monitoring** does not require treatment in an otherwise healthy individual (answer **b**). All of the other types of PVCs listed are considered dangerous under any circumstances, for they reflect pathology in the heart or may rapidly lead to life-threatening situations. A PVC falling on a T wave (answer a) can trigger ventricular tachycardia or fibrillation, for the T wave represents the heart's vulnerable period of repolarization. Three PVCs in a row (answer c) can essentially be considered ventricular tachycardia and thus can be classified as a potentially life-threatening dysrhythmia. Multifocal PVCs (answer d) indicate that there are numerous irritable foci in the myocardium and thus suggest widespread myocardial ischemia. But even unifocal PVCs occurring at rates of more than 15 per minute (answer e) are worrisome because they suggest ventricular irritability and instability.

FURTHER READING

American Heart Association. Standards and guidelines for cardiopulmonary resuscitation (CPR) and emergency cardiac care (ECC). *JAMA* 255:2905, 1986.

Baron DW et al. Protective effect of lidocaine during regional myocardial ischemia. *Mayo Clin Proc* 57:442, 1982.

Dunn HM et al. Prophylactic lidocaine in the early phase of suspected myocardial infarction. *Am Heart J* 110:353, 1985.

Harrison DC et al. Should prophylactic antiarrhythmic drug therapy be used in acute myocardial infarction? *JAMA* 247:2019, 1982.

Koster RW, Dunning AJ. Intramuscular lidocaine for prevention of lethal arrhythmias in the prehospitalization phase of acute myocardial infarction. *N Engl J Med* 313:1105, 1985.

Lie KI. Pre- and in-hospital antiarrhythmic prevention of ventricular fibrillation complicating acute myocardial infarction. *Eur Heart J* 5(Suppl B):95, 1984.

Lie KI et al. Lidocaine in the prevention of primary ventricular fibrillation. *N Engl J Med* 291:1324, 1974.

MacMahon S et al. Effects of prophylactic lidocaine in suspected acute myocardial infarction: An overview of results from the randomized, controlled trials. *JAMA* 260:1910, 1988.

A bus has collided with a passenger car on the interstate highway. There are 23 casualties, of whom 6 are critically injured, 3 are moderately injured, and 14 are only slightly injured.

How many ambulances will be required to handle these casualties efficiently (assume that each ambulance has a crew of two)?

a. 2
b. 5
c. 12
d. 16
e. 23

Among the casualties are the following patients. Arrange them in the order in which they would receive treatment:

a. A 43-year-old man with suspected spinal injury
b. A 15-year-old boy with a fractured forearm
c. A 23-year-old woman with tension pneumothorax
d. A 30-year-old man with a sucking chest wound and massive hemorrhage from the neck

1. _____
2. _____
3. _____
4. _____

A139

Approximately **16 ambulances** will be required to handle this situation efficiently (answer **d**). One can calculate that there will be a need for one vehicle and *at least* two rescuers for each critically injured patient; slightly injured patients can be accommodated two to a vehicle. Moderately injured fall somewhere in between, but it is better to assume that each moderately injured victim will require an ambulance, for one can use the additional rescuers to help out at the scene with other tasks, such as crowd control or hazard control. Hence, our estimate:

6 critically injured	= 6 ambulances (12 rescuers)
3 moderately injured	= 3 ambulances (6 rescuers)
14 slightly injured	= 7 ambulances (14 rescuers)
	= 16 ambulances (32 rescuers)

Answer **e** is also acceptable, but not necessarily optimal. More is not always better. A mob of rescuers at the scene of a mass casualty can create as much of a problem as a mob of bystanders if each of the rescuers does not have a clear task. Try as early as possible to make an estimate of how many rescuers and vehicles you will need. Give yourself a margin of error, but don't overdo it. The smaller the team, the more efficiently it will work.

Each of the patients listed in our second question belongs to a clearly defined priority group. Did you get them straight?

1. __d__ A 30-year-old man with a sucking chest wound and massive hemorrhage from the neck
2. __c__ A 23-year-old woman with tension pneumothorax
3. __a__ A 43-year-old man with suspected spinal injury
4. __b__ A 15-year-old boy with a fractured forearm

FURTHER READING

Butman AM. The challenge of casualties en masse. *Emerg Med* 15(7):110, 1983.
Caroline NL. *Emergency Care in the Streets* (4th ed.). Boston: Little, Brown, 1991, Ch. 21.
Haynes BE et al. A prehospital approach to multiple-victim incidents. *Ann Emerg Med* 15:458, 1986.
Kelly JT. Model for pre-hospital disaster response. *J World Assn Emerg Disaster Med* 1:80, 1986.
Koehler JJ et al. Prehospital index: A scoring system for field triage of trauma victims. *Ann Emerg Med* 15:178, 1986.
Mathews TP. Triage 81. *J World Assn Emerg Disaster Med* 1:153, 1985.
Rund DA, Rausch TS. *Triage*. St Louis: Mosby, 1981.
Schwartz TJ. Model for pre-hospital disaster response. *J World Assn Emerg Disaster Med* 1:78, 1986.
Yates DW. Major disasters: Surgical triage. *Br J Hosp Med* 22:329, 1979.

The call comes in at 9:30 in the evening for a "sick child." You arrive at a nice ranch house in the suburbs, and you are ushered into the child's room by the babysitter. The child is 9 years old and appears to be sleeping peacefully. The babysitter is worried because usually this particular boy is up raising hell at 9:30, and today he hasn't left the bedroom since she arrived at 5:00. When she went to check on him just now, she had trouble waking him. The babysitter says that she knows the boy has a history of asthma and that he has been having "a lot of breathing problems lately."

On physical examination, you find the child asleep and difficult to awaken. His skin is pale with a bluish tinge to it. The pulse is 130 and regular. Respirations are 30 and quiet. Pupils are slightly dilated but reactive. Neck veins are not distended. The chest is hyperresonant to percussion. Breath sounds are not well heard, but no wheezes are audible. The abdomen is soft. There are occasional twitching movements in the extremities.

Which of the following statements about this child and his management are true and which are false?

a. He should immediately be given humidified oxygen and assisted ventilation.

TRUE　　　　　　　　FALSE

b. The fact that he is able to sleep peacefully indicates that he is not having a serious asthmatic attack.

TRUE　　　　　　　　FALSE

c. The child should receive intravenous fluids, for he is probably significantly dehydrated.

TRUE　　　　　　　　FALSE

d. The absence of loud wheezes in the patient's chest indicates that he is not suffering from an asthmatic attack, and the source of his problem must be sought elsewhere.

TRUE　　　　　　　　FALSE

A140

a. He should immediately be given humidified oxygen and assisted ventilation.

TRUE. This boy is showing evidence of severe hypoxemia (bluish skin, tachycardia) and hypercarbia (sedation and muscle twitching), and he may die within minutes if this situation is not reversed.

b. The fact that he is able to sleep peacefully indicates that he is not having a serious asthmatic attack.

FALSE! He is sleeping "peacefully" because he is under the influence of a very powerful narcotic, carbon dioxide, and his somnolence should immediately indicate to you that this patient is in enormous danger. A SLEEPY ASTHMATIC IS AN ASTHMATIC IN TROUBLE!

c. The patient should receive intravenous fluids, for he is probably significantly dehydrated.

TRUE. Dehydration is often a prominent feature of status asthmaticus (prolonged, intractable asthmatic attacks) and may itself lead to a worsening of the child's condition. As the child becomes more and more dehydrated, mucus plugs obstructing his smaller bronchi become drier and more solidly impacted and are thus more difficult to cough out. Rehydration with intravenous fluids will help loosen the secretions.

d. The absence of loud wheezes in the patient's chest indicates that he is not suffering from an asthmatic attack, and the source of his problem must be sought elsewhere.

FALSE!! Wheezes are heard when air passes through constricted air passages during respiration. The absence of wheezes may indicate that the airways are not significantly constricted, but it can also indicate—as it does in the case of our 9-year-old asthmatic—that *no air is passing through the airways at all.* Our little boy has simply ceased effective ventilation. That is the reason we barely hear any breath sounds and why the carbon dioxide levels in his blood have built up to a point where they have anesthetized the child. A SILENT CHEST IN AN ASTHMATIC MEANS DANGER! It means that the airways are *so* constricted and *so* plugged up with mucus that scarcely any air can pass through them. Our therapy will be aimed at opening up the airways (with bronchodilators) and assisting the patient with his gas exchange (through assisted ventilation with supplemental oxygen).

FURTHER READING

Carden DL et al. Vital signs including pulsus paradoxus in the assessment of acute bronchial asthma. *Ann Emerg Med* 12:80, 1983.

Groth ML, Hurewitz AN. Pharmacologic management of acute asthma. *Emerg Med* 21(7):23, 1989.

Harper TB et al. Techniques of administration of metered-dose aerosolized drugs in asthmatic children. *Am J Dis Child* 135:218, 1981.

Hurwitz ME et al. Clinical scoring does not accurately assess hypoxemia in pediatric asthma patients. *Ann Emerg Med* 13:1040, 1984.

Johnson AJ et al. Circumstances of death from asthma. *Br Med J* 288:1870, 1984.

Kampschulte S, Marcey J, Safar P. Simplified management of status asthmaticus in children. *Crit Care Med* 1:69, 1973.

Kravis LP et al. Unexpected death in childhood asthma. *Am J Dis Child* 139:558, 1985.

Lee H et al. Aerosol bag for administration of bronchodilators to young asthmatic children. *Pediatrics* 73:230, 1984.

Lulla S et al. Emergency management of asthma in children. *J Pediatr* 97:346, 1980.

Mellis CM. Important changes in the emergency management of acute asthma in children. *Med J Aust* 148:215, 1988.

Nguyen MT et al. Causes of death from asthma in children. *Ann Allergy* 55:448, 1985.

Reyes de la Rocha S, Brown MA. Asthma in children: Emergency management. *Ann Emerg Med* 16:79, 1987.

Sly RM. Mortality from asthma in children 1979–1984. *Ann Allergy* 60:433, 1988.

Strunk RC et al. Physiologic and psychological characteristics associated with deaths due to asthma in childhood: A case-controlled study. *JAMA* 254:1193, 1985.

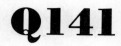

A call comes in one frigid winter day from a winter sports area about 15 miles outside of town where an 18-year-old woman has fallen while ice-skating and injured her arm. You find her sitting on a bench by the side of the pond, gingerly holding her right wrist. There is swelling and deformity in the midsection of the right forearm, and the area is very tender to palpation. The radial pulse is strong, and there is no loss of sensation in the fingers.

You put her arm in slight traction and apply an air splint, carefully inflating it just to the point where your thumb makes a slight indentation in the splint. Then you put the splinted arm in a sling and assist the patient to your ambulance.

1. About 10 minutes later, while you are en route to the hospital, the patient begins complaining of pins-and-needles sensations in her right hand. You should

   a. Inflate the air splint slightly more.
   b. Deflate the air splint slightly.
   c. Remove the patient's sling and let her arm hang dependent to improve blood flow to her hand.
   d. Do nothing; paresthesias are to be expected after a fracture to the forearm.

2. Which of the following statements about the treatment of fractures in the field is NOT true?

   a. Fractures involving joints should be straightened immediately to prevent damage to nerves and arteries.
   b. Dress wounds before splinting fractures.
   c. Immobilize fractures before moving the patient.
   d. Do not attempt to push protruding bone ends back into a wound when there is an open (compound) fracture.

A141

1. When the patient begins complaining of paresthesias in her hand, you should **deflate the air splint slightly** (answer b). "But I inflated it correctly to begin with," you protest. "I did it exactly according to the books—just to the point where I could still indent it with slight pressure by my thumb." True, true. The air splint was applied correctly. But now the situation has changed somewhat. For when you took the patient from the frigid bench by the side of the pond and put her in your nice, warm ambulance, the air inside the splint began to warm up. And as the air warmed, it expanded, causing the splint to grow tighter, to the point that it was interfering with the patient's circulation. Certainly under such circumstances, one does not want to inflate the air splint further (answer a), and to remove the sling and allow the patient's arm to hang dependent (answer c) will only encourage swelling in the distal extremity. Paresthesias are NOT to be expected after a routine fracture (answer d); their presence suggests that there has been damage to the surrounding nerves or that something is compromising peripheral blood flow. If paresthesias do occur, your first job is to make sure that they are not the result of your treatment. Recheck your splint to be certain it isn't too tight.

2. Answer **a** is NOT true. Fractures involving joints should NOT under most circumstances be straightened in the field; they should be splinted where they lie. Attempts to straighten such fractures in the field are more likely to *cause* damage to nerves and arteries than to prevent it. A rigid splint fastened above and below the involved joint will keep the area stable through transport.

   In general, the field treatment of orthopedic injuries is aimed at preventing further injury. Wounds are dressed before fractures are splinted (answer b) in order to minimize handling of an open wound during manipulation of the fracture(s). One immobilizes all fractures before moving the patient (answer c), lest one aggravate a fracture with undue motion around broken bone ends. Finally, pushing broken bone ends back into an open wound is a sure formula for infection (answer d). Cover the broken bone ends with a sterile dressing that has been moistened with sterile saline, splint the extremity securely, and transport.

FURTHER READING

Anast GT. Fractures and splinting. *Emergency* 10(11):42, 1978.

Burtzloff HE. Splinting closed fractures of the extremities. *Emerg Med Serv* 10(3):70, 1981.

Canan S. Grasping objectives of long-bone splinting. *Rescue* 2(5):45, 1989.

Caroline NL. *Emergency Care in the Streets* (4th ed.). Boston: Little, Brown, 1991, Ch. 19.

Caroline NL. *Emergency Medical Treatment: A Text for EMT-As and EMT-Intermediates* (3rd ed.). Boston: Little, Brown, 1991, Ch. 17.

Connolly JF. Fracture pitfalls:
  The ankle. *Emerg Med* 16(7):49, 1984.
  The elbow. *Emerg Med* 15(11):163, 1983.
  The femur. *Emerg Med* 15(21):51, 1983.
  The forearm. *Emerg Med* 15(13):235, 1983.
  General principles. *Emerg Med* 14(17):161, 1982.
  The knee: Bone and soft tissue. *Emerg Med* 16(1):205, 1984.
  The humerus. *Emerg Med* 15(9):170, 1983.
  Metacarpals and phalanges. *Emerg Med* 15(15):201, 1983.
  Pathologic fractures. *Emerg Med* 16(11):61, 1984.
  Tibial fractures. *Emerg Med* 16(5):43, 1984.
  The wrist. *Emerg Med* 15(14):195, 1983.

Gustafson JE. Contraindications to the repositioning of fractured or dislocated limbs in the field. *JACEP* 5:184, 1976.

Lhowe D. Basics of broken bones for the nonorthopedist: 2. Primary care for nondisplaced fractures. *Emerg Med* 19(16):89, 1987.

Menkes JS. Pitfalls in orthopedia trauma:
  Part I. The upper extremity. *Emerg Med* 21(5):64, 1989.
  Part II. The lower extremity. *Emerg Med* 21(6):108, 1989.

Rayburn BK. Prehospital care of fractures and dislocations of the extremities. *EMT J* 4(2):61, 1980.

Rector J, Phelps DB. Care of the injured hand. Part VI: Fractures and dislocations. *Emerg Med Serv* 8(1):16, 1979.

Tomford W. Basics of broken bones for the nonorthopedist: I. The fundamental principles. *Emerg Med* 19(15):25, 1987.

Wald DA, Ziemba TJ, Ferko JG. Upper extremity injuries. *Emergency* 21(3):25, 1989.

Winspur I, Phelps DB. Emergency care of the injured hand. Part XI: Hand dressings, splints, and casts. *Emerg Med Serv* 9(1):22, 1980.

This time it's in a small trailer camp on the outskirts of town that you are called upon to deliver a baby. The mother has had six previous pregnancies and informs you that her "bag of waters" broke about 10 minutes ago. She is having contractions 3 minutes apart. You set her up for delivery and notice that she is crowning and that the umbilical cord is protruding from the vagina.

    You should

a. Push the umbilical cord back into the vagina, so that the baby's head will come out first.
b. Clamp and cut the umbilical cord immediately.
c. Reach past the umbilical cord and gently push the baby's head a few centimeters back into the vagina; transport the patient immediately to the hospital, supine, with her hips elevated on a pillow.
d. Start an IV and add 10 units of oxytocin (Pitocin) to the bag.

A142

The correct answer is **c**: Reach past the umbilical cord and gently **push the baby's head a few centimeters back into the vagina.** This maneuver takes the pressure off the umbilical cord, which would otherwise be compressed by the baby's head against the vaginal wall, thereby cutting off the baby's blood supply from the placenta. Do NOT clamp and cut the umbilical cord (answer b); it is the baby's only source of oxygenated blood until he or she is out in the world breathing on his own. To cut the cord at this point is equivalent to strangling the infant. Do NOT try to push the cord itself back, for it may be damaged if it is jammed past the baby's head (answer a). Oxytocin is not indicated until the baby has been delivered, for it is used to promote contraction and shrinking of the uterus (answer d).

It is important to get this mother to the hospital as rapidly as possible. Elevation of her hips on pillows will help, by gravity, to keep the baby's head from pressing against the birth canal, but you may have to maintain some manual pressure on the baby's head as well. The knee-chest position is also effective, but it is rather difficult to maintain safely in a moving ambulance. Notify the hospital of your situation and your estimated time of arrival so the obstetric team can prepare themselves for the case.

FURTHER READING
Anderson B, Shapiro B. *Emergency Childbirth Handbook.* Albany, NY: Delmar, 1979.
Beware the prolapsed cord. *Emerg Med* 17(15):47, 1985.
Caroline NL. *Emergency Care in the Streets* (4th ed.). Boston: Little, Brown, 1991, Ch. 35.
Emergence emergencies. *Emerg Med* 4(9):89, 1972.
Kilgore JR. Management of an obstetric patient by the EMT. *EMT J* 4(2):50, 1980.
Nixon RG. Third trimester obstetric complications. Part III: Problems during fetal delivery. *Emerg Med Serv* 10(5):80, 1981.
Williams C. Emergency childbirth. *Emerg Med Serv* 14(3):100, 1985.
Wojslawowicz JM. Emergency childbirth for emergency medical technicians. *EMT J* 1(4):66, 1977.

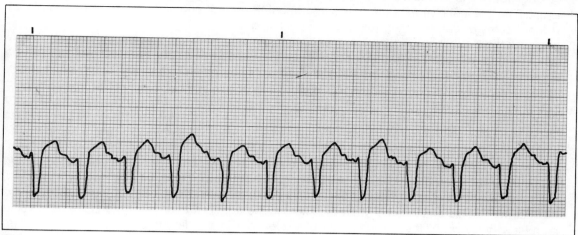

Figure 20

You are just about to parcel out the pizza with double cheese and mushrooms that you and your colleagues ordered for midnight dinner when the call comes in for "a man who can't breathe." With a last wistful glance at the pizza, you head for the outskirts of the city, to one of the more affluent neighborhoods. You are admitted into a large house by a very excited maid, who hurries you to the master bedroom. There, sitting upright in bed, is a man who appears to be in his late 50s and who is in severe respiratory distress. He is too dyspneic to give you any history, but his wife states that he woke up about half an hour ago complaining of difficulty breathing. He has a history of high blood pressure and had a previous heart attack 8 years ago. On physical examination, he is in extreme distress. He is struggling to breathe, and pink-tinged foam is coming from his mouth. His pulse is strong, and blood pressure is 190/100. You obtain the rhythm strip shown in Figure 20.

1. Examine the patient's rhythm strip:

   a. His rhythm is _____ regular _____ irregular.
   b. The rate is _____ per minute.

2. The ECG pattern is

   a. Sinus tachycardia
   b. Junctional tachycardia
   c. Paroxysmal atrial tachycardia (PAT)
   d. Ventricular tachycardia
   e. Atrial flutter

3. Which of the following is NOT part of the management of this patient?

   a. Administer oxygen at the highest possible concentration.
   b. Keep the patient sitting up with feet dangling.
   c. Start an IV lifeline with D5W.
   d. Administer morphine, 5 to 10 mg by slow IV titration.
   e. Apply rotating tourniquets to the extremities.

4. Nitroglycerin is sometimes used in the emergency treatment of the condition this patient is manifesting. It is used in these circumstances because

   a. It causes peripheral vasodilatation, thereby enabling blood to pool in the peripheral circulation and relieving congestion in the lungs.
   b. It prevents the development of chest pain.
   c. It prevents the development of life-threatening cardiac dysrhythmias.
   d. It raises the blood pressure and thereby promotes better perfusion of the brain.
   e. It slows the pulse and thereby improves cardiac output.

A143

1. The patient's rhythm is **very slightly irregular;** the rate is approximately **110 per minute.**
2. The ECG pattern is **sinus tachycardia** (answer **a**). If you look closely, you will see the P waves poking out of the downstroke of the preceding T wave (the P–R interval is about 0.16 seconds). The presence of these P waves in a fixed, normal relationship to the QRS complexes virtually rules out all of the other possibilities listed.
3. As you have doubtless deduced, our patient is suffering from fulminant pulmonary edema secondary to left heart failure. Rotating tourniquets (answer **e**) are probably not part of the appropriate management of this patient. If you chose to use them, you could not be very severely rebuked, for this matter is somewhat controversial, and rotating tourniquets remain in use in some centers. However, there are little, if any, good data in the medical literature to support their use, and on theoretic grounds at least, there are several reasons to believe that rotating tourniquets could in fact be deleterious—by periodically reintroducing a volume load of stagnant, acidotic blood into the general circulation. Pending definitive studies on the subject, the use of rotating tourniquets will remain a matter of local policy, but in any case, they should never be a substitute for more definitive measures of reducing the volume load on the heart, such as diuretics and even phlebotomy (withdrawing a quantity of blood). Nor should their use distract from basic principles of therapy, such as the administration of oxygen (answer a) and morphine (answer d), the maintenance of the patient in a sitting position with feet dangling (answer b), and the provision of an IV lifeline (answer c).
4. Nitroglycerin is sometimes administered to patients in severe cardiogenic pulmonary edema in an attempt to perform an "internal phlebotomy," i.e., to **cause peripheral vasodilatation and thereby enable blood to pool in the extremities rather than in the lungs** (answer **a**). It is unlikely to prevent the pain of myocardia ischemia if there is significant shunt and hypoxemia in an angina-prone patient (answer b), nor does it have any role in preventing cardiac dysrhythmias (answer c). One may anticipate a drop, not a rise, in blood pressure after nitroglycerin administration (answer d), for nitroglycerin decreases peripheral resistance (Remember? BLOOD PRESSURE = CARDIAC OUTPUT × PERIPHERAL RESISTANCE). And nitroglycerin would not be expected to have any direct effects on the heart rate, one way or the other (answer e).

By now, you might as well forget about the pizza. Your friends at the firehouse probably took care of it for you while you were taking care of our patient.

FURTHER READING

Abrams J. Vasodilator therapy for chronic congestive heart failure. *JAMA* 254:3070, 1985.
Bertel O, Steiner A. Rotating tourniquets do not work in acute congestive heart failure and pulmonary edema. *Lancet* 1:762, 1980.
Cohn JN, Fanciosa JA. Vasodilator therapy of cardiac failure. *N Engl J Med* 279:27, 254, 1977.
Forrester JS, Staniloff HM. Heart failure. *Emerg Med* 16(4):121, 1984.
Francis GS et al. Acute vasoconstrictor response to intravenous furosemide in patients with chronic congestive heart failure. *Ann Intern Med* 103:1, 1985.
Genton R, Jaffe AS. Management of congestive heart failure in patients with acute myocardial infarction. *JAMA* 256:2556, 1986.
Goldberg H, Nakhjavan FK. Pathophysiology, diagnosis, and treatment of heart failure. *Hosp Med* 8(7):8, 1972.
Hoffman JR, Reynolds S. Comparison of nitroglycerin, morphine and furosemide in treatment of presumed prehospital pulmonary edema. *Chest* 92:586, 1987.
Levy DB, Pollard T. Failure of the heart. *Emergency* 20(12):22, 1988.
Marantz PR et al. Clinical diagnosis of congestive heart failure in patients with acute dyspnea. *Chest* 97:776, 1990.
Markiewicz W et al. Sublingual isosorbide dinitrate in severe congestive failure. *Cardiology* 67:172, 1981.
Morgan MT. Rotating tourniquets: A critical evaluation. *STAT* 2(2):63, 1980.
Posner MD. Cardiac failure: Tourniquets vs. phlebotomy (letter). *N Engl J Med* 290:1485, 1974.
Rasanen J et al. Continuous positive airway pressure by face mask in acute cardiogenic pulmonary edema. *Am J Cardiol* 55:296, 1985.
Robin ED, Carroll IC, Zelis R. Pulmonary edema. *N Engl J Med* 288:239, 292. 1972.
Roth A. Are rotating tourniquets useful for left ventricular preload reduction in patients with acute myocardial infarction and heart failure? *Ann Emerg Med* 16:764, 1987.
Tresch DD et al. Out-of-hospital pulmonary edema: Diagnosis and treatment. *Ann Emerg Med* 12:533, 1983.
Vaisanen IT, Rasanen J. Continuous positive airway pressure and supplemental oxygen in the treatment of cardiogenic pulmonary edema. *Chest* 92:481, 1987.
Wulf-Dirk B, Schupp D. Effect of sublingual nitroglycerin in emergency treatment of severe pulmonary edema. *Am J Cardiol* 41:931, 1978.

Two backpackers were tramping through some local woods when one of them was bitten by a large snake. His companion killed the snake and then made his way to a farmhouse a few miles away to phone for help. You reach the farmhouse about 25 minutes after receiving the call and make your way on foot with the victim's companion to the victim.

You find the victim sitting on a rock, looking ruefully at his left calf. He complains of pain around the area where he was bitten and has strange pins-and-needles sensations around his mouth. Beside him is a dead snake, which your partner—who is well versed in such things—immediately identifies as a diamondback rattlesnake.

On physical examination of the patient, the only notable findings are some twitching of the facial muscles and swelling around the area of the bite.

Which of the following measures are indicated in the management of this patient? (There may be more than one correct answer.)

a. Apply a light, wide constricting band to the leg, about 5 inches above the bite, just tight enough to occlude venous circulation.
b. Splint the leg, and do not permit the patient to walk on it.
c. Use the crosscut technique to suction the venom out of the wound.
d. Apply ice compresses to the area of the bite.
e. Bring the dead snake with you to the emergency room.

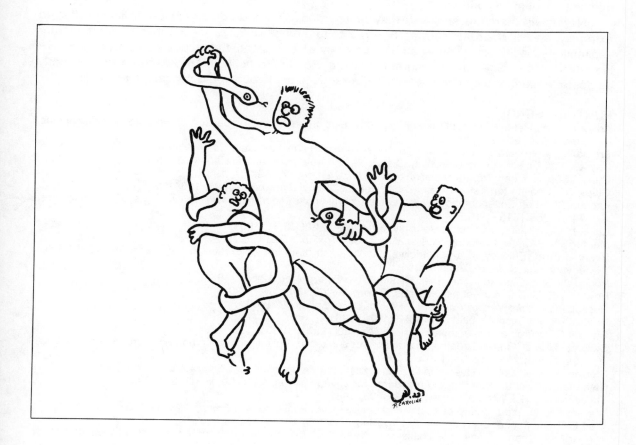

A144

In managing the victim of snakebite you should **splint the patient's leg and not permit him to walk on it** (answer **b**). A bitten extremity should be splinted just as if it were broken, to minimize motion in the extremity that might increase blood flow to the bitten area. For similar reasons, the patient should not be permitted to walk on a bitten leg, so you'll have to carry him back to the farmhouse where you left the ambulance.

If the snake is indeed dead, by all means bring it with you to the emergency room (answer **e**). While your partner may be an expert on snakes (and judging from the patient's symptoms, it appears that your partner's information was correct), it will still be useful for the emergency room staff to make their own definitive identification of the creature. Do make certain that the snake *is* really dead, though, and not just dozing, before you pick it up and toss it in the back of the vehicle with the patient.

None of the other treatments mentioned is indicated for the treatment of snakebites. Constricting bands (answer a), previously recommended as a means of slowing absorption of the snake venom, have not been shown to be effective; and all too often, swelling of a bitten extremity converts a constricting band into an arterial tourniquet and thereby jeopardizes the limb. Incision and suction (answer c) is similarly out of favor. Even proponents of the method agree that incision and suction is unlikely to be of much use if more than 15 to 20 minutes have elapsed since the time of the bite, and—taking into account the time it took the victim's companion to reach the farmhouse, your response time of 25 minutes, and the time it took all of you to get to the victim —considerably more than 15 to 20 minutes have passed since the bite was sustained.

While cooling (answer d) was previously recommended for the treatment of snakebites, that method too is now out of favor. Cooling was not found to be of any benefit, and in many cases it only aggravated the tissue damage. Furthermore, valuable time may be wasted searching for a means to cool the wound.

Nowadays, therefore, snakebite may be regarded as a load-and-go situation: Splint the affected extremity, and hit the road; start an IV en route to the hospital. The most important treatment for snakebite—specific antivenin—can be given only when the patient reaches the hospital, so there is nothing to be gained by tarrying at the scene. Be sure to notify the receiving hospital as early as possible, so that they can start making arrangements to obtain the necessary antivenin.

FURTHER READING

Anker R et al. Retarding the uptake of "mock venom" in humans: Comparison of three first aid techniques. *Med J Aust* 6(5):212, 1982.

Arnold R. Controversies and hazards in the treatment of pit viper bites. *South Med J* 72:909, 1979.

Boyden TW. Snake venom poisoning: Diagnosis and treatment. *Ariz Med* 37:639, 1980.

Curry SC et al. Death from a rattlesnake bite. *Am J Emerg Med* 3:227, 1985.

Glass TG. Cooling for first aid in snakebite (letter). *N Engl J Med* 305:1095, 1981.

Kitchen CS et al. Envenomation by the eastern coral snake (*Micrurus fulvius fulvius*): A study of 39 victims. *JAMA* 258:1615, 1987.

Kunkel DB. Treating snakebites sensibly. *Emerg Med* 20(12):51, 1988.

Mentor SA. Beware: Nonpoisonous snakes. *J Clin Toxicol* 15:259, 1979.

Pearn J et al. Efficacy of a constrictive bandage with limb immobilization in the management of human envenomation. *Med J Aust* 6(6):293, 1981.

Podgorny G. Snakebite in the United States. *Ann Emerg Med* 12:651, 1983.

Powers RD. Taking care of bite wounds. *Emerg Med* 22(13):131, 1990.

Russell FE. *Snake Venom Poisoning*. Philadelphia: Lippincott, 1980.

Russell FE. Rattlesnake bite. *JAMA* 245:1579, 1981.

Russell FE. When a snake strikes. *Emerg Med* 22(12):21, 1990.

Stewart ME et al. First-aid treatment of poisonous snakebite: Are currently recommended procedures justified? *Ann Emerg Med* 10:331, 1980.

Steuven H et al. Cobra envenomation: An uncommon emergency. *Ann Emerg Med* 12:636, 1983.

Sutherland SK et al. New first aid measures for envenomation. *Med J Aust* 1:378, 1980.

Thygerson A. Tick bites. *Emergency* 13(6):26, 1981.

Wasserman G. Wound care of spider and snake envenomations. *Ann Emerg Med* 17:1331, 1988.

Watt CW. Snakebite: Don't cool it. *Emerg Med Serv* 8(3):10, 1979.

Wingert WA, Chan L. Rattlesnake bites in southern California and rationale for recommended treatment. *West J Med* 148:37, 1988.

Winneberger TR et al. Snakebite treatment in the 80's. *NC Med J* 46:572, 1985.

You are called to one of the more run-down sections of town to attend to a "man with a headache." A middle-aged woman greets you at the door of a small, shabby house and tells you that she came this morning to check on her father, who lives here alone, and she found him very ill. You enter and house and find it quite warm and stuffy. You note that someone has recently caulked up all the cracks around the windows and in general tried to weatherproof the place. In the center of the living room, a kerosene stove is lit.

The patient is a man in his 70s complaining of a severe, throbbing headache and dizziness. He appears agitated and confused, and periodically he retches into a basin by the sofa. His skin is warm and flushed. Pulse is 110 and slightly irregular. Blood pressure is 160/100, and respirations are 20. The remainder of the physical examination is unremarkable, but meanwhile you note that you are beginning to have a headache yourself.

Which of the following is NOT part of the management of this patient?

a. Take the patient out of the house immediately.
b. Administer 100% oxygen.
c. Break a few perles of amyl nitrite into a sponge or handkerchief and hold it over the patient's nose for 20 seconds out of each minute.
d. Start an IV with D5W to keep the vein open.
e. Monitor cardiac rhythm.

A145

It's no wonder you got a headache, with all that carbon monoxide around. Our patient caulked up his house to keep winter out, but in the process, he also succeeded in keeping the products of combustion from his kerosene stove nicely locked in. Now he is suffering the consequences, and he presents a characteristic picture of carbon monoxide poisoning. Headache, confusion, irritability, dizziness, nausea, and vomiting—all of these may be symptoms of carbon monoxide intoxication. The cherry red color of the skin, while classic, is not always present.

The use of amyl nitrite (answer **c**) is NOT part of the management of this patient. Amyl nitrite is administered in cases of cyanide poisoning, not for carbon monoxide intoxication, and although the clinical presentations of those two poisonings may have certain features in common, there is nothing in this patient's history or environment to suggest that he is the victim of cyanide exposure.

The first principle of therapy in carbon monoxide poisoning is to remove the patient from the exposure environment (answer a). He should also receive 100% oxygen at the first possible moment (answer b), for he is suffering from asphyxiation at the cellular level, owing to the fact that carbon monoxide has a 200 times greater affinity for hemoglobin than oxygen has. Thus even small concentrations of inhaled carbon monoxide rapidly displace oxygen from the hemoglobin molecules, thereby interfering with the transport of oxygen from the lungs to the peripheral tissues.

An IV lifeline should be placed in the event that life-threatening cardiac dysrhythmias arise secondary to tissue hypoxia (answer d). The patient's pulse is already somewhat irregular, and one must assume that the myocardium isn't very happy about the fact that the red cells are trying to foist carbon monoxide upon it in place of oxygen. An unhappy myocardium can very quickly become an irritable myocardium, and cardiac monitoring is thus strongly indicated (answer e).

FURTHER READING

Barret L et al. Carbon monoxide poisoning: A diagnosis frequently overlooked. *J Toxicol* 23:309, 1985.

Boutros AR, Hoyt JL. Management of carbon monoxide poisoning in the absence of a hyperbaric oxygen chamber. *Crit Care Med* 4:114, 1976.

Burney RE, Wu S, Nemiroff MJ. Mass carbon monoxide poisoning: Clinical effects and results of treatment in 184 victims. *Ann Emerg Med* 11:394, 1982.

Caplan YH et al. Accidental poisonings involving carbon monoxide, heating systems, and confined spaces. *J Forensic Sci* 31:117, 1986.

Dan BB. The twilight zone: Death on a Sunday morning (editorial). *JAMA* 261:1188, 1989.

Done AK. Carbon monoxide: The silent summons. *Emerg Med* 5(2):268, 1973.

Finck PA. Exposure to carbon monoxide: Review of the literature and 567 autopsies. *Milit Med* 131:1513, 1966.

Ginsberg MD. Carbon monoxide intoxication: Clinical features, neuropathology and mechanisms of injury. *J Toxicol* 23:281, 1985.

Heckerling PS. Occult carbon monoxide poisoning: A cause of winter headache. *Am J Emerg Med* 5:201, 1987.

Heckerling PS et al. Predictors of occult carbon monoxide poisoning in patients with headache and dizziness. *Ann Intern Med* 107:174, 1987.

Jackson DL. Accidental carbon monoxide poisoning. *JAMA* 243:772, 1980.

Kirkpatrick JN. Occult carbon monoxide poisoning. *West J Med* 146:52, 1987.

Levy DB. A breath of dead air. *Emergency* 20(11):18, 1988.

Manoguerra AS. Carbon monoxide poisoning. *Emergency* 12(1):29, 1980.

Myers RAM, Linberg SE, Cowley RA. Carbon monoxide poisoning: The injury and its treatment. *JACEP* 8:479, 1979.

Myers RAM, Snyder SK, Emhoff TA. Subacute sequelae of carbon monoxide poisoning. *Ann Emerg Med* 14:1163, 1985.

Norkool DM, Kirkpatrick JN. Treatment of acute carbon monoxide poisoning with hyperbaric oxygen: A review of 115 cases. *Ann Emerg Med* 14:1168, 1985.

Olson KR. Carbon monoxide poisoning: Mechanisms, presentation, and controversies in management. *J Emerg Med* 1:233, 1984.

Poisoning without warning: The silent perils of carbon monoxide. *Emerg Med* 22(14):20, 1990.

Wharton M et al. Fatal carbon monoxide poisoning at a motel. *JAMA* 261:1177, 1989.

Zarem HA, Rattenborg CC, Harmel MH. Carbon monoxide toxicity in human fire victims. *Arch Surg* 107:851, 1973.

You are called to a nearby winter resort to join the search for a 48-year-old skier who was lost during a heavy snowstorm 2 days before. By the time you reach the resort, a search party has located the skier and is just bringing him by toboggan back to the main lodge. The head of the search party states that at the time they found the patient, about 30 minutes ago, he was unconscious and had a very weak pulse.

On examination, you find an unconscious man, apneic and pulseless. You immediately begin artificial ventilation and external cardiac compressions, while your partner attaches the monitor leads. The monitor shows that the patient is in ventricular fibrillation.

Which of the following statements about this patient and his care is NOT true?

a. If the patient has been in cardiac arrest for more than 10 minutes, there is no hope for him to regain neurologic function.

b. Defibrillation attempts are unlikely to be successful until the patient has been rewarmed, and basic life support should continue until that time.

c. One should not waste time in the field with advanced life support measures but rather should transport the patient rapidly to the hospital, with CPR continuing during transport.

d. One must be careful not to hyperventilate such a patient, since a drop in his arterial PCO_2 to levels below normal may have adverse effects on the brain.

A146

Statement **a** is NOT true. When a patient suffers cardiac arrest from cold exposure, all bets are off regarding the "magic time limit" for full neurologic recovery. The same low temperatures that put the heart into fibrillation may confer significant protection upon the brain and permit it to survive for considerable periods with inadequate or even absent perfusion. Moral: DON'T GIVE UP ON THE HYPOTHERMIC CARDIAC ARREST! Even though the patient may have been pulseless for some time and may look very dead indeed—cold, rigid, apneic, areflexic—one must assume that there is an excellent chance for full recovery and continue resuscitation efforts at least until full rewarming has been accomplished.

Stabilization in the field is an impractical goal in cases of hypothermia. Defibrillation attempts are unlikely to meet with success until the patient has been rewarmed (answer b), and the time spent searching for a vein in a cold arm will simply delay definitive therapy in the hospital. Thus one should not waste time with advanced life support measures but rather should transport the patient rapidly to the hospital, continuing CPR en route (answer c).

Extremes of hyperventilation should be avoided in a patient with possible ischemic brain injury, for a fall in arterial PCO_2 levels significantly below normal may result in a decrease in cerebral blood flow (answer d). The goal is to maintain the PCO_2 in the low normal range, best accomplished in the field by slow, steady artificial ventilation at a physiologic rate. Don't forget that our frozen patient isn't producing as much CO_2 as a normothermic individual, for his metabolic rate is considerably slower. A rate of artificial ventilation of about 8–10 inflations/min should be sufficient.

FURTHER READING

Arnold JW, Eichenberger CH. The hydraulic sarong: Emergency treatment device for accidental hypothermia. *JACEP* 4:438, 1975.

Avery WM. Hypothermia: The silent killer. *Emerg Med Serv* 8(1):26, 1979.

Bangs CC. Immersion hypothermia. *Emergency* 12(1):43, 1980.

Bangs CC. Caught in the cold. *Emerg Med* 15(21):29, 1982.

Besdine RW. Accidental hypothermia: The body's energy crisis. *Geriatrics* 34:51, 1979.

Danzl DF et al. Multicenter hypothermia study. *Ann Emerg Med* 16:1042, 1987.

DaVee TS et al. Extreme hypothermia and ventricular fibrillation. *Ann Emerg Med* 9:100, 1980.

Donner HJ. Out in the cold. *Emerg Med* 17(21):21, 1985.

Fergusson NV. Urban hypothermia. *Anaesthesia* 40:651, 1985.

Fishbeck KH, Simon RP. Neurological manifestations of accidental hypothermia. *Ann Neurol* 10:384, 1981.

Fitzgerald FT. Hypoglycemia and accidental hypothermia in an alcoholic population. *West J Med* 133:105, 1980.

Forgey WW. *Death by Exposure: Hypothermia*. Merrillville, IN: ICS Books, 1985.

Harnett RM, Pruitt JR, Sias FR. A review of the literature concerning resuscitation from hypothermia: Part I. The problem and general approaches. *Aviat Space Environ Med* 24:106, 1982.

Lathrap TG. *Hypothermia: Killer of the Unprepared*. Portland, OR: Mazamas, 1975.

Leavitt M, Podgorny G. Prehospital CPR and the pulseless hypothermic patient. *Ann Emerg Med* 13:492, 1984.

Ledingham I, Mone J. Treatment of accidental hypothermia: A prospective study. *Br Med J* 280:1102, 1980.

McClean D, Emslie-Smith D. *Accidental Hypothermia*. Philadelphia: Lippincott, 1977.

Miller JW, Danzl D, Thomas DM. Urban accidental hypothermia: 135 cases. *Ann Emerg Med* 9:456, 1980.

Mills WJ. Out in the cold. *Emerg Med* 8(1):134, 1976.

Moss JF et al. A model for the treatment of accidental severe hypothermia. *J Trauma* 26:68, 1986.

O'Keefe KM. Accidental hypothermia: A review of 62 cases. *JACEP* 6:491, 1977.

Osborne L et al. Survival after prolonged cardiac arrest and accidental hypothermia. *Br Med J* 289:881, 1984.

Romet TT, Hoskin RW. Temperature and metabolic responses to inhalation and bath rewarming protocols. *Aviat Space Environ Med* 59:630, 1988.

Sherman FT et al. Hypothermia detection in emergency departments: How low does your thermometer go? *NY State J Med* 82:374, 1982.

Siebke H et al. Survival after 40 minutes submersion without cerebral sequelae. *Lancet* 1:1275, 1975.

Southwick FS, Dalglish PH. Recovery after prolonged asystolic cardiac arrest in profound hypothermia. *JAMA* 243:1250, 1980.

Steinemann S, et al. Implications of admission hypothermia in trauma patients. *J Trauma* 30:200, 1990.

Steinman AM. Immersion hypothermia. *Emerg Med Serv* 6(4):22, 1977.

Stine RJ. Accidental hypothermia. *JACEP* 6:413, 1977.

Tacker WA et al. Transchest defibrillation under conditions of hypothermia. *Crit Care Med* 9:390, 1981.

Webb JQ. Cold to the core: Treating the hypothermic patient. *JEMS* 14(2):30, 1989.

Weyman AE et al. Accidental hypothermia in an alcoholic population. *Am J Med* 56:13, 1974.

White JD. Hypothermia: The Bellevue experience. *Ann Emerg Med* 11:417, 1982.

Wilkerson JA (ed.). *Hypothermia, Frostbite, and Other Cold Injuries*. Seattle: Mountaineers, 1986.

Zachary L et al. Accidental hypothermia treated with rapid rewarming by immersion. *Ann Plast Surg* 9:238, 1982.

Zell SC, Kurtz KJ. Severe exposure hypothermia: A resuscitation protocol. *Ann Emerg Med* 14:339, 1985.

A call comes in late at night about a "sick child" in a nearby housing project. When you arrive, a very distraught mother tells you that her 6-year-old son has been "having fits." He has been ill today with an upper respiratory infection and a high fever, and about half an hour ago he began having seizures. He has had three seizures so far. The mother didn't notice how they started.

You find the child apparently asleep on his bed. He is difficult to arouse. As you are examining him, his eyes suddenly open and deviate sharply to the right, and he rapidly develops another grand mal seizure.

Which of the following would NOT be part of the management of this child?

a. Administer oxygen at high concentration.
b. Start an IV line.
c. Wedge a bite-block between the child's teeth to prevent him from biting his tongue.
d. Administer 25% dextrose IV, 1 ml per kilogram.
e. Administer diazepam (Valium), 0.3 mg per kilogram IV.

A147

Once a patient has clamped his teeth together in the course of a seizure, attempts to jam a bite-block or any other object between the teeth are probably futile and may lead to significant damage to the teeth. Thus, answer **c** is NOT part of the treatment of this child.

Status epilepticus, i.e., repeated seizures occurring without a lucid interval in between, is a dire medical emergency and requires urgent treatment. Death occurs from hypoxemia, and for that reason the administration of oxygen has the highest priority (answer a). An IV line should be established as a route for medications (answer b), and 25% dextrose (answer d)—prepared by diluting 50% dextrose 1 : 1 in saline—should be among the first medications given. In the event that the seizures are due to hypoglycemia, the administration of dextrose will provide definitive treatment. Once an adequate airway and good oxygenation have been established, a medication like diazepam (Valium) may be given in an attempt to terminate the seizure activity (answer e).

FURTHER READING

Albano A, Reisdorff EJ, Wiegenstein JG. Rectal diazepam in pediatric status epilepticus. *Am J Emerg Med* 70:168, 1989.

Berg AT et al. Predictors of recurrent febrile seizures: A metaanalytic review. *J Pediatr* 116:329, 1990.

Camfield PR. Treatment of status epilepticus in children. *Can Med Assoc J* 128:671, 1983.

Drawbaugh RE, Deibler CG, Eitel DR. Prehospital administration of rectal diazepam in pediatric status epilepticus. *Prehosp Disaster Med* 5(2):155, 1990.

Freeman JM. Febrile seizures: A consensus of their significance, evaluation, and treatment. *Pediatrics* 66:1009, 1980.

Gabor AJ. Lorazepam versus phenobarbital: Candidates for drug of choice for treatment of status epilepticus. *J Epilepsy* 3:3, 1990.

Glass BA. To sponge or not to sponge (letter). *Ann Emerg Med* 16:607, 1987.

Knudsen FU. Effective short-term diazepam prophylaxis in febrile convulsions. *J Pediatr* 106:487, 1985.

Knudsen RU. Rectal administration of diazepam in solution in the acute treatment of convulsions in infants and children. *Arch Dis Child* 54:855, 1979.

Lacey DJ et al. Lorazepam therapy of status epilepticus in children and adolescents. *J Pediatr* 108:771, 1986.

Mitchell WG et al. Lorazepam is the treatment of choice for status epilepticus. *J Epilepsy* 3:7, 1990.

Newman J. Evaluation of sponging to reduce body temperature in febrile children. *Can Med Assoc J* 132:641, 1985.

Oppenheimer EY et al. Seizures in childhood: An approach to emergency management. *Pediatr Clin North Am* 26:837, 1979.

Rothner AD et al. Status epilepticus. *Pediatr Clin North Am* 27:593, 1980.

Sonander H et al. Effects of the rectal administration of diazepam. *Br J Anaesth* 5:578, 1985.

Tomlanovich MC, Rosen P, Mendelsohn J. Simple febrile convulsions. *JACEP* 5:347, 1976.

Vining EPG et al. Status epilepticus. *Pediatr Ann* 14:764, 1985.

Volpe JJ. Management of neonatal seizures. *Crit Care Med* 5:43, 1977.

1. A 22-year-old woman complains of profuse vaginal bleeding. She says she has used "hundreds" of sanitary napkins during the past 2 days. She denies any pain. She denies the possibility that she might be pregnant. She uses the "loop" for contraception. Her present bleeding has come at the usual time for her period, but it is much heavier than usual.

   On physical examination, she is anxious but in no acute distress. Pulse is 80 and regular and does not change when you raise her from a supine to a sitting position. Blood pressure is 130/70. You may conclude that

   a. The patient should be transported immediately to the hospital for blood transfusion.
   b. The patient's account of the extent of her bleeding may be somewhat exaggerated.
   c. The patient is suffering from an ectopic pregnancy.
   d. You should immediately start two IVs with normal saline and run in fluid as rapidly as possible.

2. Later the same day, a woman in her third trimester of pregnancy calls for an ambulance because of vaginal bleeding. She states that the bleeding started 2 hours earlier, and she has already soaked through 12 sanitary napkins. You find her pale, with clammy skin. Pulse is 120, rising to 140 when she sits up. Blood pressure is 80/60.

   Which of the following is NOT part of her management?

   a. Start an IV line with normal saline solution.
   b. Keep the patient flat, lying on her side.
   c. Pack the vagina with sterile dressings.
   d. Administer oxygen.
   e. Apply military antishock trousers and inflate the leg sections.

A148

1. The young lady who has gone through so many boxes of sanitary napkins has probably overestimated the extent of her bleeding (answer **b**), for your physical examination does not provide any evidence of significant hemorrhage. Her pulse is slow and steady, without postural changes.

   She does need to be evaluated for her problem, but precipitous transportation to the hospital for a blood transfusion is wholly unnecessary (answer a), as is massive fluid therapy (answer d). There is no evidence in the patient's history or physical examination for ectopic pregnancy (answer c), which usually presents as abdominal pain.

2. Our pregnant lady, on the other hand, has not exaggerated the extent of her bleeding. She is in shock, and she needs all the usual measures for that condition. One should NOT, however, insert *anything,* including sterile packs, into the vagina of a patient with third trimester bleeding (answer **c**). One must assume that this woman is suffering from abruptio placenta or placenta previa until proved otherwise, and the blind insertion of packs or anything else into the vagina may simply convert her slow, steady bleeding into rapid exsanguination. Administer oxygen (answer d); keep her flat, on her side (answer b); and apply the leg sections of the MAST (answer e). Start at least one IV with a large-bore cannula and normal saline (answer a) and run it wide open. And get her to the hospital promptly. Meanwhile, notify the emergency room that you are on your way so an obstetric team can be summoned.

FURTHER READING

Barber JM. EMT checkpoint: Early detection of hypovolemic states. *EMT J* 2(2):72, 1978.

Bennet BR. Shock: An approach to teaching EMTs normal physiology before pathophysiology. *EMT J* 2(1):41, 1978.

Boulton FE et al. Obstetric haemorrhage: Causes and management. *Clin Haem* 14:683, 1985.

Celebrezze EM. Third trimester predelivery hemorrhage. *Emergency* 13(10):48, 1981.

Nixon RG. Third trimester obstetric complications. Part I: Antepartum hemorrhage and fetal distress. *Emerg Med Serv* 10(3):53, 1981.

Wilson RF. Science and shock: A clinical perspective. *Ann Emerg Med* 14:714, 1985.

The call comes in as "difficulty breathing," and you and your crew rocket off to an apartment building on the east side of town. Awaiting you at the doorway is a harried young man, who explains that his roommate is very sick. He escorts you to the apartment, on the third floor, and on the way he explains that his roommate is known to suffer from AIDS and now seems to have pneumonia.

1. Armed with this information, you should:

    a. call for another ambulance to handle the case, and instruct the crew to remove all equipment from the vehicle before responding.
    b. explain politely to the roommate that your ambulance service does not transport AIDS patients, lest the infection spread to the ambulance crew and other patients.
    c. treat the case as any other, but exercise special caution in disposing of needles and the patient's bodily secretions.
    d. don surgical cap, gown, gloves, and mask before entering the patient's apartment.
    e. get the hell out of there as fast as possible.

2. Which of the following is *NOT* known to be a mode of transmission of AIDS?

    a. contaminated needles
    b. casual contact
    c. sexual intercourse
    d. placental transfer from infected mother to fetus
    e. contaminated blood products

A149

1. When called to see a patient with AIDS, you should **treat the case as any other, but exercise special caution in disposing of needles and the patient's bodily secretions** (answer c). When a person enters the medical profession—as a physician, nurse, paramedic, EMT, or whatever—that person accepts an obligation to care for the sick and injured, whatever their circumstances, whatever their affliction. To refuse to give medical service to *any* patient is not consistent with that obligation. Furthermore, medical professionals should be sufficiently knowledgeable about illnesses such as AIDS that they do not succumb to the hysteria that may be prevalent among the lay community. EMTs and paramedics who are well-informed about AIDS should know that proper precautions with needles and the patient's bodily secretions will virtually eliminate any possibility of disease transmission. There is no need to get decked out like a surgeon just to examine an AIDS patient (answer d), for that get-up will only impose a psychologic barrier between you and the patient. (If you want to wear a surgical mask to protect the immunologically compromised *patient* from germs *you* might be harboring, that is another matter; but if you do so, explain the reasons for the surgical mask to the patient.) Nor is there any need to empty the ambulance of equipment before placing the patient inside (answer a). Routine airing and cleaning procedures after the case, with disposal of the patient's secretions and soiled bedding in properly labelled biohazard containers, is sufficient. Needless to say, any form of refusal to see or transport the patient (answers b and e) is entirely unacceptable.

2. **Casual contact** (answer b) is not known to have any role in spreading the disease AIDS. Even people living in intimate daily contact with AIDS patients, such as members of their families sharing the same household, have not become infected unless they had sexual intercourse with the patient. Similarly, there have been no reported cases of hospital workers acquiring AIDS after treating AIDS patients except in instances where the hospital worker was accidently stuck with a needle that had been used for an AIDS patient. The message is clear: An ambulance crew exercising sensible precautions need have nothing to fear from transporting a patient with AIDS.

FURTHER READING

AIDS—on the front line. *Emerg Med* 18(1):24, 1986.

American College of Emergency Physicians. AIDS: Statement of principles and interim recommendations for emergency department personnel and prehospital care providers. *Ann Emerg Med* 17:1249, 1988.

Baker J. What is the occupational risk to emergency care providers from the human immunodeficiency virus? *Ann Emerg Med* 17:700, 1988.

Burrow GN. Caring for AIDS patients: The physician's risk and responsibility. *Can Med Assoc J* 129:1911, 1983.

Centers for Disease Control. Recommendations for prevention of HIV transmission in health-care settings. *JAMA* 258:1293, 1987.

Centers for Disease Control. Update: Human immunodeficiency virus infections in health-care workers exposed to blood of infected patients. *MMWR* 36:285, 1987.

Centers for Disease Control. First 100,000 cases of acquired immunodeficiency syndrome—United States. *JAMA* 262:1453, 1989.

Cueva KG. The AIDS factor. *Emergency* 21(1):48, 1989.

Curran JW et al. Acquired immunodeficiency syndrome (AIDS) associated with transfusions. *N Engl J Med* 310:69, 1984.

Friedland G. AIDS and compassion. *JAMA* 259:2898, 1988.

Gerbert B et al. Why fear persists: Health care professionals and AIDS. *JAMA* 260:3481, 1988.

Hahn RA et al. Prevalence of HIV infection among intravenous drug users in the United States. *JAMA* 261:2677, 1989.

Hardy AM et al. The incidence rate of acquired immunodeficiency syndrome in selected populations. *JAMA* 253:215, 1985.

Henderson DK et al. Prophylactic zidovudine after occupational exposure to the human immunodeficiency virus: An interim analysis. *J Infect Dis* 160:321, 1989.

Kelen GD. Human immunodeficiency virus and the emergency department: Risks and risk protection for health care providers. *Ann Emerg Med* 19:242, 1990.

Landesman SH et al. The AIDS epidemic. *N Engl J Med* 31:521, 1985.

Lemp GF et al. Survival trends for patients with AIDS. *JAMA* 263:402, 1990.

Marcus R et al. Surveillance of health care workers exposed to blood from patients infected with the human immunodeficiency virus. *N Engl J Med* 319:1118, 1988.

Nordberg M. AIDS/infection control: Critical issues for EMS. *Emerg Med Serv* 17(10):35, 1988.

Ornato JP. Providing CPR and emergency care during the AIDS epidemic. *Emerg Med Serv* 18(4):45, 1989.

Quinn T. The epidemiology of the human immunodeficiency virus. *Ann Emerg Med* 19:225, 1990.

Redfield R et al. Frequent transmission of HTLV-III among spouses of patients with AIDS-related complex and AIDS. *JAMA* 253:1571, 1985.

Rosen MJ. Acute pulmonary manifestations of AIDS. *Emerg Med* 22(1):67, 1990.

Sande MA. Transmission of AIDS: The case against casual contagion. *N Engl J Med* 314:380, 1986.

Skeen WF. Acquired immunodeficiency syndrome and the emergency physician. *Ann Emerg Med* 14:267, 1985.

Soderstrom CA et al. HIV infection rates in a trauma center treating predominantly rural blunt trauma victims. *J Trauma* 29:1526, 1989.

It's the worst kind of call: a child struck by a car. You arrive in a suburban neighborhood to find a 3-year-old boy lying in the street surrounded by a crowd of agitated bystanders. While your partner tries to deal with the loud demands that you "hurry up and get the poor kid to the hospital," you examine the boy. He is conscious but listless, and you find it odd that he isn't crying. His skin is cold, pale, and mottled. Vital signs are pulse 140, BP 90/60, and respirations 40 and shallow. There is a bruise on his forehead. Pupils are equal and reactive. The chest is stable. There are bruises on the abdomen, which looks somewhat distended (you can't adequately listen for bowel sounds because of all the noise around you). The child can move all his extremities.

For each of the following statements regarding the management of this child, indicate whether the statement is true or false.

1. Since the child's blood pressure is relatively normal for his age, it is unlikely that he has had much internal bleeding.

   TRUE   FALSE

2. A child is more likely than an adult to suffer injury to the liver and spleen after blunt abdominal trauma.

   TRUE   FALSE

3. The intravenous fluid of choice for this child is normal saline.

   TRUE   FALSE

4. If you apply a pediatric MAST to the child, you should inflate the leg sections only.

   TRUE   FALSE

5. The child should be immobilized on a backboard before he is moved.

   TRUE   FALSE

A150

1. Since the child's blood pressure is relatively normal for his age, it is unlikely that he has had much internal bleeding.

   FALSE! A child's blood vessels are capable of extreme vasoconstriction (which is evident in this case in the boy's cold, pale, and mottled skin), so a fall in blood pressure may not be evident until a child has lost a quarter of his blood volume—and you don't want to wait that long before you start treatment for shock. You need to be alert to more subtle signs of shock in a child, and this boy has several: the skin already mentioned, listless behavior, tachycardia (what is a normal pulse rate for a 3-year-old? do you remember?), and tachypnea.

2. A child is more likely than an adult to suffer injury to the liver and spleen after blunt abdominal trauma.

   TRUE. First of all, a child has less padding to absorb a blow. Furthermore, his diaphragm is lower than an adult's, and his abdominal organs are relatively larger. So all told, the child's belly is much more vulnerable to injury than the adult's, and the highly vascular liver and spleen are the most likely abdominal organs to be injured.

3. The intravenous fluid of choice for this child is normal saline.

   FALSE. The kidneys of infants and small children aren't as efficient as those of adults in handling sodium. So although a child in shock needs volume, he does not need the kind of salt load you would give an adult. D5W or D5/0.25 NS is the preferred resuscitation fluid for small children in shock.

4. If you apply a pediatric MAST to the child, you should inflate the leg sections only.

   TRUE. Inflation of the abdominal segment of the MAST compresses the abdominal contents against the child's diaphragm, so that the diaphragm is forced up into the chest cavity and therefore interferes with ventilation. Many experts advise against using the MAST at all in children.

5. The child should be immobilized on a backboard before he is moved.

   TRUE! Any severely injured child, but especially a child with evidence of head injury (this boy has a bruise on his forehead) should be assumed to have a spine injury and should be immobilized accordingly. Granted, in this situation, with the crowd clamoring for you to move on to the hospital, you will be sorely tempted to skip the backboard. Overcome the temptation. Immobilize the child rapidly and efficiently on a pediatric backboard, and *then* move promptly to the hospital.

FURTHER READING

Apple JS et al. Cervical spine fractures and dislocations in children. *Pediatr Radiol* 17:45, 1987.
Berger LR. Childhood injuries. *Public Health Rep* 100:572, 1985.
Bonadio WA, Hellmich T. Post-traumatic pulmonary contusion in children. *Ann Emerg Med* 18:1050, 1989.
Centers for Disease Control. Fatal injuries to children—United States, 1986. *MMWR* 39:442, 1990.
Frame SB, Hendrickson MF. Problem: Pediatric cervical-spine injuries. *Emerg Med* 19(19):47, 1987.
Gratz RR. Accidental injury in childhood: A literature review on pediatric trauma. *J Trauma* 19:551, 1979.
Hadley MN et al. Pediatric spinal trauma: Review of 122 cases of spinal cord and vertebral column injuries. *J Neurosurg* 68:18, 1988.
Herzenberg JE et al. Emergency transport and positioning of young children who have an injury of the cervical spine: The standard backboard may be hazardous. *J Bone Joint Surg [Am]* 71-A:15, 1989.
Huerta C, Griffith R, Joyce SM. Cervical spine stabilization in pediatric patients: Evaluation of current techniques. *Ann Emerg Med* 16:1121, 1987.
Kaufmann CR et al. Evaluation of the pediatric trauma score. *JAMA* 263:69, 1990.
Mathewson JW. Shock in infants and children. *J Fam Pract* 10:695, 1980.
McKoy C et al. Preventable traumatic deaths in children. *J Pediatr Surg* 18:505, 1983.
Myer CM. Damaged little heads and necks. *Emerg Med* 19(4):89, 1987.
Ordog GJ. Gunshot wounds in children under 10 years of age: A new epidemic. *Am J Dis Child* 142:618, 1988.
Pediatric trauma: Every minute counts. *Emerg Med* 19(11):93, 1987.
Ramenofsky ML et al. Maximum survival in pediatric trauma: The ideal system. *J Trauma* 24:818, 1984.
Rivara FP et al. Injuries to children younger than 1 year of age. *Pediatrics* 81:93, 1988.
Ruge JR et al. Pediatric spinal injury: The very young. *J Neurosurg* 68:25, 1988.
Throckmorton K, Throckmorton DW, Knight P. Number one killer. *Emergency* 20(5):20, 1988.
Wheatley J et al. Traumatic deaths in children: The importance of prevention. *Med J Aust* 150:72, 1989.
Ziegler MM. Trauma at an early age: A blow below the belt. *Emerg Med* 17(3):65, 1985.

At 1:23 A.M. on a Saturday, an explosion blasts open Reactor No. 4 at the local nuclear power station. The regional disaster plan is put into operation, and your ambulance unit is assigned to evacuating patients from the community hospital, which is situated four miles from the reactor, to another hospital 30 miles away.

1. Given the location of the community hospital, the principal danger to you and your patients will be from:

   a. alpha and beta particles carried by dust and smoke
   b. gamma rays emitted from the reactor
   c. x-rays emitted from the reactor
   d. flying debris

2. List three precautions you can take to protect yourself against that danger.

3. Those patients still awaiting evacuation would be best moved temporarily to:

   a. an area outdoors
   b. well-ventilated rooms of the hospital
   c. private homes in the neighborhood
   d. the hospital basement
   e. the reactor site

A151

1. Given the location of the community hospital, the principal danger to you and your patients will be from **alpha and beta particles carried by dust and smoke** (answer a). At a distance of four miles, gamma emissions from the reactor (answers b and c—x-rays and gamma rays are, for practical purposes, the same thing) would be negligible, and one would not expect debris (answer d) to be sailing around four miles from the explosion site either.

2. The principal methods for reducing exposure to radioactive emissions are TIME, DISTANCE, and SHIELDING:

   a. Minimize the *duration* of exposure by remaining at the exposure site for the shortest time necessary; work in shifts with other emergency personnel so that no one person has to stay in the exposure area for a long period.

   b. Put the maximum practical *distance* between yourself and the exposure area (that's why you're evacuating those patients to a more distant hospital). Needless to say, you want to head *upwind* from the accident, and the hospital to which the patients are being evacuated should have been selected on that basis.

   c. *Shield* yourself and your patient from radioactive emissions. Since the radioactivity you have to worry about in this instance comes in the form of alpha and beta particles, this means taking all possible measures to avoid ingestion, inhalation, and skin contact with these particles:

      (1) Do not eat, drink, or smoke in the exposure area.
      (2) Wear a surgical hood and mask.
      (3) Don protective clothing. If you have none, put on an extra layer of clothes. Button your shirt all the way up, and turn the collar up. Tape your shirt cuffs and pant legs closed. Tape over buttonholes and other openings in your clothing.
      (4) Wear a radiation dosimeter badge, so that your exposure can be assessed.
      (5) Stay sheltered as much as possible. Bring the ambulance right up to the ambulance bay and transfer the patients quickly into the vehicle. Don't stand around outside!
      (6) Follow the instructions of the radiation safety officer on the scene.

3. Those patients still awaiting evacuation would be best moved to **the hospital basement** (answer **d**). Earth affords good shielding, so a basement shelter is preferable to a structure above ground. Exposure to radioactive dust, steam, and smoke should, in any case, be kept to a minimum, which means staying indoors and as far as possible from the reactor site. Thus answers a, b, c, and e are all inappropriate, since all of them cause the patients greater radiation exposure.

The accident described in this question is not fictitious. At 1:23 A.M. on Saturday, April 26, 1986, an explosion ripped through Reactor No. 4 at the Chernobyl nuclear power station 130 km north of Kiev, in the Ukraine.

FURTHER READING

Adelstein SJ. Uncertainty and relative risks of radiation exposure. *JAMA* 258:655, 1987.
Beane MJ et al. Radiation primer. *EMT J* 5(4):260, 1981.
Becker DV. Reactor accidents: Public health strategies and their medical implications. *JAMA* 258:649, 1987.
Deluca SA et al. Radiation exposure in diagnostic studies. *Am Fam Physician* 36:101, 1987.
English WE. Radioactive contamination. *Emergency* 14(1):43, 1982.
Fabrikant JI. Health effects of the nuclear accident at Three Mile Island. *Health Phys* 40:151, 1981.
Gale RP. Immediate medical consequences of nuclear accidents: Lessons from Chernobyl. *JAMA* 258:625, 1987.
Geiger HJ. The accident at Chernobyl and the medical response. *JAMA* 256:609, 1986.
Goldstein HA. Radiation accidents and injuries. *Emerg Med* 14(15):195, 1982.
Huebner KF. Decontamination procedures and risks to health care personnel. *Bull NY Acad Med* 59:1119, 1983.
In the shadow. *Emerg Med* 19(2):68, 1987.
Keller PD. A clinical syndrome following exposure to atomic bomb explosions. *JAMA* 131:504, 1946.
Ketchum LE. Lesson of Chernobyl: Health consequences of radiation released and hysteria unleashed. *J Nucl Med* 28:413, 1987.
Leaning-Link J. Emergency response to nuclear accident and attack. *Disaster Med* 1:386, 1983.
Leonard RB, Ricks RC. Emergency department radiation accident protocol. *Ann Emerg Med* 9:462, 1980.
Linnemann RE. Soviet medical response to the Chernobyl nuclear accident. *JAMA* 258:637, 1987.
Loken MK. Physicians' obligations in radiation issues. *JAMA* 258:673, 1987.

Lushbaugh CC, Huebner KF, Ricks RC. Medical aspects of nuclear radiation emergencies. *Emergency* 10(10):32, 1978.

MacLeod GK. Some public health lessons from Three Mile Island: A case study in chaos. *AMBIO* 10:18, 1981.

MacLeod GK. The Three Mile Island (TMI) accident. *Disaster Med* 1:399, 1983.

MacLeod GK, Hendee WR, Schwarz MR. Radiation accidents and the role of the physician: A post-Chernobyl perspective. *JAMA* 256:632, 1986.

Merz B. Physicians' reaction to Chernobyl explosion: Lessons in radiation—and cooperation. *JAMA* 256:559, 1986.

Merz B. REAC/TS handles "hot topics." *JAMA* 256:569, 1986.

Messerschmidt O. Combined radiation injuries and medical injuries. *Disaster Med* 1:398, 1983.

Mettler FA. Emergency management of radiation accidents. *JACEP* 7:302, 1978.

Mettler FA, Rocco FG, Junkins RL. The role of EMTs in radiation accidents. *Emerg Med Serv* 6(4):22, 1977.

Miller KL, Demuth WE. Handling radiation emergencies: No need for fear. *J Emerg Nursing* 9:141, 1983.

Milroy WC. Management of irradiated and contaminated casualty victims. *Emerg Clin North Am* 2:667, 1984.

Reid D. The Three Mile Island nuclear accident: Revisited. *Disaster Med* 1:402, 1983.

Richter LL et al. A systems approach to the management of radiation accidents. *Ann Emerg Med* 9:303, 1980.

Ricks RC. Radiation response. *Emergency* 21(2):28, 1989.

Trott KR. Nuclear power plant disasters: Health consequences and need for subsequent medical care. *Lancet* 2:32, 1981.

REAC/TS (the Radiation Emergency Assistance Center/Training Site) in Oak Ridge, Tennessee, has produced a 25-minute film, available on videotape, and an accompanying training manual, *Prehospital Management of Radiation Accidents*, available for $75. For information, contact Office of Information Services, Oak Ridge Associated Universities, PO Box 117, Oak Ridge, TN 37831-0117.

It's nearly midnight on a Saturday when you get a call to a well-to-do suburban neighborhood for a man having a seizure. You arrive to find a party in full swing at the address in question, most of the participants appearing to be in their late twenties and early thirties. The host asks you to please come in through the back door, so you oblige and go around to the rear of the house. From there, you're escorted to a downstairs bedroom, where a man of about 30 is having a grand mal seizure on the floor. The embarrassed host mumbles something to you about "he was just freebasing some gold dust, and suddenly he had a fit." The seizure stops, and you quickly examine the patient. His skin is very hot. His vital signs are: pulse 160, with frequent extra beats; BP 180/120; and respirations 36 per minute and deep. The pupils are dilated but reactive. As you are conducting the head-to-toe survey, the patient has another grand mal seizure.

1. The patient is showing toxic effects of

   a. heroin
   b. marijuana
   c. cocaine
   d. LSD
   e. barbiturates

2. Which of the following would NOT be part of the treatment of this patient?

   a. naloxone
   b. diazepam
   c. lidocaine
   d. propranolol
   e. oxygen

A152

1. This patient is showing toxic effects of **cocaine** (answer **c**). In fact, the patient's host told you so—"gold dust" is one of the street names for cocaine, and "freebasing" refers to smoking a purified (and more potent) form of cocaine. So it pays to know the local street slang. But even if you didn't catch that clue from the bystander, the patient's clinical picture told the story: the combination of seizures, fever, dilated pupils, tachycardia, PVCs, hypertension, and hyperpnea. A heroin overdose (answer a) would be expected to produce *constricted* pupils and cardiorespiratory depression (hence possible *hypo*tension and slow, shallow breathing). Marijuana (answer b) rarely produces severe toxicity and cardiovascular signs. LSD intoxication (answer d) usually manifests itself in frightening hallucinations, with a minimum of physiologic disturbance. And barbiturate overdose (answer e), like heroin overdose, causes marked cardiorespiratory *depression,* not the kind of stimulation evident in this patient.

2. **Naloxone** (answer **a**) would NOT be part of the treatment of this patient. Naloxone is a specific antagonist for narcotic overdose, and this patient has not taken a narcotic. Diazepam (answer b) will be needed to try to control the patient's seizures, for he is in status epilepticus, which is a serious and immediate threat to life. Lidocaine (answer c) is indicated for the PVCs, while propranolol (answer d) will be used to try to bring the blood pressure down (it may help calm the PVCs as well). Oxygen (answer e) is required for *any* patient having seizures, especially a patient in status epilepticus. Remember, most deaths from seizures are hypoxic deaths.

FURTHER READING

Caruana DS et al. Cocaine packet ingestion: Diagnosis, management and natural history. *Ann Intern Med* 100:73, 1984.

Cocaine out of control. *Emerg Med* 16(16):65, 1984.

The deadly delights of cocaine. *Emerg Med* 15(4):67, 1983.

Fishbain DA. Wetli CV. Cocaine intoxication, delirium, and death in a body packer. *Ann Emerg Med* 10:531, 1981.

Gay GR. Clinical management of acute and chronic cocaine poisoning. *Ann Emerg Med* 11:562, 1982.

Gay GR. An old girl: Flyin' low, dyin' slow, blinded by snow: Cocaine in perspective. *Int J Addict* 8:1027, 1973.

Howard RE, Hueter DC, Davis GJ. Acute myocardial infarction following cocaine abuse in a young woman with normal coronary arteries. *JAMA* 254:95, 1985.

Kunkel DB. Cocaine then and now, Part I: Its history, medical botany and use. *Emerg Med* 18(11):125, 1986.

Kunkel DB. Cocaine then and now, Part II: Of pharmacology and overdose. *Emerg Med* 18(12):168, 1986.

McCarron MM. The cocaine 'body packer' syndrome: Diagnosis and treatment. *JAMA* 250:1417, 1983.

Mittleman RE, Wetli CV. Death caused by recreational cocaine use: An update. *JAMA* 252:1889, 1984.

Rothenberg R. Cocaine. *Emerg Med Serv* 13(2):29, 1984.

Schachne JS, Roberts BH, Thompson PD. Coronary artery spasm and myocardial infarction associated with cocaine use. *N Engl J Med* 310:1665, 1984.

Turner BM. Drug use: Myths, reality, and problems for EMS. *Emerg Med Serv* 12(4):49, 1983.

Washton AM, Gold MS. Crack (letter). *JAMA* 256:711, 1986.

The call comes in from a local factory, 10 miles out of town, as "severe headache," and the patient turns out to be a 36-year-old black man, in obvious distress. He says the headache came on fairly rapidly during the morning and that now it's excruciating. He feels very nauseated, he says, and has vomited before your arrival. On examination, he appears in severe pain. His skin is warm and moist. Vital signs are: pulse 64, BP 230/146, and respirations 32. Pupils are equal and reactive. The neck is supple. The chest is clear. The abdomen is nontender. Sensation and movement are intact in all extremities.

1. This patient is most likely suffering from:

   a. migraine
   b. subdural hematoma
   c. acute hypertensive crisis
   d. cerebrovascular accident
   e. sinus headache

2. The drug that your medical director is most likely to order, if he decides you should begin treatment in the field, is

   a. ergotamine
   b. dexamethasone
   c. nifedipine
   d. diazepam
   e. diphenhydramine

A153

1. This patient is most likely suffering from **acute hypertensive crisis** (answer **c**). The rapidly developing headache in the context of extremely high blood pressure is the tip-off. Neither migraine (answer a) nor sinus headache (answer e) would be likely to produce such extreme elevations of blood pressure. There is no history of trauma, so a subdural hematoma (answer b) is unlikely. And at the moment, the patient shows no obvious signs of a cerebrovascular accident (answer d), or stroke—although if he's not treated expeditiously, he may well suffer a stroke very soon.

2. The drug used for rapid lowering of the blood pressure in severe hypertension is **nifedipine** (answer **c**). None of the other drugs mentioned is appropriate in this case. It is given by making several pinholes in a 10-mg capsule and popping the capsule under the patient's tongue.

   Previously, the drug recommended for lowering dangerously high blood pressure in the field was diazoxide. There were several drawbacks to diazoxide for field use, among them the fact that it often produced a precipitous drop in blood pressure. Nifedipine has proved a safer alternative and has the advantage that it can be given by mouth. Another good drug for lowering the blood pressure in hypertensive emergencies is the beta blocker, labetalol. Labetalol can provide safer blood pressure reduction than that induced by diazoxide; its only disadvantage is that it must be given by titrated infusion, which is difficult to manage in the field.

FURTHER READING

Bannon LT et al. Single dose oral atenolol for urgent blood pressure reduction. *Drugs* 25 (Suppl 2):84, 1983.

Bertel O et al. Nifedipine in hypertensive emergencies. *Br Med J* 286:19, 1983.

Blesdoe BE. Hypertensive emergencies. *JEMS* 15(4):67, 1990.

Cressman MD et al. Intravenous labetalol in the management of severe hypertension and hypertensive emergencies. *Am Heart J* 107:980, 1984.

Ferguson RK, Vlasses PH. Hypertensive emergencies and urgencies. *JAMA* 255:1607, 1986.

Finnerty FA. Hypertensive emergencies. *Hosp Med* 10(4):8, 1974.

Garrett BN, Kaplan NM. Efficacy of slow infusion of diazoxide in the treatment of severe hypertension without organ hypoperfusion. *Am Heart J* 103:390, 1982.

Haft JI. Use of the calcium-channel blocker nifedipine in the management of hypertensive emergency. *Am J Emerg Med* Suppl 3(6):25, 1985.

Haft JI, Litterer WE. Chewing nifedipine to rapidly treat hypertension. *Arch Intern Med* 144:2357, 1984.

Huey J et al. Clinical evaluation of intravenous labetalol for the treatment of hypertensive urgency. *Am J Hypertens* 1(3, Part 3):284S, 1988.

Huysmans FTM, Thien T, Koene RA. Acute treatment of hypertension with slow infusion of diazoxide. *Arch Intern Med* 143:882, 1983.

Lebel M et al. Labetalol infusion in hypertensive emergencies. *Clin Pharmacol Ther* 37:615, 1985.

O'Mailia JJ et al. Nifedipine-associated myocardial ischemia or infarction in the treatment of hypertensive urgencies. *Ann Intern Med* 107:185, 1987.

Phillips RA. Nifedipine and hypertensive emergencies. *Emerg Med* 22(15):91, 1990.

Rahn KG. How should we treat a hypertensive emergency? *Am J Cardiol* 63:48C, 1989.

Segal JL. A primer on hypertensive emergencies. *Emerg Med* 10(8):23, 1975.

Wright S. Use of nifedipine in hypertensive emergencies. *J Emerg Med* 6:584, 1988.

At 1:15 A.M., your dispatcher receives a call via 911 from a sobbing woman who can manage only to say, "Please, please help me." The dispatcher does manage to find out that the woman is calling from a phone booth downtown, at the corner of Fifth and Main, and you head for the address without really having a clear idea of what the problem is. At the phone booth, you find a woman, about 25 years old, sobbing violently. Her hair is in disarray, and her clothes are torn and mud-spattered. All she can tell you between sobs is, "He raped me."

Which of the following statements about the management of this patient are true and which are false?

1. You should try to obtain as many details as possible from the patient regarding the circumstances of the attack.

   TRUE   FALSE

2. You should do a thorough head-to-toe assessment of the patient before transporting her to the hospital.

   TRUE   FALSE

3. You should discourage the patient from making any attempt to "clean up" before going to the hospital.

   TRUE   FALSE

4. You should indicate on your trip sheet that the diagnosis in this case is rape.

   TRUE   FALSE

A154

1. You should try to obtain as many details as possible from the patient regarding the circumstances of the attack.

   FALSE. You are not there to conduct a criminal investigation; you're there to render urgent medical care. The patient will in all probability have to tell her story in all its detail at least once, in the emergency room, and possibly again to the police—and each time it will be painful enough. If she *wants* to talk about it, by all means listen sympathetically. But otherwise, confine your questions to those that will reveal any urgent medical problems that may need attention in the field (e.g., "Where does it hurt?").

2. You should do a thorough head-to-toe assessment of the patient before transporting her to the hospital.

   FALSE. Limit your physical examination to a search for immediately life-threatening injuries. (Do not examine the vaginal area unless there is obvious bleeding that must be controlled.) Many rape victims regard a physical examination as yet another assault on their privacy, as if they were being raped all over again. As is, the patient will be subjected to one very thorough physical exam in the emergency room. One is enough.

3. You should discourage the patient from making any attempt to "clean up" before going to the hospital.

   TRUE. If at all possible, it is desirable to preserve evidence, which means the patient should be discouraged from changing clothes, showering, using the toilet, gargling, or drinking any fluids before being examined in the emergency room. But respect the patient's feelings. If she feels she *must* wash up, and gentle persuasion cannot convince her otherwise, let her do so.

4. You should indicate on your trip sheet that the diagnosis in this case is rape.

   FALSE. Your trip sheet is a legal document. It should contain facts, not opinions. And at this point, the only fact you know for sure is that the patient *says* she was raped. So that is what you write down: "The patient states she was raped," not "The patient was raped."

FURTHER READING

Cryer L et al. Crisis management: The EMT and the sexual assault victim. *EMT J* 3(4):42, 1979.
Evrard JR, Bold EM. Epidemiology and management of sexual assault victims. *Obstet Gynecol* 53:381, 1979.
Hunt GR. Rape: An organized approach to evaluation and treatment. *Am Fam Physician* 15:154, 1977.
Mills P. *Rape Intervention Resource Manual.* Springfield, IL: Thomas, 1977.
Podgorney G. Rape: A crime and a trauma. *Emerg Med Serv* 6(5):37, 1977.
Santiago JM et al. Long-term psychological effects of rape in 35 rape victims. *Am J Psychiatry* 142:1338, 1985.
Schloss B. Sexual assault. *Emergency* 11(2):47, 1979.
Tintinalli J, Hoelzer M. Clinical findings and legal resolution in sexual assault. *Ann Emerg Med* 14:447, 1985.

WHY DON'T YOU PICK ON SOMEONE YOUR OWN SIZE?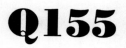

You are called at 6 o'clock one evening to a two-story house in a suburban neighborhood to see a 3-year-old child who fell down the stairs. A man, apparently the child's father, answers your ring at the door and escorts you into the living room, where the child is sitting listlessly, showing no interest in your arrival. "He was playing on the stairs and fell down or something," the father tells you.

"When did this happen?" you ask.

"Uh, I think it was this morning," the father says.

You go over to examine the child, who just stares at you blankly. You notice that his clothes are dirty, as are his face and hands. He offers no resistance as you undress him. On physical examination, you find bruises over the right temple, back, buttocks, abdomen, and anterior thighs. Some of the bruises look more recent than others. The child's right arm appears to be angulated, and he whimpers a little when you move it.

You tell the father that you'll have to take the child to the emergency room. He says, "That's O.K. I'll meet you there later. I'm waiting for an important phone call." So you are constrained to take the child to the hospital unaccompanied by a parent. When you reach the emergency room, the charge nurse takes one look at the child and says, "Is this kid here *again*?"

1. List at least 5 clues in the above story that should make you suspect this child is the victim of abuse.

2. Given that you suspect child abuse, you should:

   a. confront the father with your suspicions.
   b. notify the police of the case as soon as you are out of the house.
   c. notify the emergency room staff of your suspicions, in private, when you reach the hospital.
   d. keep your suspicions to yourself; you could get sued for false allegations.

A155

1. Clues to child abuse in this case:

   a. vague history from the parent
   b. an injury occurring some time before you were called
   c. the child's apathy: he doesn't cry; he doesn't show the normal fear of strangers; he doesn't turn to his father for comfort.
   d. evidence that the child is poorly cared for
   e. a pattern of injury that doesn't match up with the history
   f. the combination of old and fresh bruises
   g. extremity fracture
   h. the father's lack of interest in accompanying the child to the emergency room
   i. previous emergency room visits

2. Given that you suspect child abuse, you should **notify the emergency room staff of your suspicions, in private, when you reach the hospital** (answer c). Confronting the father (answer a) is unlikely to be a useful exercise, and it could endanger both you and the child. As to calling the police (answer b), let the emergency room physician make that decision after he's heard your story and examined the child. What about keeping your suspicions to yourself (answer d)? If you're worried about a legal problem (not to mention about the welfare of the child), you'd better *not* keep your suspicions to yourself. For if that child returns home and gets beaten up again and dies, then you certainly *will* have legal problems; in many states, you can be liable to criminal prosecution for keeping silent. So whenever you have reason to suspect child abuse, report your suspicions to the emergency room physician, and note that you have done so on your trip sheet for the call.

FURTHER READING

AAP Committee on Hospital Care. Medical necessity for the hospitalization of the abused and neglected child. *Pediatrics* 79:300, 1987.

Akbarnia B et al. Manifestations of the battered-child syndrome. *J Bone Joint Surg [Am]* 56A:1159, 1974.

Beals RK et al. Fractured femur in infancy: The role of child abuse. *J Pediatr Orthop* 3:583, 1983.

Bergman AB et al. Changing spectrum of serious child abuse. *Pediatrics* 77:113, 1986.

Buchanan MFG. The recognition of non-accidental injury in children. *Practitioner* 229:815, 1985.

Christoffel KK et al. Should child abuse and neglect be considered when a child dies unexpectedly? *Am J Dis Child* 139:876, 1985.

Council on Scientific Affairs. AMA diagnostic and treatment guidelines concerning child abuse and neglect. *JAMA* 254:796, 1985.

Henry GL. Legal Rounds. Problem: Suspecting child abuse. *Emerg Med* 18(19):129, 1986.

Hobbs CJ. When are burns not accidental? *Arch Dis Child* 61:357, 1986.

Kaplan JM. Pseudoabuse: The misdiagnosis of child abuse. *J Forensic Sci* 31:1420, 1986.

King J et al. Analysis of 429 fractures in 189 battered children. *J Pediatr Orthop* 8:585, 1988.

Kottmeier PK. The intricacies of abuse. *Emerg Med* 17(3):75, 1985.

Ledbetter DJ et al. Diagnostic and surgical implications of child abuse. *Arch Surg* 123:1101, 1988.

Lipton H. Stepping into child abuse. *Emergency* 22(9):23, 1990.

Ludwig S, Warman M. Shaken baby syndrome: A review of 20 cases. *Ann Emerg Med* 13:104, 1984.

Millmire ME et al. Serious head injury in infants: Accident or abuse? *Pediatrics* 75:340, 1985.

Montrey JS et al. Nonaccidental burns in child abuse. *South Med J* 78:1324, 1985.

A protocol for managing the sexually abused child. *Emerg Med* 17(10):59, 1985.

Purdue GF et al. Child abuse by burning: An index of suspicion. *J Trauma* 28:221, 1988.

Reynolds EA, Davidson L, Dierking BH. Delivering and documenting care in child abuse cases. *JEMS* 14(10):71, 1989.

Ricci R. Child sexual abuse: The emergency department response. *Ann Emerg Med* 15:711, 1986.

Robertson DM et al. Unusual injury? Recent injury in normal children and children with suspected non-accidental injury. *Br Med J* 285:1399, 1982.

Rosenberg N, Bottenfield G. Fractures in infants: A sign of child abuse. *Ann Emerg Med* 11:178, 1982.

Silverman FN. Child abuse: The conflict of underdetection and overreporting. *Pediatrics* 80:441, 1987.

Solomons G. Trauma and child abuse: The importance of the medical record. *Am J Dis Child* 134:503, 1980.

Vey PK. Child abuse: Your standard of care. *Emerg Med Serv* 13(2):89, 1984.

It's the afternoon of the playoffs in your local softball league, and you and your partner are sitting in the stands, enjoying a day off (although you've got your portable transceiver with you, just in case). It's the eighth inning, your team is 3 runs ahead, and heavy, black clouds hang over the field. Suddenly there is a deafening crash amidst a flash of white light. When you recover from the unexpected explosion, you notice that the air smells funny and that there are softball players strewn all over the field. Some of them are moving, some of them aren't. You quickly radio for every available ambulance to come to the scene, and meanwhile you and your partner dash out onto the field to start triage and treatment of the victims.

For each of the following statements about this situation, indicate whether the statement is true or false.

1. If you find any victim not breathing, the first thing you should do is open his airway by head tilt-chin lift.

   TRUE   FALSE

2. Cardiac arrest caused by a direct lightning hit is most likely to take the form of ventricular fibrillation.

   TRUE   FALSE

3. Persons struck by lightning are apt to suffer temporary paralysis.

   TRUE   FALSE

4. Lightning burns usually show a bull's eye entrance wound and cause massive thermal damage to internal organs.

   TRUE   FALSE

5. Persons sustaining a direct hit from lightning may suffer contusion to internal organs and massive internal bleeding.

   TRUE   FALSE

A156

1. If you find any victim not breathing, the first thing you should do is open his airway by head tilt-chin lift.

   FALSE. By all means, open the airway—but NOT by head tilt-chin lift. Spinal injury due to violent muscle spasms is not uncommon in victims of lightning injury; so use *jaw thrust* to open the airway, and avoid any unnecessary movement of the patient's head and neck.

2. Cardiac arrest caused by a direct lightning hit is most likely to take the form of ventricular fibrillation.

   FALSE. Cardiac arrest caused by a direct lightning hit is most likely to take the form of *asystole*. Nonetheless, unlike most other patients found in asystole, victims of lightning injury found in asystole have an excellent chance of being successfully resuscitated—if someone starts CPR in time.

3. Persons struck by lightning are apt to suffer temporary paralysis.

   TRUE. Temporary leg paralysis is seen in as many as 70 percent of lightning victims, and temporary arm paralysis occurs in about 30 percent. Thus paralysis in a lightning victim is not necessarily a sign of permanent spinal injury. To be on the safe side, you'd still better immobilize the lightning victim on a long backboard. But you can honestly reassure the paralyzed patient that in all probability, he or she will regain the function of the paralyzed limbs.

4. Lightning burns usually show a bull's eye entrance wound and cause massive thermal damage to internal organs.

   FALSE. Unlike electric burns from household current or utility lines, lightning burns are usually quite superficial and have a spidery, feathery, or zigzag appearance.

5. Persons sustaining a direct hit from lightning may suffer contusion to internal organs and massive internal bleeding.

   TRUE. The enormous concussive force of a lightning strike can rupture eardrums and hollow organs and can contuse solid organs. So be alert for signs of shock in the victim of lightning injury.

FURTHER READING

Amey BW et al. Lightning injury with survival in five patients. *JAMA* 253:243, 1985.
Caroline NL. *Emergency Care in the Streets* (4th ed.). Boston: Little, Brown, 1991, Ch. 15.
Caroline NL. *Emergency Medical Treatment: A Text for EMT-As and EMT-Intermediates* (3rd ed). Boston: Little, Brown, 1991. Ch. 13.
Cooper MA. Lightning injuries: Prognostic signs for death. *Ann Emerg Med* 9:134, 1980.
Cooper MA. Of volts and bolts. *Emerg Med* 15(8):99, 1983.
Craig SR. When lightning strikes: Pathophysiology and treatment of lightning injuries. *Postgrad Med* 79:109, 1986.
Kirstenson S et al. Lightning-induced acoustic rupture of the tympanic membrane. *J Laryngol Otol* 99:711, 1985.
Kotagal S et al. Neurologic, psychiatric and cardiovascular complications in children struck by lightning. *Pediatrics* 70:190, 1982.
Moran KT et al. Lightning injury: Physics, pathophysiology, and clinical features. *Irish Med J* 79:120, 1986.
Ravitch MM et al. Lightning stroke. *N Engl J Med* 264:36, 1961.
Taussig HB. "Death" from lightning—and the possibility of living again. *Ann Intern Med* 68:1345, 1968.
Taylor CO, Carr JC, Rich J. EMS system in action: Survival of two girls after direct lightning strikes. *EMT J* 5(6):419, 1981.

"Sick baby" is the way the call comes in early one morning. When you reach the address in question, you find a distraught woman, who leads you immediately to a bedroom and points to the crib inside. As you go over to the crib, the woman hangs back at the door. You find a baby, who looks to be about 2 months old, lying pale and motionless in the crib. The baby's skin is cold to the touch. There is no pulse.

You should:
a. start CPR, and continue CPR all the way to the hospital.
b. ask the mother why she didn't call earlier.
c. wrap the baby in a blanket and transport it to the morgue.
d. tell the mother there is nothing you can do, and advise her to call a funeral home to transport the baby.

A157

Probably there is no absolutely "right" answer to this question, but this author favors answer **a**: you should **start CPR and continue CPR all the way to the hospital.** Granted, it is not going to do any good for the baby. This baby is the victim of sudden infant death syndrome (SIDS), or crib death, and has apparently been dead for some time before you arrived. So you will not succeed in resuscitating the infant. But you may help the mother, by making her feel that everything possible has been done to try to save the life of her child. Certainly you should not do anything to make her feel guilty (answer b), for she doubtless already has enormous guilt feelings, which are not, in any case, warranted. Nor is it consistent with professional behavior simply to abandon a bereaved parent at the scene (answer d), leaving her without comfort or emotional support under such tragic circumstances. To wrap the baby up like a package and deliver it to the morgue (answer c) is also a rather insensitive course of action under the circumstances. The important thing to keep in mind in such cases is that when you can no longer help the dead, the needs of the living have first priority. Put yourself in the mother's place, and try to imagine how *you* would feel if you found *your* child dead in its crib. What would *you* want from an emergency medical team that came to the house in response to your call for help?

FURTHER READING

Brown KR. Sudden infant death syndrome: Part 1, Update for EMS providers. *Emerg Med Serv* 12(5):52, 1983.

Brown KR. Sudden infant death syndrome: Part 2, General theories of SIDS development. *Emerg Med Serv* 12(7):31, 1983.

Carpenter RG et al. Identification of some infants at immediate risk of dying unexpectedly and justifying intense study. *Lancet* 2:343, 1979.

Gould JB et al. Management of the near-miss infant. *Pediatr Clin North Am* 26:857, 1979.

James TN. Crib death. *Am Coll Cardiol* 5:1185, 1985.

Kleinberg F. Sudden infant death syndrome. *Mayo Clin Proc* 59:352, 1984.

Peterson DR. Evolution of the epidemiology of sudden infant death syndrome. *Epidemiol Rev* 2:97, 1980.

Premature mortality due to sudden infant death syndrome. *JAMA* 255:1992, 1986.

Shannon DC, Kelly DH. SIDS and near-SIDS. *NEJM* 306:959 and 306:1022, 1982.

Stanton AN. Overheating and cot death. *Lancet* 2:1199, 1984.

Strimer R, Adelson L, Oseasohn R. Epidemiologic features of 1,134 sudden unexpected infant deaths. *JAMA* 209:1493, 1969.

Weinstein SE. SIDS: The role of the EMT. *Emerg Prod News* 9(9):35, 1977.

It's one of those nights when a batch of uncut heroin hits the streets, and you get half a dozen calls to minister to local addicts suffering from overdose. The last call comes around 3:30 in the morning, by which time you feel like *you've* had some kind of an overdose. The patient is a 26-year-old man who is deeply comatose, breathing shallowly 6 times a minute. His pupils are constricted, his sclerae are very yellow, and there are needle tracks on both arms. It takes you quite a while to find a usable vein, but finally you manage to get your needle into a patent vein on the man's left hand, and you quickly squirt in a dose of naloxone. The patient wakes up with a jerk and flings out his arm, sending you and the hypodermic flying across the ambulance to the crew bench, where you land painfully on top of the hypodermic needle. Uttering a few expletives, you extract the needle from your thigh, and start to pitch it away, but then suddenly you remember those yellow eyes.

You should:

a. get a gamma globulin shot as soon as you reach the emergency room.
b. get a hepatitis B vaccination as soon as you reach the emergency room.
c. start a course of penicillin right away and continue it for two weeks.
d. take no immediate treatment measures, but stay in touch with the emergency room physician at the receiving hospital regarding the patient's final diagnosis and any follow-up treatment you will need.
e. take no treatment measures, but burn all the equipment in the ambulance to prevent the hepatitis from being spread to other patients.

A158

If you've been exposed by needle-stick to hepatitis in an IV drug user, you should **stay in touch with the emergency room physician at the receiving hospital regarding the patient's final diagnosis and any followup treatment you may need** (answer **d**). Gamma globulin (answer a) probably won't help, for an IV drug user is most likely to be suffering from hepatitis B, and gamma globulin is principally effective against hepatitis A. As to hepatitis B vaccination (answer b), now is not the time to think about that. You *should* have been immunized against hepatitis B as a prerequisite to starting your employment as an EMT or paramedic. Penicillin (answer c) and other antibiotics have no activity against viral illnesses like hepatitis, so there's no point in popping pills for two weeks. And if you want to burn down the ambulance (answer e), that's your business; but it's a rather extreme way to prevent hepatitis transmission. A thorough airing and disinfection of the vehicle interior, along with careful disposal of any needles used for the patient, are really all that's required.

FURTHER READING

Bader T. A protocol for needle-stick injuries. *Emerg Med* 18(2):36, 1986.

Centers for Disease Control. Recommendations of the immunization practices advisory committee update on hepatitis B prevention. *MMWR* 36(23), 1987.

Clawson JJ et al. Prevalence of antibody to hepatitis B virus surface antigen in emergency medical personnel in Salt Lake City, Utah. *Ann Emerg Med* 15:183, 1986.

Francis DP et al. The safety of the hepatitis B vaccine: Inactivation of the AIDS virus during routine vaccine manufacture. *JAMA* 256:869, 1986.

Hollinger FB. Factors influencing the immune response to hepatitis B vaccine, booster dose guidelines, and vaccine protocol recommendations. *Am J Med* 87 (Suppl 3A):3A. 1989.

Iserson KV, Criss EA. Hepatitis B prevalence in emergency physicians. *Ann Emerg Med* 14:119, 1985.

Kunches LM. Hepatitis B exposure in emergency medical personnel: Prevalence of serologic markers and need for immunization. *Am J Med* 75:269, 1983.

Maddrey WC. Viral hepatitis today. *Emerg Med* 21(16):124, 1989.

Maniscalco PM. Hepatitis B. *Emerg Med Serv* 19(3):37, 1990.

Moss WD. Hepatitis B. *Emerg Med Serv* 12(5):48, 1983.

Pepe PE et al. Viral hepatitis risk in urban emergency medical services personnel. *Ann Emerg Med* 15:454, 1986.

Schwartz, JS. Hepatitis B vaccine. *Ann Intern Med* 100:149, 1984.

Snyder M. Management of health care workers remotely vaccinated for hepatitis B who sustain significant blood and body fluid exposures. *Infect Control Hosp Epidemiol* 9:462, 1988.

Valenzuela TD. Occupational exposure to hepatitis B in paramedics. *Arch Intern Med* 145:1976, 1985.

West KB. Non-A, non-B and delta hepatitis: Hepatitis C and D. *Emerg Med Serv* 19(3):37, 1990.

A 28-year-old man was the driver of a car that was struck broadside by another vehicle. You find him semiconscious, with bruises about his head. Pulse is 120 and feeble. There is an open wound of the chest, through which air is being sucked in when the patient attempts to breathe. The right hip is obviously fractured, and there is moderate bleeding from an open wound on the right thigh.

1. What is your *first* step in managing this patient?

    a. Start an IV with normal saline.
    b. Put a pressure dressing over the wound on the right leg.
    c. Close the sucking chest wound with any available means.
    d. Give 10 mg of morphine for pain.
    e. Remove the patient from the car on a long backboard.

2. Having accomplished the first step, what would you do *next*?

A159

Yes, we're back to our old refrain: ABC.

1. The most immediate threat to this patient's airway, not to mention his breathing, is his sucking chest wound. Apparently the area of the wound is larger than that between the vocal cords, for when the patient makes an effort at inhalation, air is being preferentially drawn in through the wound, rather than through the airway. Thus the first step in managing this patient is to restore his normal airway and permit more efficient breathing, i.e., to **close the sucking chest wound with any available means** (answer **c**).
2. Having accomplished that, we move on to the circulation, which is being jeopardized by hemorrhage from the right thigh. The bleeding must be stopped, so our next step is to **put a pressure dressing over the wound on the right leg** (answer **b**).

Where do we go from here? Since an open chest wound is a load-and-go situation, we now need to remove the patient from the car with a long backboard (answer **e**) and then start transport. We can whip in the IV (answer **a**) en route to the hospital. Do NOT give morphine (answer **d**)! The patient has a depressed state of consciousness and is probably in shock, two excellent reasons to keep the morphine locked up in the vehicle for some other patient.

FURTHER READING

Caroline NL. *Emergency Care in the Streets* (4th ed.). Boston: Little, Brown, 1991, Ch. 17.

Caroline NL. *Emergency Medical Treatment: A Text for EMT-As and EMT-Intermediates* (3rd ed.). Boston: Little, Brown, 1991, Ch. 15.

Ferko JG, Singer EM. Injuries to the thorax. *Emergency* 22(4):20, 1990.

Frame SB, McSwain NE. Chest trauma. *Emergency* 21(7):22, 1989.

Gauthier RK. Thoracic trauma. *Emerg Med Serv* 13(3):28, 1984.

Ivatury RR et al. Penetrating thoracic injuries: In-field stabilization vs. prompt transport. *J Trauma* 27:1066, 1987.

Neclerio EA. Chest trauma. *Clin Symp* 22:75, 1980.

Smith MG. Penetrating the complexities of chest trauma. *JEMS* 14(8):50, 1989.

Thoracic trauma. *Emerg Med* 12(19):69, 1980.

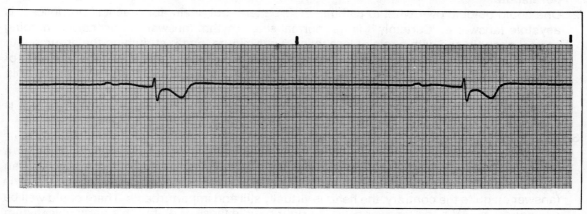

Figure 21

You are called to attend to a 57-year-old man who collapsed at home. Your response time is 10 minutes, and you find the patient lying in the living room of his suburban home. His wife is too agitated to give you very much information, save for the fact that "he was fine, he didn't complain of anything, and then he just collapsed." The patient is apneic, and you cannot palpate any pulse. His face is quite blue.

1. Examine the patient's rhythm strip in Figure 21:

    a. The rhythm is _____ regular _____ irregular.
    b. The rate is _____ per minute.

2. The ECG pattern is

    a. Normal sinus rhythm
    b. Sinus bradycardia
    c. Junctional rhythm
    d. Complete heart block
    e. Asystole

3. The rhythm is indicative of

    a. Widespread ventricular irritability
    b. Damage to the AV node
    c. Multiple ectopic foci in the atria
    d. Damage to the right bundle
    e. A dying heart

4. Which of the following would NOT be part of the initial management of this patient?

    a. Start artificial ventilation and external cardiac compressions.
    b. Administer oxygen.
    c. Countershock at 200 joules.
    d. Start an IV with D5W.
    e. Administer epinephrine, 5 to 10 ml of a 1:10,000 solution IV.

A160

1. With only two beats on the rhythm strip, it is **impossible to determine whether the rhythm is regular or irregular;** for all practical purposes, there is no rhythm, and the rate is **less than 20 per minute.**

2. One could quibble over what to call this ECG pattern, but again, for practical purposes it is **asystole** (answer **e**). Certainly it is not normal sinus rhythm (answer a), for there is nothing normal about it, and with a rate of less than 20 per minute, one is stretching the argument to call it a sinus bradycardia (answer b); bradycardia is slow, but not *that* slow! The presence of P waves rules out the possibility of junctional rhythm (answer c), and their fixed relationship to the QRS complexes precludes complete heart block (answer d).

   A rhythm like that shown in Figure 21 is also referred to as an agonal rhythm, and it is often the last rhythm seen on the ECG prior to complete asystole and biologic death.

3. The rhythm is indicative of a **dying heart** (answer **e**)—the last blips of a ventricle saying its farewells to the world. In all probability, these electrical events are not accompanied by a pulse, for there is generally little or no muscular activity associated with complexes of an agonal rhythm. Certainly there is no irritability of either the ventricles (answer a) or the atria (answer c); quite the contrary, the heart is virtually still and imperturbable. There could well be damage to the AV node (answer b) or the right bundle (answer d), but this particular rhythm strip does not furnish the evidence to support these conclusions.

4. Countershock at 200 joules is NOT part of the initial management of this patient (answer **c**). There is nothing to defibrillate! If after oxygenation and the administration of epinephrine the rhythm becomes ventricular fibrillation, that is another matter. But in asystole, 200 joules will accomplish nothing save possible additional damage to the myocardium.

FURTHER READING

Adelson L, Hoffman W. Sudden death from coronary disease. *JAMA* 176:129, 1961.

Bass E. Cardiopulmonary arrest: Pathophysiology and neurologic complications. *Ann Intern Med* 103(Part 1):920, 1985.

Caroline NL. *Emergency Care in the Streets* (4th ed.). Boston: Little, Brown, 1991, Ch. 23.

Clinton JE et al. Cardiac arrest under age 40: Etiology and prognosis. *Ann Emerg Med* 13:1011, 1984.

Cobb LA. Cardiac arrest during sleep. *N Engl J Med* 311:1044, 1984.

Eisenberg MS et al. Out-of-hospital cardiac arrest: Significance of symptoms in patients collapsing before and after arrival of paramedics. *Am J Emerg Med* 4:116, 1986.

Goldberg AH. Cardiopulmonary arrest. *N Engl J Med* 290:381, 1974.

Goldstein S et al. Analysis of cardiac symptoms preceding cardiac arrest. *Am J Cardiol* 58:1195, 1986.

Medendorp GS et al. Analysis of cardiac symptoms preceding cardiac arrest. *Am J Cardiol* 58:1195, 1986.

USEFUL REFERENCES IN EMERGENCY CARE

BIBLIOGRAPHY

Baldwin GA (ed.). *Handbook of Pediatric Emergencies*. Boston: Little, Brown, 1989.

Bassuk EL, Fox SS, Prendergast KJ. *Behavioral Emergencies: A Field Guide for EMTs and Paramedics.* Boston: Little, Brown, 1983.

Caroline NL. *Emergency Care in the Streets* (4th ed.). Boston: Little, Brown, 1991.

Caroline NL. *Emergency Medical Treatment: A Text for EMT-As and EMT-Intermediates* (3rd ed.). Boston: Little, Brown, 1991.

Caroline NL. *Study Guide for Emergency Care in the Streets*. Boston: Little, Brown, 1991.

Caroline NL. *Workbook for Emergency Medical Treatment: Review Problems for EMTs* (3rd ed.). Boston: Little, Brown, 1991.

Copass MK, Eisenberg MS. MacDonald SC. *Paramedic Manual* (2nd ed.). Philadelphia: Saunders, 1987.

Copass MK, Soper RG, Eisenberg MS. *EMT Manual* (2nd ed.). Philadelphia: Saunders, 1991.

Eisenberg MS, Copass MK. *Manual of Emergency Medical Therapeutics* (2nd ed.). Philadelphia: Saunders, 1982.

Eisenberg MS, Cummins RO, Ho MT. *Code Blue: Cardiac Arrest and Resuscitation*. Philadelphia: Saunders, 1987.

Jenkins JL, Loscalzo J. *Manual of Emergency Medicine*. Boston: Little, Brown, 1990.

MacDonald MG, Miller MK (eds.). *Emergency Transport of the Perinatal Patient*. Boston: Little, Brown, 1989.

McNeil EL. *Airborne Care of the Ill and Injured*. New York: Springer-Verlag, 1983.

Mills K, Morton R, Page G. *A Color Atlas of Accidents and Emergencies*. London: Wolfe Medical, 1984.

Safar P, Bircher NG. *Cardiopulmonary Cerebral Resuscitation* (3rd ed.). Philadelphia: Saunders, 1988.

Stine RJ, Marcus RH (eds.) *A Practical Approach to Emergency Medicine*. Boston: Little, Brown, 1987.

INDEX FOR INSTRUCTORS

The following index is arranged by topic according to the organization of *Emergency Care in the Streets*, Fourth Edition, a textbook that follows the general sequence of and covers all the objectives of the National Training Course for Emergency Medical Technician–Paramedic of the United States Department of Transporation. If this book is used as an instructional aid for that course, questions relating to any given unit may be assigned by consulting this index. **All entries refer to question numbers.**

The following subject index is keyed to the questions and answers in this book. A number preceded by *QA* indicates that the topic is dealt with in both the question and the answer of that number. A number preceded by *A* indicates that the topic is mentioned only in the answer to the question of that number. For example,

Asystole, calcium for, A29

indicates that a discussion of calcium for asystole can be found in Answer 29. Entries in boldface indicate questions that are illustrated with an electrocardiogram.

Trauma. *See also under specific area of the body*
  in children, QA150
    multiple, QA105, QA107, QA131, QA159
Triage, QA99, QA108, QA139

Umbilical cord, prolapse of, A126, QA142
Unconscious patient, QA3. *See also* Coma
Urinary output, in shock, QA12

Vaginal bleeding, QA148
Vagus nerve, stimulation of, A20
Valium. *See* Diazepam
Valsalva maneuver, QA20
Vasoconstriction, QA56
Vasopressor drugs, A102, A120, A124, A132, A137
Ventilation, assisted and controlled, A15, QA114
Ventricular fibrillation
  defibrillation for, A49

  in hypothermia, QA146
    management of, A25, A91
Ventricular irritability, oxygen and, A25
Ventricular tachycardia, A32, **QA65, QA134**
Venturi mask, QA38
Violent patient, QA115
Vital signs, in head injury, QA104
Vomiting, induction of, QA98, QA123

Wenckebach rhythm, A95, **QA110**
Wheezes
  in asthma, A33, QA63, QA140
  definition of, QA7
  differential diagnosis of, A71
  in infants, QA77
  significance of, QA140
Wounds, priorities in treating, QA3

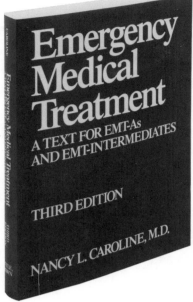

Little, Brown books cover the field!

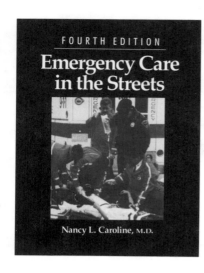

NO POSTAGE
NECESSARY IF
MAILED IN THE
UNITED STATES

BUSINESS REPLY MAIL
FIRST CLASS   PERMIT NO. 2117   BOSTON, MA

POSTAGE WILL BE PAID BY ADDRESSEE

Little, Brown and Company
Distribution Center
Medical Division
200 West Street
P.O. Box 9131
Waltham, MA 02254-9931

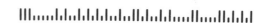